Speech-Language Pathologists in Public Schools

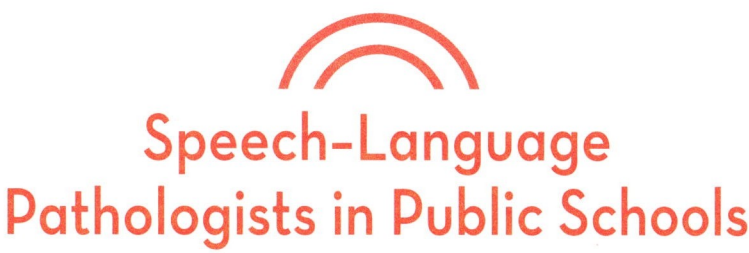

Speech-Language Pathologists in Public Schools

MAKING A DIFFERENCE FOR AMERICA'S CHILDREN

THIRD EDITION

Barbara J. Moore

Judy K. Montgomery

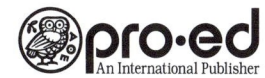

pro·ed
An International Publisher

8700 Shoal Creek Boulevard
Austin, Texas 78757-6897
800/897-3202   Fax 800/397-7633
www.proedinc.com

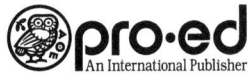

© 2018, 2008, 2001 by PRO-ED, Inc.
8700 Shoal Creek Boulevard
Austin, Texas 78757-6897
800/897-3202   Fax 800/397-7633
www.proedinc.com

Library of Congress Cataloging-in-Publication Data

Names: Moore, Barbara J., 1957- author. | Montgomery, Judy K., 1947- author.
Title: Speech/language pathologists in public schools : making a difference
    for America's children / Barbara J. Moore, Judy K. Montgomery.
Other titles: Making a difference for America's children
Description: Third Edition. | Austin, Texas : PRO-ED, Inc., [2018] | Includes
    bibliographical references and index.
Identifiers: LCCN 2017020612 (print) | LCCN 2017030023 (ebook) | ISBN
    9781416410706 (e-book PDF) | ISBN 9781416410690 (print)
Subjects: LCSH: Speech therapy for children—United States. | Communicative
    disorders in children—United States. | Children with
    disabilities—Education—United States.
Classification: LCC LB3454 (ebook) | LCC LB3454 .M66 2018 (print) | DDC
    618.92/85506—dc23
LC record available at https://lccn.loc.gov/2017020612

Art Director: Jason Crosier
Designer: Lissa Hattersley
This book is designed in Minion and Neutra Text.

Printed in the United States of America
1 2 3 4 5 6 7 8 9 10   26 25 24 23 22 21 20 19 18 17

CONTENTS

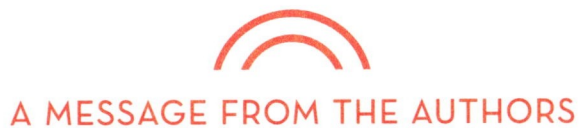

A MESSAGE FROM THE AUTHORS

Welcome to the third edition of this publication. If you are a student or a university professor, this may be your textbook. If you are a beginning speech–language pathology clinician in the schools, this book may be your guide to understanding your work setting. If you are an accomplished speech–language pathologist or a supervisor, it may be your opportunity to match your skills with the latest school-based research and "up your game." All of these possibilities were in our thoughts as we composed each page.

As speech–language pathologists who have worked in the public schools of this country for many decades, we have marveled at the exciting changes that have taken place in school-based speech–language pathology. Sweeping new federal legislation in public education has marked each edition of our book: Elementary and Secondary Education Act/No Child Left Behind in 2001, Individuals With Disabilities Education Improvement Act of 2004, and Every Student Succeeds Act in 2015. Implementation at the state and local levels followed, and speech–language pathologists were there, side by side with their general education colleagues, supporting literacy, response to intervention, Common Core State Standards, accountability, access to the curriculum, and interprofessional collaboration. We are proud to have played a role in journaling this educational adventure.

This third edition maintains the structure of our previously organized 10 chapters as a lens to appreciate the roles and responsibilities of speech–language pathologists in public school life. Though states vary in their models for providing speech and language services, they are more alike than different. This is due in no small way to the powerful influence of the American Speech–Language–Hearing Association (ASHA) guiding the work of speech–language pathologists in America's schools. Its many documents, professional development programs, conferences, and consistent presence in the halls of Congress have firmly established assessment and intervention services in public schools for students with communication disabilities. We are grateful for the vigilance that ASHA has displayed nationally on our behalf. A powerful and well informed national professional association has resulted in a strong state educational credentialing process, state licensing expansion, and national accreditation of university training programs, which preserves our role in public schools. These protections do not come without great effort. We discuss their considerable value in these pages. As busy clinicians, we can overlook their importance.

With regard to examining previous laws, regulations, and research, we would like to note that certain terms used throughout the book are not the currently preferred terms. Specifically, terms such as *mental retardation, mentally retarded, backward,* and the like are ones we would not have used ourselves, but because these were accepted terms at the time in the sources quoted, we could not change them and thus change the quoted material. The authors do not condone or encourage the use of these terms. *Intellectual disability* is the currently preferred term. We ask that our readers bear this in mind as they encounter the older nonpreferred terms.

With this book, we have endeavored to share our great love for the public schools in our nation. As speech–language pathologists, we have the privilege to work with children and families to build communication skills so tomorrow's citizens learn to read, write, understand, analyze, and eventually advance the knowledge in their country. Our role in increasing literacy and cognitive development has expanded tenfold since the turn of the century. As Margaret Mead reminded us, "Children must be taught how to think; not what to think." Speech–language pathologists are part of that educational challenge!

Speech–language pathologists in many states provided us with ideas, models, rubrics, sample goals, schedules, and implementation plans that they have found successful as they serve the needs of children with communication disabilities. We have included many of these contributions and are thankful that we have such generous colleagues and friends. Although there remain many obstacles to what we wish to accomplish with our young charges, and not every day ends in victory, our speech–language pathologist colleagues find great joy in their work in schools. We share this feeling. Problems remain. We have set our goals high—doing all we wish to do will tax our energy, resources, and resolve. Pursuing these goals may spur us on to do more. "Watch for big problems. They disguise big opportunities" (H. Jackson Brown, Jr.). Recognizing our colleagues' joy has propelled us to create the third edition of this book. We set out to share needed information and to underscore the value of evidence-based practices; our connection with families; and the thrill of resolving problems, using technology, and ever more tightly linking our speech and language profession with our nation's public schools. It is a worthwhile journey.

—Barbara J. Moore, EdD, CCC-SLP
—Judy K. Montgomery, PhD, CCC-SLP

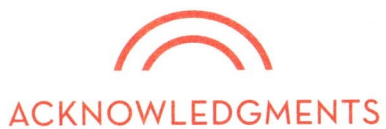

ACKNOWLEDGMENTS

We would like to thank and acknowledge the following individuals and organizations.

Portions of Chapters 4, 5, 6, and 7 were adopted and modified from an unpublished document prepared for the Louisiana Department of Education. We gratefully acknowledge the department's interest and support of speech–language pathologists and of this work.

Patricia Harriman, who skillfully assisted in the preparation of this document. We are grateful for her final eye on this manuscript.

Beth Rowan, for her patience and advice throughout this process.

The many, many speech–language pathologists and audiologists who inspire our work—our friends, colleagues, and coworkers. You make a difference every day for America's children, and it is our humble honor to stand shoulder to shoulder with you in this work.

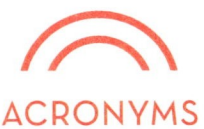

ACRONYMS

AAC	augmentative and alternative communication
ADA	Americans With Disabilities Act of 1990
ADR	alternative dispute resolution
ASCD	Association for Supervision and Curriculum Development
ASD	autism spectrum disorder
ASHA	American Speech–Language–Hearing Association
AT	assistive technology
BIP	behavioral intervention plan
CCC	Certificate of Clinical Competence
CCSS	Common Core State Standards
C.F.R.	Code of Federal Regulations
CLD	culturally and linguistically diverse
DD	developmental disability
DLL	Dual-Language Learners
EAA	Educational Audiology Association
EAHCA	Education for All Handicapped Children Act
EBP	evidence-based practice
ELL	English-language learners
ESEA	Elementary and Secondary Education Act
ESSA	Every Student Succeeds Act
FAPE	free appropriate public education
FBA	functional behavioral assessment
FERPA	Family Educational Rights and Privacy Act
HIPAA	Health Insurance Portability and Accountability Act
ICT	instructional consultation team
IDEA 2004	Individuals With Disabilities Education Improvement Act of 2004
IEE	Independent Educational Evaluation
IEP	Individualized Education Program
IFSP	Individualized Family Service Plan
IST	instructional support team
ITP	Individualized Transition Plan
LEA	local education agency
LRE	least restrictive environment
MDAT	multidisciplinary assessment team

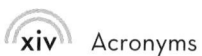

MTSS	Multi-Tiered System of Supports
NBPTS	National Board for Professional Teaching Standards
NCES	National Center for Education Statistics
NCLB	No Child Left Behind
NEA	National Education Association
OCR	Office for Civil Rights
OSEP	Office of Special Education Programs
OSERS	Office of Special Education and Rehabilitative Services
PBIS	positive behavioral intervention and supports
PBS	positive behavioral supports
PLC	professional learning community
PWN	prior written notice
REI	Regular Education Initiative
RTI	response to intervention
SEA	state education agency
SIG	special interest group
SLPA	speech–language pathology assistant
UDL	universal design for learning
UNHS	universal newborn hearing screening
USDE	U.S. Department of Education
YRE	year-round education

CHAPTER 1

Speech–Language Services in the Educational System

Trends and Considerations

● *In This Chapter*

This chapter introduces issues surrounding the educational system within which school-based speech–language pathologists work—including the impacts of school reform for both general and special education, characteristics of children and families of the 21st century, and incidences of children with disabilities who are identified as needing special education (e.g., speech–language) services in the schools. The chapter concludes with a consideration of trends in school reform and the corresponding roles of professionals.

● *Chapter Questions*

1. How has the role of the school-based speech–language pathologist evolved since the implementation of special education in this country?
2. What is meant by "educational reforms"? Why is it important for speech–language pathologists in public schools to be aware of general and special education reforms?
3. How have school reform movements affected the delivery of speech–language services in schools?
4. Discuss why the information presented about children and their environments is important to speech–language pathologists in schools.
5. Discuss how educational trends will influence your work.

Speech–Language Services in Public Schools

Many people work together to make the American educational system successful for children. Among the talented and dedicated people who make a difference for children in America's public schools are speech–language pathologists, who specialize in speech, language, and communication development and disorders. The discipline of communication sciences and disorders is composed of two professions: speech–language pathology and audiology. The primary focus of this book is on the practice and contributions of speech–language pathologists providing services in America's public schools and the difference that these services, and those who provide them, make for children whose communication needs hinder their accomplishments in reading, writing, listening, and speaking.

Speech–language services in public schools serve vital functions for students with communication disorders, and the provision of such services has grown and evolved significantly in the past 50 years. Accordingly, the roles of speech–language pathologists in public schools are nearly unrecognizable compared to the work of speech–language pathologists in the late 1960s and early 1970s. This change is due to a combination of factors. First, schools, as institutions, are not the same as they were 50 years ago. Public expectations and the demands placed on the educational system are greater now than at any time in the history of the country. This is most dramatically illustrated in the legislative mandates placed on schools and their employees.

Second, the children of the 21st century have different needs and different futures and bring more diverse life experiences to the school setting. Third, the profession of speech–language pathology has evolved, along with its scientific research base, which consequently affects school practice. For speech–language pathologists to work effectively in the public school setting, they must not only be competent in the treatment of communication disorders, delays, and disabilities but also understand the educational system in which they work.

In the past, university programs for communication disorders taught that speech–language pathologists in the school setting were predominantly separated from the general education system that employed them. This is no longer true or desirable. Educational systems (used here to refer to public school systems) are increasingly dynamic and interactive institutions. Speech–language pathologists in either preservice or in-service situations must be able to view their work within the context of the larger dynamic, interactive, and responsive educational system. The educational system of the 21st century now meaningfully connects general and special education.

Educational Reforms That Shaped the Profession

The United States and Europe have a long history of programs for certain types of communication disabilities, such as deafness (Hardman, Drew, & Egan, 2011), although such programs were generally found only in special schools. School programs to address the issue of "stammering" were first introduced into public education in 1910. Teachers of English literature were frequently given some training to provide "speech correction" to their students, and between the 1920s and the 1940s, university programs for specialists in the area of "speech improvement" or "speech correction" developed.

Legislation was passed in 45 states to provide funding for speech and hearing programs by the mid-1960s. Since then, speech–language programs have evolved as a vital part of public school services.

From the early titles of *speech teacher* or *speech correctionist*, a variety of titles have since been used to describe the professional who is responsible for the treatment of communication disorders in schools: *speech–language specialist, communication specialist, language–speech and hearing specialist, speech therapist,* and *speech–language pathologist.* The title *speech–language pathologist* will be used in this book to refer to a specialist who operates a speech–language program addressing communication disorders in a public school setting.

The professional organization of speech–language pathologists and audiologists is the American Speech–Language–Hearing Association (ASHA). School-based speech–language services have received increasing recognition within ASHA since 1925, when the organization was founded under the original name of the American Society of Speech Correction. Over half of the members of ASHA work in the school setting.

Speech–language services in schools are provided as part of the continuum of special education services, which exist through the mandates created by state and federal legislation during the wave of civil rights reforms in the 1970s. Special education is designed to support the general education program. Consequently, special education programs have been affected by the long history of educational reforms that have unfolded with increasing intensity since the early 1980s.

As these reforms are reviewed, the reader should keep asking the question "How do these changes affect speech–language services?"

General and Special Education Reforms

Institutional change is a part of American culture in nearly every segment of society, responding to forces on many levels: economic, demographic, political, and social. Educational reforms reflect change in these areas as well, reacting to issues that occur inside and outside the school system (Fullan, 2001). In a classic example, the nation was caught off guard in the 1950s when the then Soviet Union launched Sputnik, the first satellite, into space. The United States reacted by dramatically increasing the focus on science education in the early 1960s. Thus, politics, economics, and world public opinion influence educational reform in the United States.

Current reform movements in general education began with the infamous report from the National Commission on Excellence in Education in 1983 titled *A Nation at Risk: The Imperative for Educational Reform* (National Commission on Excellence in Education, 1983). This report announced the dismal performance of America's children on reading, writing, and math testing compared to that of their peers from other countries. The report rocked the educational system and set off waves of reform movements in every state legislature, school district, and neighborhood school. Since the 1980s, business leaders have criticized the public schools for failing to prepare an adequate workforce. Education has continued to be part of the political agenda in presidential elections and administrations. Consequently, significant changes have occurred in how school systems are governed, how instruction is delivered and measured, and how business is conducted in schools across the country.

Reforms have occurred in general and special education for different reasons. Although the reform of general education programs was prompted by national concerns about the skills and potential competitiveness of American students in a global economy, the reform of special education programs occurred as part of the ongoing mission to provide students with disabilities access to general education. Historically, general and special education reform movements have evolved and changed independently. Separate, parallel reform efforts in funding streams, administrative structures, accountability demands, curricula, personnel training, certification requirements, and even facilities have existed; all of these have dramatically changed through legislation and now are more closely aligned.

In 1986, the Regular Education Initiative (REI)—led by Madeline Will, assistant secretary for special education and rehabilitative services, with her report *Educating Students With Learning Problems: A Shared Responsibility* (Will, 1986)—criticized the dual system of general and special education and contained a set of proposals that called for general and special educators to share responsibilities for the education of students with disabilities. In the late 1980s and 1990s, the REI evolved into the Inclusion Movement, which reflected a philosophy that students with special needs should be fully integrated into general education classrooms and not removed from the classroom to receive supports and services necessary for their educational success (Friend & Bursuck, 2012). By the late 1990s, the original goal of special education, to provide access to general educational services, had been successfully achieved, according to Congress (IDEA Amendments of 1997).

There are many commonalities in the reform movements of general and special education on which a unified system can be built. The call was to work together and resolve the differences, not as general or special educators but as educators of all children. As speech–language pathologists provided services within school settings, understanding the issues of reform (see Chapter 2) and the demands of the educational system was necessary to support students within the context of reform programs.

Education continues to play a unique role in the transmission and perpetuation of values that seek to rectify political and social inequalities. The early reform movements of general education did not address children with disabilities, but this was vastly different under consequent reform movements. Schools had the opportunity to demonstrate how educators and students can live in a world of diversity.

Standards-Based Reform and Accountability

During the 1990s, legislative mandates reflected a movement toward standards-based education and accountability, which established expectations for what students needed to learn and know at each grade level. In a standards-based system, all students and teachers of any given grade level, anywhere in the district or state, worked toward common educational goals and provided for consistency from one grade level to the next.

In addition, in a standards-based system, students, parents, and the public were aware of the requirements of each grade level. Many districts established pacing guides so that teachers knew how to regulate their lessons to ensure that the information was covered in a consistent manner in all classrooms. Each state adopted its own set of standards for all grade levels. Schools were held accountable for what students were expected to learn through statewide assessment systems. Under these systems, state tests were designed to assess what was taught. Standards, curriculum, and testing had to be aligned.

Nolet and McLaughlin (2000) described standards-based reform as the philosophy of a systematic method of measuring student achievement. Standards were meant to apply to all students. In terms of students with disabilities, this approach represented a significant shift in the educational system's thinking about student learning and programming. Special education was built on the design of an individualized plan for each student—an Individualized Education Program (IEP). The Individuals With Disabilities Education Act (IDEA) of 1997 called for a shift from access to quality education demonstrating results. Sitting in a classroom with peers without disabilities was no longer considered enough for students with disabilities. Until this time, there were no expectations or requirements that students with disabilities would master the same curriculum as their general education peers or that the educational system should realize quantifiable educational results for these students. Under the new system, these students had to learn and the system had to be responsible for ensuring that this learning took place. In a system seeking results, individualized performance was no longer the only consideration for students with disabilities. The performances of special education students alongside other learners in the school were considered.

For special educators, expanding their view to include the bigger picture of the educational system is no small task. Speech–language pathologists realized how the philosophy of standards-based reform shaped their own view of working with students with communication disabilities, and so they needed to be knowledgeable about the school curriculum. Curriculum and instruction were recognized as the core of the educational process. Real change in education came with changes in the content and in the instructional methods used.

The late 1990s, known as the Era of Standards-Based Instruction, evolved into the Era of Accountability. With this shift in focus, schools and districts were held accountable for the first time—by law—for student learning as measured by statewide testing of standards. Students with disabilities were, and still are, expected to perform like all other students in terms of results. Chapter 2 fully describes the accountability systems established under the federal laws, the Elementary and Secondary Education Act (ESEA, previously known as No Child Left Behind [NCLB, 2002]), and the Individuals With Disabilities Education Improvement Act of 2004. This high-stakes environment brought special education to the forefront of discussions about instructional improvement and change, blending the reform movements of general and special education.

The implications were apparent for all educators: We must work together toward effective practices that positively affect student learning. Accountability in this era was not only for students but for educators as well, and it significantly affected our practice. Notably, literacy, curriculum, and statewide testing became tools of speech–language pathologists, making our practice educationally relevant to meet the needs of students on the school caseload, as well as the requirements of the law.

In a constant climate of change, education goals focused next on access to the curriculum described so carefully in state standards. But why did states, part of a single nation, have state expectations? Through the action of a governors' summit, Common Core State Standards were drawn up in 2012, and state curriculum goals were set aside for national expectations, with 15% variance overall. The remainder of this text will focus on these changes and how speech–language pathologists play a key role in advancing the educational reforms of standards-based instruction, accountability, and access to this common core.

Children and Families in the 21st Century

In the early decades of television, the traditional nuclear family was frequently portrayed as two parents and two children, usually one boy and one girl. Not surprisingly, educators often came to expect that children in their classes came from such families. The realities of children and families in the 21st century have changed; not only has the family structure changed, but the economic circumstances of families and communities have changed as well.

Indicators of Children's Well-Being

Despite media characterizations, even in 1950, only 47% of children in the United States lived in traditional families in which the father worked full-time and the mother was not in the workforce; by 1990, this number had shifted to a mere 17.9%. A difference also existed between White and Black families. In the 1940s to 1960s, 45% to 50% of White children and less than 30% of Black children lived in traditional families. These numbers shifted to only 20% for White children and only 5% for Black children in 1990 (U.S. Department of Commerce, 1993).

National Center for Education Statistics

The National Center for Education Statistics (NCES) (Kena et al., 2013) reports annually to Congress on the condition of education. These selected indicators were reported in 2013, representing information about the conditions of children in the United States in key areas of interest to school-based personnel (Federal Interagency Forum on Child and Family Statistics, 2013, pp. vii–vii).

Indicator 1: Educational attainment. In 2013, some 34% of 25- to 29-year-olds had earned a bachelor's or higher degree. Between 1990 and 2013, the size of the White–Black gap at this education level widened from 13 to 20 percentage points, and the White–Hispanic gap widened from 18 to 25 percentage points (p. 2).

Indicator 5: Children living in poverty. In 2012, approximately 21% of school-age children in the United States were in families living in poverty. The percentage of school-age children living in poverty ranged across the United States from 11% in North Dakota to 32% in Mississippi (p. 20).

Indicator 7: Preprimary enrollment. From 1990 to 2012, the percentage of 3- to 5-year-olds enrolled in preprimary programs increased from 59% to 64%. The percentage of these children who attended full-day programs increased from 39% to 60% during this period (p. 32).

Indicator 8: Public school enrollment. From school years 2011–2012 through 2023–2024, overall public elementary and secondary school enrollment is projected to increase by 5% (from 49.5 million to 52.1 million students), with changes across states ranging from an increase of 22% in Nevada to a decrease of 11% in West Virginia (p. 36).

Indicator 11: Racial–ethnic enrollment in public schools. From fall 2001 through fall 2011, the number of White students enrolled in prekindergarten through 12th grade in U.S. public schools decreased from 28.7 million to 25.6 million, and their share of public school enrollment decreased from 60% to 52%. In contrast, the number of Hispanic students enrolled during this period increased from 8.2 million to 11.8 million students, and their share of public school enrollment increased from 17% to 24% (p. 48).

Indicator 12: English-language learners. The percentage of public school students in the United States who were English-language learners (ELLs) was higher in school year 2011–2012 (9.1%) than in 2002–2003 (8.7%). Seven of the eight states with the highest percentages of ELL students in their public schools were located in the West (p. 52).

Indicator 13: Children and youth with disabilities. The number of children and youth ages 3–21 years receiving special education services was 6.4 million in 2011–2012, or about 13% of all public school students. Some 36% of the students receiving special education services had specific learning disabilities (p. 54).

Indicator 17: Concentration of public school students eligible for free or reduced-price lunch. In school year 2011–2012, 19% of public school students attended a high-poverty school, compared with 12% in 1999–2000. In 2011–2012, 28% of public school students attended a low-poverty school, compared with 45% in 1999–2000 (p. 74).

An awareness of the conditions of the families in a community and in the country is important for speech–language pathologists and other educators, especially when school teams are asked to consider children's learning challenges. In addition to the previous information, consider the following information reported by the Federal Interagency Forum on Child and Family Statistics (2013). When reviewing this information, think of the impact each condition might have on normal child development, including language that affects learning, and whether these children might be referred for, or in need of, special services.

Profiling America's Children: Selected Key Indicators of Well-Being

America's Children: Key National Indicators of Well-Being, 2013 (Federal Interagency Forum on Child and Family Statistics, 2013) continues a series of annual reports to the nation on conditions affecting children in the United States. Highlights from each section follow.

Demographic background. There were 73.7 million children ages 0–17 years in the United States in 2012, accounting for almost 24% of the population. Racial and ethnic diversity among America's children ages 0–17 years continues to grow. By 2050, about half of the American population ages 0–17 years is projected to be composed of children who are Hispanic, Asian, or of two or more races. Specifically, it is projected that 36% of the American population ages 0–17 years will be Hispanic (up from 24% in 2012), 6% will be Asian (up from 5% in 2012), and 7% will be of two or more races (up from 4% in 2012).

Family and social environment. In 2012, 64% of children ages 0–17 years lived with two married parents, down from 65% in 2011. Four percent of children lived with their own unmarried, cohabiting parents, 24% lived with only their mothers, 4% lived with only their fathers, and 4% lived with neither of their parents in 2012.

Among the 2.6 million children not living with either parent in 2012, about 55% lived with grandparents, 22% lived with other relatives, and 22% lived with nonrelatives.

There were 46 births for every 1,000 unmarried women ages 15–44 years in 2011, down from 48 per 1,000 in 2010; 40.7% of all births were to unmarried women, a percentage that has remained quite stable since 2008.

Overall, the percentage of all children living in the United States with at least one foreign-born parent has risen from 15% in 1994 to 24% in 2012.

In 2011, the adolescent birth rate was 15 per 1,000 adolescents ages 15–17 years. The rate has fallen for four consecutive years, continuing a decline, briefly interrupted in 2005–2007, that began in 1991–1992.

The number of substantiated child maltreatment reports declined to just fewer than 10 per 1,000 children ages 0–17 years in 2011.

Economic circumstances. In 2011, 22% of all children ages 0–17 years (16.1 million) lived in poverty, which was not significantly different from the percentage in 2010. The percentage of children who had at least one parent working year-round, full-time rose from 71% in 2010 to 73% in 2011.

Health care. The percentage of children who had health insurance coverage at some point during the year was essentially unchanged at 91% in 2011. The number of children without health insurance at any point during 2011 was 7 million (9% of all children).

The percentage of children ages 0–17 years who did not have a source of health care declined from 5% in 2010 to 4% in 2011.

Physical environment and safety. In 2011, about 66% of children lived in counties with measured air pollutant concentrations above the levels of one or more of the primary National Ambient Air Quality Standards at least once during the year, compared with 67% in 2010.

The percentage of children ages 4–11 years with any detectable level of blood cotinine, an indicator of recent exposure to secondhand smoke, declined from 53% in 2007–2008 to 42% in 2009–2010.

The percentage of U.S. households with children who had one or more of three housing problems—physically inadequate housing, crowded housing, or cost burden resulting from housing that costs more than 30% of household income—rose from 45% in 2009 to 46% in 2011.

Behavior. In 2012, about 2% of 8th graders, 5% of 10th graders, and 9% of 12th graders reported smoking cigarettes daily in the past 30 days, the lowest reported percentages among these students in the history of the survey.

Binge drinking—consuming five or more alcoholic beverages in a row in the past 2 weeks—among 12th graders rose from 22% in 2011 to 24% in 2012.

Education. The average National Assessment of Educational Progress (NAEP) (Federal Interagency Forum on Child and Family Statistics, 2013, p. 194) mathematics scores for 4th and 8th graders were 1 point higher in 2011 than in 2009 and higher in 2011 than in all previous assessments.

The percentage of high school graduates who had completed Algebra II rose from 70% to 76% between 2005 and 2009.

In 2011, 91% of young adults ages 18–24 years had completed high school, either with a diploma or with an alternative credential such as a general equivalency diploma (GED).

About two thirds (68%) of high school completers enrolled immediately in a 2-year or 4-year college in 2011; this percentage is unchanged from 2010 but down from the percentage in 2009 (70%).

Health. The percentage of infants born preterm declined for the fifth straight year in 2011, to 11.7%, down from a high of 12.8% in 2006.

The infant mortality rate of 6.0 deaths per 1,000 live births in 2011 was not statistically different from the rate of 6.1 per 1,000 in 2010.

In 2007–2008, the average diet-quality score for children ages 2–17 years was 50 out of a possible 100 and was not statistically different from that in 2003–2006.

In 2009–2010, 18% of children ages 6–17 years were obese, which was not statistically different from the percentage in 2007–2008.

Special feature: The kindergarten year. The kindergarten year marks a key transition in children's development. Even at kindergarten entry, children differ in their cognitive, social–emotional, and learning skills.

Three and a half million children entered kindergarten for the first time in the fall of 2010. Eighty-nine percent attended public kindergartens, and 11% attended private ones. In addition, 55% of children had attended center-based care as a primary care arrangement in the year prior to kindergarten.

Girls received higher scores than boys on kindergarten entry assessments in reading and approaches to learning; however, there was no measurable difference in performance between boys and girls in mathematics and science.

Multiple differences in children's performance were observed among students in the various racial and ethnic groups. In most cases, Asian and White, non-Hispanic kindergartners had higher scores than their peers.

Reading, mathematics, science, and approaches-to-learning scores were lower for kindergartners in households with incomes below the federal poverty level and for those at 100%–199% of the federal poverty level than for those in households with incomes at or above 200% of the federal poverty level.

Significance of Child and Family Statistics

Why should speech–language pathologists attend to statistics such as these? Simply put, language and other learning issues that arise out of the conditions mentioned in the previous section strongly influence which children are more likely to be referred for special education services. Concerns were raised by Congress during the reauthorization of IDEA in both 1997 and 2004 about the rate of increase in the number of racial and ethnic minority students who were identified as requiring special education services. Between 1980 and 1990, the rates of special education identification grew 53% for Hispanic children, 13.2% for Black children, and 107.8% for Asian children. Compare this to an increase of 6% for White children.

Despite the attention given to this topic in 1997, the Individuals With Disabilities Education Improvement Act of 2004 (IDEA 2004) focused greater attention and mandates on the overidentification of minority children in special education. In the latest reauthorization, Congress included a new section on "over-identification and disproportionality" (IDEA 2004, Section 1412 [c][24]) because of the finding that Black children were identified disproportionately with intellectual disabilities and emotional disorders and that, in general, minority children in schools with predominantly White students and teachers are disproportionately placed in special education. Children and family statistics help educators understand the conditions that may contribute to learner challenges; these children may or may not require special education but likely will need extra attention and/or assistance from the public education system. Having academic difficulties does not necessarily mean that an individual has an educational disability. It is contingent on educators, especially speech–language pathologists, to understand the difference between struggles and true disabilities and assess and intervene appropriately. A child's upbringing can significantly affect classroom performance. Language growth and development depend on many factors, both constitutional (nature) and experiential (nurture). Cognitive development, working memory, and vocabulary size all influence success in the classroom (Biemiller, 1999). Oral language development, which begins in infancy, lays the foundation for reading, writing, and other school experiences. Speech–language pathologists in schools must understand the implications of differences in the language development of children from all types of backgrounds and experiences.

In a seminal work on this topic, Biemiller (1999) referenced several studies and noted that children from low-income families had been found to have "smaller vocabularies and less advanced language development than their more advantaged peers" (p. 13). A longitudinal study of the language and achievement differences between advantaged and disadvantaged children by Hart and Risley (as cited in Biemiller, 1999) found that "advantaged children were found to have twice the vocabulary of welfare children and were adding vocabulary at twice the rate" (p. 14). Intriguingly, Hart and Risley (1995) reported:

> The longitudinal data showed that in the everyday interactions at home, the average (rounded) number of words children heard per hour was 2,150 in the professional families, 1,250 in the working-class families, and 620 in the welfare families. . . . Given the consistency we saw in the data, we might venture to extrapolate to the first 3 years of life. By age 3, the children in professional families would have heard more than 30 million words, the children in working-class families 20 million, and the children in welfare families 10 million. (p. 132)

Children who come to school with a primary language other than English or from a different cultural background will also bring different linguistic experiences. These experiences can be varied, from realizing the benefits of bilingualism to having limited opportunities to develop language skills and school-type experiences. The linguistic abilities that a child brings to school lay the foundation on which the child will build his or her academic knowledge.

In addition to the educational differences and challenges that may come from cultural and linguistic differences, speech–language pathologists and educators are becoming increasingly aware of the impact of poverty on student performance, including an impact on cognitive development, student achievement, social and behavioral development, academic achievement, and health and wellness. Social justice advocates, along with education leaders, are pushing educational systems to reach out to these students and their families by using strategies to mitigate the impact of poverty and close both the opportunity and achievement gaps for these students (Dill, 2015; Howard, 2010; Milner, 2012).

Roseberry-McKibbin (2012) reported that poverty and homelessness also have an impact on children's oral and literate language development. Speech–language pathologists must understand the variables affecting children who are from low-socioeconomic circumstances and how this might impact these students' performance. She cautioned to never equate poverty with dysfunction.

Since 2001, homeless children have had the right to receive an education in public schools and cannot be turned away because of lack of residency in the school's residence zone. The circumstances of these children are often unstable and uncertain, potentially causing anxiety and inattention in school for children who do not know where they are going to sleep at night. Homeless children may live in parks, hotels, abandoned buildings, or other public places. Their circumstances may lead to lack of nutrition and poor medical care. School attendance can also be a problem. Roseberry-McKibbon (2012) reviewed potential psychological and physical effects, which could include the following:

- Malnutrition
- Illness
- Hearing and vision problems

- Housing problems (e.g., lead poisoning, frequent moving, crowded conditions, no place to play outside)
- Neighborhood problems (e.g., violence)
- Family stress
- Fewer learning resources
- Lack of cognitive and linguistic stimulation

Being poor does not cause children to have language and behavioral impairments. However, certain language and behavioral characteristics are associated with being from a low-socioeconomic-status (SES) background.

Limited access to health care may affect language skills. Brain development can be affected if the mother is malnourished during pregnancy. If there is a lack of health care, children may be sick more often and miss school. When children are sick or hungry, they have difficulty learning and concentrating on schoolwork. Parents may not have the skills to help or may not be the ones caring for the children after school because of their need to find work. A stimulating language environment and interaction may not be occurring because of low education levels of parents or caregivers. The factor most highly related to SES is the mother's educational level (Roseberry-McKibbon, 2012).

The Condition of Education

To appreciate the broader institution in which speech, language, and audiology services are provided, information about the education system as a whole is presented throughout this text. The National Center for Educational Statistics (NCES) is charged with reporting to Congress information about the condition and progress of education. In the 2013 report, a special feature on kindergarten students was included. Noting that kindergarten is a pivotal year for students, the NCES reported the following indicators. The data were drawn from the *Early Childhood Longitudinal Study, Kindergarten Class of 2010–2011* (ECLS-K:2011) (NCES, 2015), which is a longitudinal study of young children conducted by the NCES:

- Older first-time kindergartners tended to score higher on the reading assessment than younger first-time kindergartners in the fall of kindergarten. For instance, kindergartners who were older than 6 years of age in the fall of kindergarten had higher fall reading scores than children in younger age groups, and children who were younger than 5 years old in the fall of kindergarten had the lowest reading scores on average.
- Girls typically scored higher than boys on the reading assessment.
- Asian kindergartners had higher fall reading scores than their peers in all of the other racial–ethnic groups. In addition, White non-Hispanic kindergartners had higher fall reading scores than their Black non-Hispanic, Hispanic, Native Hawaiian/Pacific Islander, and American Indian/Alaska Native classmates, and Black non-Hispanic kindergartners outscored Hispanic kindergartners.

- Fall reading scores increased with each level of parental education. For example, kindergartners whose parent(s) had not completed high school had the lowest fall reading scores, on average, and kindergartners whose parent(s) had completed some graduate education had the highest fall reading scores.
- First-time kindergartners' fall reading skills also differed with respect to their primary care arrangements in the year prior to kindergarten. Children who had not received any nonparental care on a regular basis and those whose primary care arrangement was home-based care with a relative had lower fall reading scores than children who attended home-based nonrelative care, attended center-based care, or had multiple care arrangements.
- In addition, first-time kindergartners whose primary home language was English scored higher on the reading assessment than their peers who had a non-English primary home language.

Reading scores were also lower for children in households with incomes below the federal poverty level and for those in households at 100%–199% of the federal poverty level than for those in households with incomes at or above 200% of the federal poverty level (NCES, 2015, p. 71). Key indicators from the NCES 2014 report are highlighted in Table 1.1.

As members of a building, district, or regional support team, speech–language pathologists are called on to build strong school-wide programs to develop the linguistic, cognitive, academic, and behavioral skills of students with and without disabilities. They are in a unique position to work as members of multidisciplinary teams that serve children school-wide to help them develop the language and communication skills needed for school success. Knowing what we know about language development, poverty, and the impact of cultural and linguistic difference, consider what predictions

TABLE 1.1 America's Children at a Glance for 2014

Indicator	2013 value
Children ages 0–17 years in the United States	73.6 million
Children as a percentage of the population in the United States	23.3
Children ages 0–17 years living with two married parents	64%
Children ages 5–17 years who speak a language other than English at home	22.3%
Children ages 5–17 years who speak a language other than English at home and who have difficulty speaking English	5% (2012)
Children ages 0–17 years in poverty	22% (2012)

Note. From *The Condition of Education 2014* (NCES 2014-083), by G. Kena et al., 2014, Washington, DC: U.S. Department of Education, National Center for Education Statistics. Retrieved from http://nces.ed.gov/pubsearch.

you might make about the kindergartners who arrive at the schoolhouse door with differences in their background experience. The challenge for public education is to ensure educational equity for all of these children—for all of America's children.

Incidence of Children With Disabilities

IDEA 2004 requires that services be provided to children who are identified as having a disability from birth to 21 years of age. Annually, the U.S. Department of Education (USDE) reports to Congress on the latest issues and information about the children served under IDEA. During the 2011–2012 school year, 6.4 million children received services under IDEA 2004, approximately 13% of the total school population. This number reflects a decline in the number of students served under this program since 2005–2006 (Kena et al., 2014). The eligibility categories of specific learning disability and speech–language impairment represent the two largest eligibility categories (40.1% and 18.2%, respectively) nationally for children ages 6–21 years. For children ages 3–5 years, speech–language impairment is the most common disability category, followed by developmental delays (37.2%) and autism (7.8%) (U.S. Department of Education, 2014).

The statistics and numbers reported here, in terms of both the conditions in which children live and the identified number of children served through special education programs, give a sense of the sometimes daunting nature of the issues that are faced and must be considered by school-based speech–language pathologists. Throughout the training program in communication sciences and disorders and throughout a speech–language pathologist's working career, it will be critical for the speech–language pathologist to have refined clinical skills in all areas of the field. However, when working with children in a school setting, speech–language pathologists must recognize that one of the foremost tasks is to understand the circumstances in which a child lives. Speech–language pathologists must seek information regarding a student's living situation and then understand the ecological impact this has on his or her language and learning development in order to design appropriate diagnostic practices, intervention protocols, or both. This awareness marks the beginning of seeing the student as a whole child and as a member of a family, classroom, and school community.

Predictions for the Future

This first chapter presents a broad view of the issues facing educational systems, particularly as they apply to the education of children with disabilities and the provision of special education, specifically speech–language services, in the public schools. While reading the chapters in this book, consider the application of points of law or the provision of assessment and intervention services within the context of the forces and issues that affect the educational system and the children and families served. Also consider the evolving roles for speech–language pathologists in schools and how these roles embrace system change and invite speech–language pathologists to be a part of building the systems of the future while providing services to students and working in concert with educators and interested others.

Schools are dynamic and changing institutions. Change is constant, which can be both energizing and frustrating. System change, however, is vital as we respond to new research, the needs of society, and legislative requirements. To consider the future as it is currently defined, consider the following information as it relates to all educators.

Twenty-First-Century Learners

Just as educators and parents become familiar with standards, accountability, access, and the Common Core, the education world continues to change. Speech–language pathologists play an increasingly critical role in these changes. Importantly, our work is to consider the future that students will be facing when they leave our school buildings. Our mission is to ensure that students are prepared to enter the world of work in a future that is still undefined. In the work world of the Digital Age, workers will need to have 21st-century skills that extend beyond the mastery of standards. The base competency that workers will need to compete in a global economy and a digital world is more sophisticated and technological than it has ever been. The North Central Regional Educational Laboratory and the Metiri Group (2003) described the importance of educational systems preparing students for the future:

> In order to thrive in a digital economy, students will need Digital Age proficiencies. It is important for the educational system to make parallel changes in order to fulfill its mission in society, namely the preparation of students for the world beyond the classroom.

Twenty-first-century skills are reflected in the Common Core State Standards and in many other education reform initiatives in order to focus on the skills that students need to develop so they are prepared for their future work world (Common Core State Standards, n.d.-b).

Top Trends in Special Education

The work that speech–language pathologists will do in schools will be driven by the same forces that are creating change in general education. Assessment and intervention trends are identified as follows. Assessment will be

- Based on response to intervention (RTI) models
- Performance based
- Curriculum driven
- Considerate of the demands of statewide and classroom assessments
- Limiting use of standardized measures
- Presented through technology
- Easier to link to goal writing

Intervention will be

- Focused on helping students master curriculum—the work of school
- Focused on outcomes and student achievement
- Provided through blended service delivery models
- Provided within networks
- Linked to the Common Core State Standards
- Measured by academic success
- Presented through technology

As speech–language pathologists familiarize themselves with the 21st-century skills that students need, trends in reading and literacy, and trends in assessment and intervention for special education, they will be at the center of building stronger schools and more effective programs for students. Speech–language pathologists working in public schools will be a part of these trends and ask "What role will I play?" and "How will these programs, initiatives, movements, and predictions influence my work?" While speech–language pathologists in public schools in every state consider these questions, let us say, "Welcome to the public schools!"

CHAPTER 2

The Legislative Foundation of Educational Services for Special Student Populations

● *In This Chapter*

This chapter provides an overview of the legislative history of educational mandates in the United States for learners who are struggling or have disabilities, describes the foundations of the laws, reviews the development of special education legislation for students with disabilities, and discusses the impact and interface of the Elementary and Secondary Education Act (ESEA), (ESEA was reauthorized in 2015 as the Every Student Succeeds Act [ESSA, 2015]) and the Individuals With Disabilities Education Improvement Act of 2004 (IDEA 2004), including the implications of standards-based reform and accountability. This chapter introduces the cornerstone concepts of *free appropriate public education* (FAPE) and *least restrictive environment* (LRE) and discusses the relevance of these for speech-language and audiology services in schools.

● *Chapter Questions*

1. Explain how the legislative history of special education led to laws that are considered to be civil rights protections.
2. Discuss how the concepts of free appropriate public education (FAPE) and least restrictive environment (LRE) apply to speech, language, and hearing programs.
3. Review some of the significant mandates in the Individuals With Disabilities Education Improvement Act of 2004 (IDEA 2004). Discuss why you think these aspects are required in federal law.
4. Discuss the importance of the Elementary and Secondary Education Act (ESEA) and its requirements for both general and special education.
5. Consider what knowledge speech-language pathologists will need to assist students in accessing Common Core State Standards and the general education curriculum.
6. What are the similarities and differences among the provisions of IDEA 2004, Section 504, and the Americans With Disabilities Act of 1990 (ADA)?

The Legislative History of Education for Struggling Learners

Special education and other educational programs are governed by a combination of federal, state, and local laws and regulations. Both general and special education laws are extensive and encompass broad requirements. At the federal level, a framework is set forth of what is required in a law passed by Congress and signed by the president. The law is then interpreted and administered by the U.S. Department of Education (USDE), which sets forth federal rules, known as the *Code of Federal Regulations*. States then pass legislation that incorporates their interpretation and application of the federal law and regulations. Counties, administrative units, and school districts can adopt detailed procedures directing their implementation of state and federal laws. State laws may grant greater rights to children and their parents than federal laws do, but they must at least meet the federal requirements. In some cases, the federal law leaves procedures to be set by states and local entities.

Chapter 1 described how the reform issues of general and special education historically existed in parallel but not in a coordinated fashion. To some degree, this was reflected in the legislation that was put forth during these times. Currently, the laws of general and special education are intended to be coordinated and encompass all learners in the United States. The history of our democracy is deeply rooted in equal opportunity, which is grounded in the public education system. The role of the federal government in education has been historically questioned yet is now firmly established. The central focus of the educational system in the United States is ensuring that all citizens have access to the American Dream. The viability of our nation rests on the development and perpetuation of an educated citizenry. To this end, important legislation governs education, particularly as it applies to individuals who may not have the advantages of others in accessing educational benefits. These learners include children who are underprivileged economically, those who come from culturally and linguistically diverse backgrounds, and those with educational disabilities.

General Education

The role of the federal government has expanded significantly over the past 100 years, certainly in the past 50. In 1965, as part of the War on Poverty and the civil rights movement, President Lyndon B. Johnson signed the Elementary and Secondary Education Act (ESEA) into law, which broadened both the federal influence and the legislative intent for educational programs in the United States. Title I of ESEA was specifically intended to support economically underprivileged children and to address the inequalities in the educational system experienced by these children, particularly those in poor and rural areas.

As with special education, general education laws have been expanded and transformed through considerable revisions since the original enactment. This is reflected in reform movements and is the result of public and political pressure, as well as advancements in the field. While parents and teachers of children with disabilities were fighting for programs and the right to an appropriate education for these children, others were concerned about the overall educational picture for all children in the United States.

On December 10, 2015, President Barack Obama signed into law the Every Student Succeeds Act (ESSA), the long-awaited reauthorization of ESEA, known previously as the No Child Left Behind Act of 2001 (NCLB, 2001). Prior to the implementation of NCLB, speech–language pathologists and special educators had infrequently attended to ESEA's remedial programs for students who were economically disadvantaged, the largest of which was Title I. In fact, students who had been eligible for services under Title I were often subsequently denied access to such services once they became eligible as students with a disability. NCLB completely revamped all educational programs under its purview and expanded the scope of its role beyond any previously realized. Most importantly, NCLB included requirements for students with disabilities, forging stronger bonds between general and special education. The passage of NCLB in 2001 created a joint responsibility for accountability of the educational outcomes of struggling learners, including students with disabilities. The integration of efforts to provide resources and support for these students has not been without challenge, and it most certainly has affected the practice of all educators, including speech–language pathologists. The ESSA continues some of the provisions put in place under NCLB but also changed many of the main requirements, specifically those related to accountability. What has not changed is the requirement for school systems to be accountable for the educational progress of students with disabilities.

Special Education

On December 3, 2004, President George W. Bush signed the reauthorization of IDEA 2004 into law. This updating of the nation's special education law again reaffirmed the legislative and political commitment to the education of children with disabilities, strongly emphasizing the need for aligning special education practices and outcomes with those of general education and ESEA/NCLB 2001. The road to this ceremony in room 350 of the Dwight D. Eisenhower Office Building was long, beginning before the implementation of the Education for All Handicapped Children Act (EAHCA) in 1975, which established the framework for special education as it is known today. In his signing statement, President Bush acknowledged this embattled history as he set the vision of what the law would mean for children with disabilities:

> America's schools educate over 6 million children with disabilities. In the past, those students were too often just shuffled through the system with little expectation that they could make significant progress or succeed like their fellow classmates. Children with disabilities deserve high hopes, high expectations, and extra help.

The history of special education has been characterized by controversy, encountering debate over subjects ranging from philosophical to fiscal issues. Critics of special education, including general educators and politicians, have become increasingly vocal about their concerns regarding expense (see "Funding" in Chapter 9), lack of adequate results, and a dual system for disciplining students (see "Positive Behavior Supports and Student Discipline" in Chapter 8).

IDEA 2004 strongly established that the national mandate regarding the education of students with disabilities must include academic achievement at the same level as expected for children in general education. This agenda can be seen with the statement of findings in the introduction to the bill (see following). Congress acknowledged the impressive history that led to the establishment of special education and not only emphasized that these issues should never be forgotten but also presented the challenge to educators and those involved with students with disabilities to improve educational results for these children. Speech-language pathologists and other special educators who work under IDEA 2004 should be ever mindful of the long, hard-fought battle and historic events that led to the current special education system.

IDEA 2004 Statement of Findings

(c) FINDINGS. Congress finds the following:

(1) Disability is a natural part of the human experience and in no way diminishes the right of individuals to participate in or contribute to society. Improving educational results for children with disabilities is an essential element of our national policy of ensuring equality of opportunity, full participation, independent living, and economic self-sufficiency for individuals with disabilities.

(2) Before the date of enactment of the Education for All Handicapped Children Act of 1975 (P.L. 94-142), the educational needs of millions of children with disabilities were not being fully met because—

(A) the children did not receive appropriate educational services;

(B) the children were excluded entirely from the public school system and from being educated with their peers;

(C) undiagnosed disabilities prevented the children from having a successful educational experience; or

(D) a lack of adequate resources within the public school system forced families to find services outside the public school system.

(3) Since the enactment and implementation of the Education for All Handicapped Children Act of 1975, this title has been successful in ensuring children with disabilities and the families of such children access to a free appropriate public education and in improving educational results for children with disabilities.

(4) However, the implementation of this title has been impeded by low expectations, and an insufficient focus on applying replicable research on proven methods of teaching and learning for children with disabilities.

(5) Almost 30 years of research and experience has demonstrated that the education of children with disabilities can be made more effective by—

(A) having high expectations for such children and ensuring their access to the general education curriculum in the regular classroom, to the maximum extent possible, in order to—

(i) meet developmental goals and, to the maximum extent possible, the challenging expectations that have been established for all children; and

(ii) be prepared to lead productive and independent adult lives, to the maximum extent possible;

(B) strengthening the role and responsibility of parents and ensuring that families of such children have meaningful opportunities to participate in the education of their children at school and at home.

Source. IDEA 2004, § 601[c].

Until the mid- to late 1960s, the federal government played virtually no role in the education of children with disabilities, with the exception of providing some assistance between the 1820s and 1870s in creating special schools for children who were blind, deaf, or mentally ill (Friend & Bursuck, 2012). Most of the responsibility for educating children with disabilities previously fell to states or to private individuals and organizations. By 1911, a U.S. Bureau of Education survey found "6% of cities reporting special classes (i.e., 11% for gifted; 25% for backward; 10% for physically exceptional [non-English speaking]; and 17% for morally exceptional, delinquent, and incorrigible")" (Council for Exceptional Children, 1997, p. 11). In 1930, "the White House Conference on Special Education reported the following statistics of handicapped children in the United States: 300,000 crippled; 18,212 deaf; 3,000,000 hard of hearing; 14,000 blind; 50,000 partially seeing; 1,000,000 defective speech; 450,000 mentally retarded; and 1,500,000 gifted" (CEC, 1997, p. 20).

After both World War I and World War II, the U.S. government recognized the need for vocational-type training for veterans, especially those who returned with disabilities from war. Federal involvement in the education of children with disabilities was slow to follow. Some states provided education to students who entered public education with a variety of difficulties, including intellectual disabilities or cognitive limitations. Notably, states such as Illinois, New York, Florida, California, and Wisconsin implemented programs that followed functionally based (called *occupational education* or *vocational education*) curricula, focusing on job skills, community skills, living skills, and some academically related skills. The need for federal involvement in mandating and regulating the education of children with disabilities began to emerge with a growing parent movement and with the assistance of President John F. Kennedy, who established the President's Committee on Mental Retardation in the early 1960s (CEC, 1997; Friend & Bursuck, 2012).

In 1958, President Dwight D. Eisenhower signed P.L. 85-926, the Education of Mentally Retarded Children Act, which was a bill that provided financial assistance to colleges educating teachers of children with intellectual or cognitive disabilities. The first direct subsidy for services to special populations, including children with disabilities, came in 1966, the second year of ESEA (P.L. 89-10). This act established the system of remedial education for economically disadvantaged students, known as Title I, and provided some entitlements to state-supported or state-operated schools for children with disabilities.

Roots of Special Education in Civil Rights Legal Action

The lack of federal assistance was apparent not just in the education of children with disabilities but also pertaining to other educational and social issues. The Supreme Court case that dramatically changed the nation's course was *Brown v. Board of Education* (1954). The Supreme Court ruled unanimously that the doctrine of "separate but equal" was inherently unequal and therefore unconstitutional. While *Brown* specifically dealt with racial segregation, it laid the foundation for the education of children with disabilities and other disenfranchised groups because the right-to-education issue was argued on the principles of equal protection under the law for all citizens.

Brown clarified that although the U.S. Constitution never once refers to public education, the principles of equal protection and due process under the Fifth and Fourteenth Amendments apply to public education. For all groups who have experienced segregation or discrimination, the foundation of *Brown* is solid. Equal opportunity, equal protection, and the right to an education are founded in the Constitution and apply to all groups, regardless of race, color, creed, gender, disability, or national origin. In this decision, the court established that "integration into public education was the only way in which students' constitutional rights to equal opportunity could be protected when diverse student groups learned together"; integration was the only way to achieve equal opportunity for groups of diverse learners by ensuring that all students learned together (Friend & Bursuck, 2012).

Equal protection and due process are foundational to special education law. Two major court cases solidified the connection between equal protection and due process under the Fourteenth Amendment: *Pennsylvania Association for Retarded Children (PARC) v. Commonwealth of Pennsylvania* (1972) and *Mills v. D.C. Board of Education* (1972).

The *PARC* case challenged a state law in Pennsylvania that allowed public schools to deny an education to children whom examiners determined to be below the mental age of 5 years. *PARC* was settled on a consent decree that (a) provided full access to an education for children with mental retardation, (b) established the standard of appropriateness, and (c) established a standard for least restrictive environment (LRE).

On the heels of the *PARC* case, *Mills v. D.C. Board of Education* was a case brought by students with varying types of disabilities who had been excluded from school and denied an education in the District of Columbia schools. The basis of their exclusion from school was the disabilities of these children. In its ruling, the District Court ordered the following:

- The District of Columbia shall provide to each child of school age a free and suitable publicly supported education regardless of the degree of the child's mental, physical, or emotional disability or impairment. Furthermore, defendants shall not exclude any child resident in the District of Columbia from such publicly supported education on the basis of a claim of insufficient resources.
- Defendants shall not suspend a child from the public schools for disciplinary reasons for any period in excess of 2 days without affording him or her a hearing pursuant to the provisions of Paragraph 13.f. and without providing for his or her education during the period of any such suspension.

With the strength of *Brown*, *PARC*, and *Mills*, court cases continued to be brought forward, yet estimates showed that millions of children with disabilities still were not receiving a public education. Most states had some form of special education programs, but these varied dramatically from state to state. Ultimately, during the 1970s, states joined with existing advocacy groups to seek federal legislation that would provide financial assistance and guidance for the provision of education to children with disabilities (Friend & Bursuck, 2012; New America Foundation, 2012). Interestingly, some 60 years later, after the nation has observed the 60th anniversary of *Brown*, many still question whether full equity has been reached for racial desegregation (American Civil Liberties Union, 2014; Maxwell, 2014). This conversation is powerful because it pertains to services to others from disenfranchised groups, including students with disabilities and children of impoverished or low-SES backgrounds. (See the discussion in "Significance of Child and Family Statistics" in Chapter 1.)

Legislative Response: Special Education as a Federal Mandate

In 1970, Congress passed the Education of the Handicapped Act (P.L. 91-230). This law established minimum requirements for states to follow in order to receive federal assistance. Following *PARC* and *Mills*, Congress acted by enacting laws in the area of nondiscrimination and also providing some funding. In Section 504 of the Rehabilitation Act of 1973 (P.L. 93-112), discrimination against those with disabilities was prohibited in any system that received federal funding. (See "Parental Notification and Involvement" in Chapter 8.) Additional federal financial assistance for states came in the amendments to the Elementary and Secondary Education Act of 1974 (ESEA, P.L. 93-380).

These dramatic changes to the ESEA clearly laid the foundation for what was soon to come. In 1975, Congress amended the Education of the Handicapped Act by passing the Education for All Handicapped Children Act (EAHCA, P.L. 94-142). This law established special education as it is known today, with requirements for the provision of services, procedural safeguards, and funding mechanisms to support the programs. The federal mandate for special education has been revised and updated several times since 1975. The 1990 amendments (P.L. 101-476) renamed the law to be the Individuals With Disabilities Education Act, commonly referred to as IDEA, which is how the law is now known. In addition, the Americans With Disabilities Act of 1990 (ADA, P.L. 101-336) was signed into law by President George H. W. Bush in 1990, further expanding the scope of discriminatory practices identified as illegal in all public accommodations. The 2004 reauthorization of IDEA kept the acronym IDEA but added the word *improvement* to the full name of the law, so that it is known as P.L. 108-446, the Individuals With Disabilities Education Improvement Act of 2004 (IDEA 2004).

Federal mandates, including those for special education, provide guidance through legislation but then require states to develop their own programs to implement the federal regulations. It is for this reason that the provision of services may look different from state to state. Monitoring how states implement their special education programs is the responsibility of the Office of Special Education Programs (OSEP). OSEP works closely with the state education agencies (SEAs) to ensure that federal requirements are being met in each state and uses a continuous improvement-monitoring model that focuses on student outcomes.

States work to maintain their own identity in the provision of special education services. Issues such as the provision of free appropriate public education (FAPE), least restrictive environment (LRE), student discipline, funding, and service delivery to students in correctional facilities have provided arenas for the struggle between state and federal interpretations of special education procedures. The history of special education reflects a recurring pattern of a series of legal cases, followed by revisions to the law, followed by another series of legal cases that interpret the revisions and also deal with emerging areas of practice.

The Education for All Handicapped Children Act

In 1975, the EAHCA established the system under which special education has operated since its origination. The act described a complex set of procedures designed to rectify the issues that had been brought forward by the courts, parents, educators, and states. Congress was concerned with the number of children who remained unserved by the public school systems, so Child Find, a mandate that requires local education agencies (LEAs) to establish a system designed to locate, evaluate, and serve children with disabilities, was enacted. The history of court decisions leading up to the establishment of the EAHCA was reflected in the law's key components, including

- providing federal funding for special education programs;
- establishing procedures to ensure the provision of special education services;
- establishing conceptual parameters under which the procedures were to be followed, including FAPE, LRE, procedural safeguards, and zero reject; and
- requiring the provision of services to children ages 0–21 years, identified through Child Find activities, resulting in an evaluation process and qualifying for the program according to certain criteria.

Eligibility Criteria

Following the passage of EAHCA in 1975, states were allowed 3 years to establish a state plan for the implementation of the law. The federal law provided the outline of a process for developing an Individualized Education Program (IEP) that would be based on an evaluation to determine the child's eligibility. (See Chapter 4 for a full description of IEP processes and procedures, including eligibility requirements.)

One of the most critical features of the EAHCA (1975) was the institution of procedural safeguards or due process protection for children and parents, which provided full partnership for parents in the decision-making processes in special education. In special education, the term *due process* refers to the procedural rights, protections, and safeguards for parents and children and also refers to procedures involving appeal procedures including hearings and mediation. Procedural safeguards provide (a) timelines for evaluations, (b) access to and review of records, (c) parental involvement and consent, (d) parental input into program development, and (e) procedures for complaints and disagreements. If parents and school districts are unable to agree on identification, evaluation, or any other aspects of the IEP or placement (including goals and short-term objectives or benchmarks), then either party may request a *due process hearing*. A due process hearing involves presentation of evidence by both parties before an impartial hearing officer. Prior to the hearing, a resolution session, mediation, or other methods to resolve a dispute may be requested or required. (See Chapter 8 "Resolution Sessions, Mediation, Due Process Hearings, and State IDEA Complaints.")

Over the years, several amendments have been added to the EAHCA (1975), increasing the requirements under this law. Two important changes occurred in 1986: the Preschool Amendments to the Education of the Handicapped Act (P.L. 99-457) and the addition of Part H (now Part C), which extended the age of eligibility to include infants and toddlers who may receive services under less intensive eligibility criteria. This change came as a result of professionals and parents lobbying Congress to fund early intervention services, with the belief that early intervention would prevent or reduce the need for lifelong special services. Another important addition to the law came in 1986 with the passage of the Handicapped Children's Protection Act (known as the Attorneys' Fees Bill, P.L. 99-372). This act authorized awarding attorneys' fees to families who prevailed in lawsuits under the due process provisions of the law. (See "Impartial Due Process Hearings" in Chapter 8.)

The Individuals With Disabilities Education Act: EAHCA 1990 and 1997 Revisions

The evolution of legislative mandates under the law demonstrates how legal requirements are implemented in response to societal and political circumstances and advances in research. In this way, change becomes an ever-occurring situation in schools, as educators must adjust to the latest changes in the law. It takes time to implement changes that occur in the law. However, when legislation is enacted, the time to implement is typically short, challenging school districts to bring their systems quickly into compliance, even if the new requirements are not philosophically or fiscally easy to implement. The lesson for practitioners in schools is this: Expect change to occur on a regular basis.

The 1990 revisions to the EAHCA (1975) included a new name: the Individuals With Disabilities Education Act (IDEA). This name reflected the consciousness of the

"People First" movement, which emphasized that persons with disabilities should be recognized as individuals first, replacing the label as a name.

American Psychological Association's Guidelines for "People First" Language

The overall principle for "nonhandicapping" language is to maintain the integrity (worth) of individuals as human beings (see the *Publication Manual of the American Psychological Association* by the American Psychological Association, 2010, p. 76). Avoid language that objectifies a person by his or her condition (e.g., *autistic, neurotic*), that uses pictorial metaphors (e.g., *wheelchair bound* or *confined to a wheelchair*), that uses excessive and negative labels (e.g., *AIDS victim, brain damaged*), or that can be regarded as a slur (e.g., *cripple, invalid*). Use people first language, and do not focus on the individual's disabling or chronic condition (e.g., *person with paraplegia, youth with autism*). Also use people first language to describe groups of people with disabilities. For instance, refer to *children with autism* rather than *autistic children*.

Avoid euphemisms that are condescending when describing individuals with disabilities (e.g., *special, physically challenged, handi-capable*). Some people with disabilities consider these terms patronizing and offensive.

Source. From *Publication Manual of the American Psychological Association* (6th ed., p. 76), by the American Psychological Association (APA), 2010, Washington, DC: Author. ©2010 by the APA.

Examples of People First Language (K. Snow, 2017)

Do the words used to describe *you* have an impact on your life? *You bet!* Contrary to the age-old "sticks and stones" lesson we learned as children, *words do matter!*

For too long, people who happen to have conditions we call "disabilities" have been subjected to devaluation, marginalization, prejudice, and more. And the first way to devalue someone is through language, by using words or labels to identify a person/group as "less than," as "the other," "not like us," and so forth. Once a person/group has been identified this way, it makes it easier to justify prejudice and discrimination. Our language shapes out attitudes; our attitudes shape our language; they're intertwined. And our attitudes and language *drive our actions!*

Using People First Language—putting the person before the disability—and eliminating old, prejudicial, and hurtful descriptors, can move us in a new direction. People First Language is not political correctness; instead, it demonstrates good manners, respect, and the Golden Rule, and more—it can change the way we see a person, and it can change the way a person sees herself!

The modifications to EAHCA (1975) in IDEA (1990) provisions reflected changes in the communities of persons with disabilities and special education, as highlighted in Table 2.1.

TABLE 2.1. Modifications to the Education for All Handicapped Children Act in the Individuals With Disabilities Education Act (1990)

Legislative change	Societal, research, or practice advancement or influence
Changed the name of the special education law to the Individuals With Disabilities Education Act (IDEA)	This change reflects the impact of the "People First" movement, which emphasized that persons with disabilities are individuals first and should not be referred to as a label.
Added the new eligibility category of *autism*	By 1990, much controversy existed regarding the education of students with autism. Other eligibility categories such as *speech or language impairment* or *intellectual disability* did not accurately describe characteristics that were unique to children with autism.
Added the new eligibility category of *traumatic brain injury* (TBI)	By 1990, medical technology enabled higher survival rates from accidents, evidenced by an increase in students with TBI in schools. These children showed a different pattern of recovery, in that their special needs did not result from a developmental condition, as did all other eligibility areas. Identifying these students under the categories of *speech or language impairment*, *intellectual disability*, and/or *other health impairment* did not accurately identify these students' learning needs.
Added a requirement for transition planning for students beginning at the age of 16 years	Students who had been receiving special education and related services were not successful in the world of work after exiting the public education system. It became apparent that as part of their special education services, Individualized Education Program (IEP) teams needed to specifically address the development of skills that students needed to master to hold a job. As a result, a statement of needed transition services, often called an Individualized Transition Plan (ITP), was required for students beginning at the age of 16 years (changed to age 14 years under the IDEA Amendments of 1997 and then back to 16 years under IDEA 2004).
Added new requirements under IDEA (1990) that called for greater integration of students with even the most significant disabilities into their communities and schools	This focus was consistent with the Regular Education Initiative and the Inclusion Movement (discussed in "Educational Reforms That Shaped the Profession" in Chapter 1) that fought against the isolation and segregation of students with disabilities.
Added the requirement for the consideration of assistive technology as part of the IEP process	This requirement mandated the consideration and purchase of assistive technology devices if the IEP team found that the student was in need of such equipment and services.

Requirements of the IDEA Amendments of 1997

With the reauthorization of IDEA in 1997, Congress identified the lack of positive educational results as a major concern for the education of students with disabilities. IDEA shifted the focus of special education from educational access to accountability for educational results.

While acknowledging that the mandate for special education had resulted in progress, Congress (IDEA Amendments of 1997) stated that there was a need to do much more. To accomplish this, reauthorization focused on five areas (OSERS, 1999). These focus areas and resulting requirements are described in Table 2.2.

The Interface of General and Special Education:
The Elementary and Secondary Education Act and the Individuals With Disabilities Education Improvement Act of 2004

The Every Student Succeeds Act (ESSA, 2015) reflected the fundamental precepts of the previous Elementary and Secondary Education Act (ESEA) reauthorization known as the No Child Left Behind Act (NCLB, 2001). (*Note.* ESEA was originally passed in 1965 and established federal programs for serving underprivileged students. Like special education laws, ESEA has been reauthorized and expanded throughout its legislative history.) In 2001 and 2004, when the major laws that directed federal education programs for general and special education were reauthorized, they became integrated in ways previously unknown in the education system. This section will review the substantial changes brought to the educational system through ESEA and NCLB, as well as IDEA 2004.

We have all been taught in civics classes how laws are made. For the purpose of understanding the application of education law to our work, speech–language pathologists and special and general educators need to have knowledge of how laws and requirements are established. Federal laws are passed by Congress and signed into law by the president, just as we have been taught. Federal laws are known as public laws (P.L.). The numbers of the laws represent the session of Congress when the law was passed and a bill number. So, P.L. 94-142, the Education for All Handicapped Children Act (EAHCA), was passed and signed into law in the 94th session of Congress and was the 142nd bill to be passed in 1975. After a bill is signed into law, it is sent to the federal regulatory office for that type of bill for development of the *Code of Federal Regulations*, which outlines more details about how to implement the law. In the case of education law, including ESEA and IDEA, the federal agency responsible for oversight and establishing the *Code of Federal Regulations* is the U.S. Department of Education (USDE). The establishment of the *Code of Federal Regulations* follows another process involving public input, before the regulations are finalized. The next step is for states to pass laws to comply with the federal law and then go through a similar process for the state to establish education code that will bring the state into compliance with the federal law. States must comply

TABLE 2.2. Individuals With Disabilities Education Act (IDEA) Focus Areas

IDEA Amendments of 1997: Focus area	Legislative change	Societal, research, or practice advancement or influence
Raising expectations for children with disabilities	This change included new requirements to describe how the student accesses the general education curriculum and how the student's disability affects his or her ability to access the curriculum.	There is clear indication that speech–language pathologists, audiologists, and other special educators must know the curriculum and the demands for learning across grade levels and content areas.
	This change included new requirements to include students with disabilities in state testing and the accountability system to demonstrate they are making progress in the general education curriculum.	The goal of achieving general education expectations challenged special educators to identify methods that would allow students to access the curriculum.
Increasing parents' involvement in the education of their children	These new requirements include greater parental involvement in the Individualized Education Program (IEP) process, including an active role in which the parents (a) provide critical information regarding the strengths of their child and express their concerns for enhancing the education of their child, (b) participate in discussions about the child's need for special education and related services and supplementary aids and services, and (c) join with the other participants in deciding how the child will be involved in and progress in the general curriculum, how the child will participate in district- and statewide assessments, and what services the agency will provide to the child, as well as the setting of those services.	Parents' complaints about the IEP process include concerns that IEP teams predetermine placement and services or do not solicit parental input or ignore what parents say. These requirements are set to ensure solicitation of parental involvement in the IEP process.
Ensuring that general education teachers are involved in planning and assessing children's progress	These new requirements state that general education teachers must participate in the development, review, and revision of IEPs. The IDEA Amendments of 1997 instituted the following for the participation of general education teachers in the IEP process: • The student's teachers must have access to the IEP document. • Teachers must be informed of their specific responsibilities related to implementing the IEP. • Teachers must be informed of the specific modifications and supports that must be provided to the student. • Teachers must participate in the development, review, and revision of the IEP, including assisting in developing positive behavioral interventions and determining supplementary aids, services, and program modifications.	General education teachers play a central role in the education of children with disabilities and have important expertise regarding the general curriculum and the general education environment. With the emphasis on involvement and progress in the general curriculum added by the IDEA Amendments of 1997, general education teachers have a critical role (together with special education and related services personnel) in implementing free appropriate public education for most children with disabilities. The requirement for participation of general education teachers on IEP teams brought a new dimension to the IEP. This provision reinforced the reality that children with disabilities are part of a school system. The services provided by the *(continues)*

TABLE 2.2. *(continued)*

IDEA Amendments of 1997: Focus area	Legislative change	Societal, research, or practice advancement or influence
(row continues)	• Services to assist the teacher, such as consultation or training, may be included under supplemental aids and services. • Attendance and participation of a regular education teacher is required if the student is, or may be, participating in the regular education environment.	speech–language pathologist, audiologist, or any other special educator must be designed to assist the child in benefiting from the core curriculum. The general education teacher brings this focus to the IEP team. The intent of these regulations is to guarantee that special education is not a "place" or a separate system but rather a support to general education. Consequently, speech–language pathologists and audiologists must know the workings of the general education classroom and the expectations for teachers and students in order to provide support to both. General education teachers may need guidance in terms of their role and responsibilities as team members and at IEP meetings.
Including children with disabilities in assessments, performance goals, and reports to the public	In addition to including students with disabilities in the district- and statewide accountability program, IDEA Amendments of 1997 also required states to have performance goals and indicators established for children with disabilities. These goals were required to be consistent to the maximum extent appropriate with the performance goals and standards for children without disabilities.	Students with disabilities were typically excluded from statewide assessments until the mid-1990s, when reform movements in both general and special education called for educational systems to be responsible and accountable for the learning of all students.
Supporting quality professional development for all personnel who are involved in educating children with disabilities	Professional development would be necessary for individuals working with children with disabilities and may be provided in a variety of different ways, including workshops, conferences, specialized trainings, mentoring, staff meetings, professional study groups, professional journals, and others. These trainings might focus on an identified need area in the school or district. State and regional trainings could also be available to both general and special education professionals.	Individuals may obtain professional development from professional associations, such as the American Speech-Language-Hearing Association or state-level speech and hearing associations, local education agencies, or other agencies that provide workshops and trainings.

with federal law, but they will interpret the law according to the systems and parameters of each state, which is why there is some variation in how states define and implement laws. After the state law and education code are established, local education agencies (LEAs) (i.e., school districts) will adopt board policy and administrative regulations for the implementation of federal and state laws. Finally, special education departments and local consortia will provide handbooks and guidance to staff and parents regarding the procedural implementation of all these requirements in the local area. Parents and staff are often confused by all these levels of requirements and sometimes confuse local policy with federal or state mandates. The school district administration can help with these clarifications, as can guidance from federal and state agencies and state and national professional associations.

Levels of Laws and Regulations

Federal
Public law
Code of Federal Regulations
▼

State
State law
Education code
▼

Local education agency or school district
School board policy
Administrative regulations

Elementary and Secondary Education Act and Every Student Succeeds Act

The passage of the Every Student Succeeds Act came 14 years following the tumultuous history of its predecessor, NCLB, which had clearly established a strong federal role in education, igniting widespread reform in instructional programs throughout the nation. Most importantly, NCLB, along with the subsequent reauthorization of IDEA 2004, put accountability for the learning of students with disabilities in the forefront by establishing requirements that tracked the progress of these students. Prior to this, general and special educators were not truly being held accountable for producing results with target populations, including students with disabilities. With the arrival of ESSA, there has been a shift to reduce the federal role in decisions related to accountability and instruction, shifting decisions to the states and local entities. Federal requirements for accountability and improvement are still in place; however, how districts get there is up to the state and local education agencies.

Key Principles and Programs of the Every Student Succeeds Act

The White House (2015) reacted positively to the passage of ESSA, reporting that the new law would fix problems that created challenges for state and local agencies under NCLB. The foundations of the new law were consistent with ESEA's commitment to providing educational programs to support underprivileged and underrepresented student groups, including children from low socioeconomic backgrounds, students with disabilities, English Learners, and children of color. The major provisions embraced the administration's reform tenets (The White House, 2015):

- College and career-ready standards for America's learners
- Rigorous accountability for all students
- Reform and resources for America's struggling schools and students
- New incentives to improve opportunities and outcomes for students
- A smart and balanced approach to testing
- Promoting equity in state and local funding

Table 2.3 reflects the various programs defined and operated under ESSA. Notable enhancements have occurred in the education of English Learners, as well as changes in reading and literacy programs. Speech–language pathologists should review this list to understand the scope of what is funded and addressed under ESSA. Many students may be eligible for services under both ESSA and IDEA. In addition, with the reauthorization of ESEA as ESSA, it is anticipated that IDEA reauthorization will come soon. Likewise, it is anticipated that IDEA reauthorization will reflect some of the changes seen in ESSA, which is why it is of interest to know and understand the provisions in this law.

School districts (i.e., local education agencies) with a high proportion of students who are economically disadvantaged are eligible for Title I funds. Funding flows to school districts and buildings based on complex formulas (which will not be described here). Funds may be used for either school-wide programs, such as before- or after-school programs or summer programs, or targeted assistance programs, such as instruction in reading or math. ESSA creates greater opportunity for flexibility in funding, meaning that although funds are designated for certain projects, there is flexibility to use funds across categories to address specific needs, within the guidelines set (New America Foundation, 2014b; Ujifusa, 2016).

Special education programs and the programs funded through ESEA are considered "categorical" programs (see "Funding" in Chapter 9). This means that dollars allocated to these programs must be spent for the specific purposes intended under each category. In years past, students who met the criteria for both special education and Title I were allowed to participate in only one program or the other because of strict spending requirements. However, in recent years, greater flexibility has been built into the funding systems in order to extend services of both programs to eligible students. Title I resources are used by school districts to provide a variety of extra and expansive services to students in general or special education. In fact, the federal government encourages joining resources through multifunding services and programs under these two statutes. ESSA Title I grants and IDEA Special Education grants represent the largest education programs provided by the federal government, with allocations of $14.9 billion for ESSA in 2016 and $11.6 billion for IDEA grants in the fiscal year 2016. (Note that used in this context, grants are funding allocations to states based on eligibility, not competitive grants.)

TABLE 2.3. Every Student Succeeds Act Programs at a Glance

Section	Example programs
Title I Improving Basic Programs Operated by State and Local Education Agencies	• State Assessment • Education of Migratory Children • Prevention and Intervention Programs for Children and Youth Who Are Neglected, Delinquent, or at Risk
Title II Preparing, Training, and Recruiting High Quality Teachers, Principals, or Other School Leaders	• Teacher and Principal Training and Recruiting • Enhancing Education Through Technology
Title III Language Instruction for English Learners and Immigrant Students	• English Language Acquisition, Language Enhancement, and Academic Achievement
Title IV 21st Century Schools	• Student Support and Academic Enrichment • 21st Century Community of Learning Centers
Title V State Innovations and Local Flexibility	• Funding Transferability for State and Local Education Agencies • Innovation in Education • Rural Education Initiative
Title VI Indian, Native Hawaiian, and Alaska Native Education	• Indian Education • Native Hawaiian Education • Alaska Native Education
Title VII Impact Aid Program	• Impact Aid
Title VIII General Provisions	• Consolidation of Administrative Funds • Maintenance of Effort • State Control Over Standards • Sense of Congress on Protecting Student Privacy and Early Learning and Child Care
Title IX Education for the Homeless and Other Laws	• Amends the McKinney-Vento Assistance Act • Homeless Children and Youths

Note. From Every Student Succeeds Act (P.L. 114-95). Retrieved from https://www.congress.gov/bill/114th-congress/senate-bill/1177/text#toc-HAE78B8E4C4BE40149D58383C87450C5C

Accountability Programs: Assessment and Standards

ESSA shifts the decisions for accountability components to the states, who are charged with making the choices about challenging academic standards and achievement assessments. The NCLB legislation stated, "The purpose of this title is to provide all children significant opportunity to receive a fair, equitable, and high-quality education, and to close educational achievement gaps" (NCLB § 1001). ESSA carries this same spirit. States are required to provide assurance to the federal government that they have adopted challenging academic content and aligned academic achievement standards, known collectively as *challenging academic achievement standards.* Academic content standards are required in math, reading and language arts, science, and any other subject that the state deems necessary. The aligned achievement standards must have three levels, at least, that will align with credit-bearing courses in institutions of higher education and relevant career technical education course work (ESSA § 1111 [b][1]). ESSA also provides that states may provide alternate academic achievement standards for students with significant cognitive disabilities, provided that the standards

(I)   are aligned with the challenging State academic content standards under subparagraph (A);

(II) promote access to the general education curriculum, consistent with the Individuals With Disabilities Education Act (20 U.S.C. § 1400 et seq.);

(III) reflect professional judgment as to the highest possible standards achievable by such students;

(IV) are designated in the individualized education program developed under section 614(d)(3) of the Individuals With Disabilities Education Act (20 U.S.C. § 1414[d][3]) for each such student as the academic achievement standards that will be used for the student; and

(V) are aligned to ensure that a student who meets the alternate academic achievement standards is on track to pursue postsecondary education or employment, consistent with the purposes of Public Law 93-112, as in effect on July 22, 2014.

States are also required to have standards for English-language proficiency, including the four domains of speaking, listening, reading, and writing, at various levels of proficiency and aligned to challenging academic achievement standards.

Both ESEA/ESSA and IDEA 2004 require the participation of students with disabilities in statewide assessments and standards-based programs. ESEA/ESSA specifically tracks the performance of students with disabilities to monitor annual progress. ESSA allows for alternate achievement assessment of students with the most significant cognitive disabilities. The alternate achievement assessment must be aligned with the alternate achievement standards. The alternate achievement standards and assessments must be discussed with parents at the student's IEP meeting. The number of students whose scores are reported from alternate achievement assessment is capped at 1% of all students in the state who are tested.

ESSA does not allow a federal mandate of specific standards and gives this obligation to the states. The new law allows for states to use existing standards that have already been adopted.

Prior to, or subsequent to, the passage of NCLB, all states established their own state standards to be in compliance with the federal law. States also developed state testing systems, which were aligned with their standards. What evolved was concern that there were disparities between states in standards and assessment systems, making it difficult to compare student performance in various states but also representing concerns about how state standards were comparing internationally.

In 2010, the National Governors Association and the Council of Chief State School Officers launched Common Core State Standards (CCSS) (www.corestandards.org). The mission statement of the CCSS states the following:

> The Common Core State Standards provide a consistent, clear understanding of what students are expected to learn, so teachers and parents know what they need to do to help them. The standards are designed to be robust and relevant to the real world, reflecting the knowledge and skills that our young people need for success in college and careers. With American students fully prepared for the future, our communities will be best positioned to compete successfully in the global economy.

The Web site for the CCSS reported that 43 states, the District of Columbia, four territories, and the Department of Defense Education Activity have adopted the CCSS, as of April 2016. The following states have not adopted the CCSS: Alaska, Indiana, Nebraska, Oklahoma, Texas, and Virginia. Minnesota has adopted English-language arts only, and the territory of Puerto Rico has not adopted CCSS.

ESSA (§ 1111 [c][2]) requires that states disaggregate their data and report on the following subgroups:

a. Students from major racial and ethnic subgroups
b. Economically disadvantaged students
c. Students with disabilities
d. English Learners

Including students with disabilities in the state testing system is fundamental to the accountability movement. Most students with disabilities spend most of their time in the general education classroom. The importance of ensuring that the educational system is responsible for the achievement of these learners is noteworthy. Inclusion of students with disabilities and the mandates for academic results are also being emphasized in the new accountability framework for special education, known as *results driven accountability*, announced in June 2014 (USDE, 2014). Further information for speech–language pathologists and other special educators on the practice implications of including students with disabilities in statewide assessments is included in Chapter 3.

With the advent of new standards, new assessment systems were also needed. Because CCSS provided common standards that can be used in every state, new assessments were also being developed to assess how students were meeting the common core. The ESSA also allows states to determine which assessments to use, in addition to which standards to use. However, prior to the law's enactment, assessment consortia were established to develop new assessment systems. These included the following:

General Assessment Systems
• Partnership for Assessment of Readiness for College and Careers (PARCC) (www.parcconline.org)
• Smarter Balanced Assessment Consortium (SBAC) (www.smarterbalanced.org)

Alternate Assessment Systems:

For Students With Significant Cognitive Disabilities

- National Center and State Collaborative (NCSC) (www.ncscpartners.org)
- Dynamic Learning Maps (DLM) (http://dynamiclearningmaps.org)
- Alternate assessment systems for students who are English-language learners
- Assessment Services Supporting English Language Learners through Technology Systems (ASSETS) consortium (http://assets.wceruw.org)
- English Language Proficiency Assessment for the 21st Century (ELPA21) (www .elpa21.org/) (Doorey, 2014)

The NCSC and DLM have also developed alternate achievement assessments for students who are using alternate achievement standards.

The new standards and new generation of assessments represent a shift in instructional approaches and a shift in the focus on what students understand and are able to do versus what they can remember (Methaney, 2013). This also means a shift in how all educators approach instruction and intervention, including speech–language pathologists and audiologists. (See more on CCSS in Chapters 3 and 5.) ESSA also calls for the use of universal design for learning (UDL) principles in their response to address the needs of the subgroups identified.

Staff Qualifications

The area of teacher qualifications is another area where ESSA sends responsibility for establishing criteria to the state. NCLB had contained the requirement for teachers and paraprofessionals to be highly qualified. ESSA now shifts to the states the determination of what it is to be an "effective" teacher. States must still report on efforts to address disparities that result in poor and minority students being taught by inexperienced or unqualified teachers or in the assignment of teachers who are not qualified to teach in core subject areas. Title II funds of ESSA can be used for professional development of teachers. States are required to report on methods or criteria determined to measure educator effectiveness and equitable distribution of high-quality teachers. ESSA also affects the requirement in the IDEA for special education teachers to be highly qualified under the NCLB rules.

Some states may choose to continue with the regulations set forth under the NCLB. Controversy rose around these provisions when the Obama administration allowed for states to apply for waivers if they included teachers' ability to raise test scores in their evaluation systems (a method known as *value added*). Under ESSA, this provision can be included but does not need to be.

For speech–language pathologists and other special education personnel, it will be important to monitor closely the requirements of their state. Speech–language pathologists are trained in programs that meet accreditation of ASHA and the state. The authors highly recommend that all speech–language pathologists attain their Certificate of Clinical Competence (CCC) through ASHA, to demonstrate their competency, in addition to the required certification and licensure required in their state. This topic is further discussed in Chapter 9.

Focus on Closing the Achievement Gap

ESSA asserts the major focus on closing the achievement gap in the purpose stated previously. Accountability indicators will measure these efforts. Indicators must include nonacademic factors and those selected by the state. In the new law, accountability systems are established to focus on certain subgroups and low-performing schools. States will identify their accountability goals with required indicators for proficiency in content subject areas, English-language proficiency, and graduation rates. In addition, one additional indicator, selected by the state, will include some indicator such as student engagement, educator engagement, access to and completion of advanced course work, postsecondary readiness, school climate and safety, or whatever else the state thinks makes sense.

States are required to have methods to identify and intervene in the bottom 5% of performing schools. In addition, states are required to intervene in high schools with graduation rates less than 67%. Finally, states must have plans to intervene where subgroups are struggling. School interventions are required, based on an evidence-based plan established by the teachers and school staff. The state and districts are required to monitor the plans.

A key aspect of the ESSA is to allow for innovation and continuous improvement. Increased focus on subgroups will be seen. This includes students with disabilities and English Learners.

Alignment and Conflicts Between ESEA/ESSA and IDEA Requirements

Although the reforms of general and special education are no longer separate or parallel, there may be conflicts between laws. Part of the reason for the conflict between the laws is that they are intended for two fundamentally different purposes, which lie in the establishment of entitlement under each law. IDEA 2004 provides individual entitlement, such as individualized assessment, individualized instruction, and individualized education programs, whereas ESEA/ESSA establishes group entitlement, such as ensuring academic achievement regardless of disability, English proficiency, socioeconomic status, or living conditions.

Assessment of students with disabilities and the inclusion of their scores in the reporting system are required. Educational systems must be responsible and held accountable for the growth and progress of students with disabilities. Since the beginning of the mandates for students with disabilities to participate in statewide testing, teachers and parents have expressed concerns about their participation. The inclusion of students with disabilities as a specific subgroup in the accountability system has led to greater attention to these learners' needs and also to effective practices for improving academic achievement.

The federal focus on ensuring that students with disabilities are educated to the fullest extent in the general education classroom, with access to the general education curriculum, is certainly connected to requirements for closing the achievement gap. With the exception of students with significant cognitive disabilities, all other students will be receiving education in the general curriculum, and therefore schools are held account-able for their learning. ESSA specifically notes the use of universal design for learning and technology as methods to create needed access for students with diverse learning needs, specifically English Learners and students with disabilities (Samuels, 2016).

The definition of "in need of special education" appears to conflict with the expec-tation for closing the achievement gap. Students receiving special education services are identified because of an academic deficiency resulting from their educational disability. If these students were performing at or near grade level, they would not be identified for special education services. Related to this, the turnover of students in the disability sub-group means that new students who are performing lower academically will be added to the disability group, whereas students who improve in their academic achievement may be dismissed from special education. Once students approach grade-level skills (i.e., near the proficient range), they are most likely dismissed from special education, as they should be. New students who are struggling academically enter special education and are counted in the disability subgroup's performance. This is one of the major conflicts between the requirements of ESEA/ESSA and those of IDEA 2004. New interpretations of growth models under ESSA will hopefully address some of these conflicts.

ESSA also includes options for the use of personalized learning as a method to close the achievement gap. Educators are familiar with Individualized Education Programs. According to KnowledgeWorks (2016, p. 2), *personalized learning* is defined as a teaching and learning framework in which

- instruction is aligned to rigorous college- and career-ready standards and the social and emotional skills students need to be successful in college and career;
- instruction is customized, allowing each student to design learning experiences aligned to his or her interests;
- the pace of instruction is varied based on individual student needs, allowing students to accelerate or take additional time based on their level of mastery;
- educators use data from formative assessments and student feedback in real time to differentiate instruction and provide robust supports and interventions so that every student remains on track to graduate; and
- students and parents have access to clear, transferable learning objectives and assessment results so they understand what is expected for mastery and advancement.

With each reauthorization of ESEA and IDEA, more overlaps and fewer conflicts are seen. As new models for accountability develop, and education adopts systematic interventions and personalized learning, many of the features of special education are now being incorporated into the general program, while at the same time broader ac-countability for the learning of students with disabilities, including students with sig-nificant cognitive disabilities, is now part of the special education world.

Implications for Speech–Language Pathologists

Speech–language pathologists working in schools must understand curricula, stan-dards, and how the statewide assessment system works in their state. Students with disabilities represent a distinct subgroup under ESEA/ESSA, which means that high-stakes testing is part of the work of school-based speech–language pathologists.

Because this testing is part of the school experience for all students, speech–language pathologists should learn as much as they can about the testing experience, how the test is constructed, and what content students will be expected to know.

Academic content and performance standards should be emphasized during intervention, because this is the information that will form the foundation of the classroom and testing experience. This does not mean that speech–language pathologists or teachers should be teaching to the test. What it does mean is this: As related service providers, speech–language pathologists should provide services in concert with the academic expectations of the classroom. Because students are expected to learn in the classroom, speech–language pathologists are expected to support students so that they can achieve an educational benefit. Speech–language pathologists should also support students in developing learning strategies to become more effective learners by turning their academic content into a vehicle for practicing strategies (Moore & Nishida, 2014; Ukrainetz, 2006; Wallach, 2008). Speech–language pathologists and all special educators must include information about statewide assessment results when preparing reports and IEPs. They should participate in all meetings at the school and district related to testing and Common Core State Standards (CCSS) to keep up with new requirements and mandates. In addition, speech–language pathologists must continue to actively examine their practices to provide services designed to assist students in meeting the demands of the classroom. The following five recommendations for becoming proficient in the lessons of ESEA/NCLB (2001) remain relevant (Moore-Brown, 2004):

1. Understand how the statewide testing system works.
2. Understand the distinction between the statewide accountability system and the national accountability system.
3. Understand that conflicts exist in the system between ESEA and IDEA 2004.
4. Examine speech–language pathologists' practice and service delivery in relation to support of students in the climate of accountability.
5. Move quickly to adjust practices and decision making in accordance with school accountability mandates.

The Individuals With Disabilities Education Improvement Act of 2004

IDEA (P.L. 108-446) was signed into law in 2004. Policy makers' goal for this reauthorization was to align IDEA 2004 with the provisions of No Child Left Behind. The final *Code of Federal Regulations*, which provides guidance on how states and local education agencies are to implement the law, was released on August 3, 2006, with implementation required on October 13, 2006.

In preparation for the reauthorization of the IDEA, the President's Commission on Excellence in Special Education (2002) made three strong recommendations for changes in the IDEA Amendments of 1997 and alignment with ESEA/NCLB:

1. Focus on results, not on process.
2. Embrace a model of prevention, not a model of failure.
3. Consider children with disabilities as general education children first.

The President's Commission specifically noted the following concerns related to the status of students with disabilities at the time: (a) the dropout rates of students with disabilities, (b) the lower enrollment rate of students with disabilities in higher education compared to that of their general education counterparts, (c) how unprepared general education teachers were to work with students with disabilities in their classrooms, and (d) the growth of the students identified as having a specific learning disability and the disproportionality of the number of students who are of minority status in special education.

The President's Commission also posed this challenge:

> We will succeed if we work to create a culture of high expectations, accountability, and results that meet the unique needs of every child. (pp. 8–9)

Requirements of IDEA 2004

The Individuals With Disabilities Education Improvement Act of 2004 is often referred to by the approved acronym *IDEA 2004*. IDEA 2004 updated the purposes of the law, which are identified as follows (IDEA 2004, § 601 [d]):

(1)(A) To ensure that all children with disabilities have available to them a free appropriate public education that emphasizes special education and related services designed to meet their unique needs and prepare them for further education, employment, and independent living;

(B) To ensure that the rights of children with disabilities and parents of such children are protected; and

(C) To assist states, localities, educational service agencies, and federal agencies to provide for the education of all children with disabilities;

(2) To assist states in the implementation of a statewide, comprehensive, coordinated, multidisciplinary, interagency system of early intervention services for infants and toddlers with disabilities and their families;

(3) To ensure that educators and parents have the necessary tools to improve educational results for children with disabilities by supporting system improvement activities; coordinating research and personnel preparation; coordinated technical assistance, dissemination, and support; and technology development and media services; and

(4) To assess and ensure the effectiveness of efforts to educate children with disabilities.

Under IDEA 2004, the foundational principles that have historically guided special education law remain the same, including the following:

1. Free appropriate public education
2. Full educational opportunity (zero-reject philosophy)
3. Child Find
4. Procedural safeguards
5. Least restrictive environment
6. Individualized Education Program (IEP)

The contents of the IEP include the following:

1. A statement of the student's present levels of achievement (IDEA 2004 specifies that this include academic achievement and functional performance, including how the child's disability affects the child's progress in the general education curriculum or preschool activities)
2. A statement of measurable annual goals that meet the child's needs resulting from the disability and that enable the child to be involved in, and make progress in, the general education curriculum
3. A description of how progress toward annual goals will be measured and when periodic progress reports will be provided
4. A statement of special education, related services, and supplementary aids and services
5. An explanation of the extent to which the child will not participate with peers who are not disabled in the regular class and activities
6. Modifications in achievement assessments, if needed
7. A projected date for beginning services, with anticipated frequency, location, and duration
8. A plan for postsecondary transition

The following themes arise from IDEA 2004:

1. A focus on the general education curriculum and academic achievement for students with disabilities
2. Decisions based on scientifically based research to the extent practicable
3. Alignment with ESEA/NCLB
4. A focus on prevention services, including early intervening and response-to-intervention models as part of eligibility determination for specific learning disability

These themes are realized in the implementation expected with this law.

Free Appropriate Public Education and Least Restrictive Environment

The intent of Congress to provide free appropriate public education (FAPE) was set forth in 1975 under the EAHCA and has been reinforced through subsequent amendments and reauthorizations. State educational agencies (i.e., state departments of education) and local educational agencies (i.e., school districts) are required to establish policies and procedures to ensure that each child with a disability has available FAPE through both procedural and regulatory conditions. These are designed to avoid the possibility of functional exclusion when students are unintentionally excluded from services or "fall through the cracks."

The *Code of Federal Regulations* defined *FAPE* as special education and related services that

(a) Are provided at public expense, under public supervision and direction, and without charge;

(b) Meet the standards of the SEA;

(c) Include an appropriate preschool, elementary school, or secondary school education in the state involved; and

(d) Are provided in conformity with the individualized education program (IEP) that meets the requirements of § 300.320 through 33.324. (34 C.F.R. § 300.17)

Fundamentally, the provision of FAPE is what special education is all about. Special education is intended to meet a child's unique educational needs, and the requirements for FAPE have been litigated, argued, and debated since the inception of P.L. 94-142. The *Rowley* decision described in the next section is a Supreme Court decision that sets the standard for IEP teams in the determination of FAPE. The judicial and legislative interpretation of FAPE continues to evolve as seen in the *Endrew F.* decision by the Supreme Court in March 2017. Nevertheless, each day across our country IEP teams set out to conduct the business of designing an IEP that will satisfy the requirements of the law, but this is not always easy because of the complexities of student needs, limited or constrained resources, or differing opinions of parents and educators and sometimes even between the educators themselves. The obligation of the IEP team is to first identify the student's needs in all areas of suspected disability either through assessment or through updating information on the student's functioning level, establish goals for the student, and then recommend supports and services that will enable the student to meet those goals. The standard of *Rowley* and *Endrew F.* requires that the IEP be designed to confer educational benefit in light of the child's unique circumstances. How this is done will be further discussed in Chapter 4. Functionally, FAPE means that students receive the services they need, but not more than they need, to attain educational benefit. One way to think about FAPE is as the umbrella under which all other requirements exist in order to lead to a FAPE for the student.

Like FAPE, the interpretation of least restrictive environment may create challenges for IEP teams. The regulations require the following:

(i) That to the maximum extent appropriate, children with disabilities, including children in public or private institutions or other care facilities, are educated with children who are not disabled; and

(ii) That special classes, separate schooling, or other removal of children with disabilities from the regular education environment occurs only when the nature or severity of the handicap is such that education in regular classes with the use of supplementary aids and services cannot be achieved satisfactorily. (34 C.F.R. § 300.114 [2])

The underlying principle of LRE is that children with disabilities will be, to the fullest extent possible, educated alongside their peers who are not disabled. Before federal legislation, it was common practice to segregate children with disabilities from their nondisabled peers. The findings of Congress in IDEA 2004 strongly emphasized the intention of Congress to have students with disabilities be taught in the general education classroom through specific referent.

The requirements for LRE call for a continuum of alternative placements (34 C.F.R. § 300.115) for children who are in need of special education and related services. Under the provisions of FAPE, these program options, if needed, would be provided at no cost to children or their families. The LRE requirements also outline what is meant by "placement" and define the responsibilities of the IEP team to ensure this provision.

In determining the educational placement of a child with a disability, including a preschool child with a disability, each public agency must ensure the following:

(a)   The placement decision—

(1) Is made by a group of persons, including the parents, and other persons knowledgeable about the child, the meaning of the evaluation data, and the placement options; and

(2) Is made inconformity with the LRE provisions of this subpart . . .

(b)   The child's placement—

(1) Is determined at least annually;

(2) Is based on the child's IEP; and

(3) Is as close as possible to the child's home.

(c)   Unless the IEP of a child with a disability requires some other arrangement, the child is educated in the school that he or she would attend if nondisabled;

(d)   In selecting the LRE, consideration is given to any potential harmful effects on the child or on the quality of services that he or she needs; and

(e)   A child with a disability is not removed from education in age-appropriate regular classrooms solely because of needed modifications in the general education curriculum. (34 C.F.R. § 300.116)

The *Code of Federal Regulations* includes clarification about the extension of LRE into nonacademic settings as established by IDEA 2004 as follows:

In providing or arranging for the provision of nonacademic and extracurricular services and activities, including meals, recess periods, and the services and activities set forth in § 300.107 (nonacademic services), each public agency must ensure that each child with a disability participates with nondisabled children in the extracurricular services and activities to the maximum extent appropriate to the needs of that child. The public agency must ensure that each child with a disability has the supplementary aides and services determined by the child's IEP Team to be appropriate and necessary for the child to participate in nonacademic settings. (34 C.F.R. § 300.117)

Often, one section of the code refers to another section. In this case, Section 300.117 refers to Section 300.107, which defines nonacademic services. It is clear that it is the intent of Congress and the USDE to extend the provisions of LRE to these settings and activities. This section states the following:

(a) Each public agency must take steps, including the provision of supplementary aids and services determined appropriate and necessary by the child's IEP team, to provide nonacademic and extracurricular services and activities in the manner necessary to afford children with disabilities an equal opportunity for participation in those services and activities;

(b) Nonacademic activities and extracurricular services and activities may include counseling services, athletics, transportation, health services, recreational activities, special interest groups or clubs sponsored by the public agency, referrals to agencies that provide assistance to individuals with disabilities, and employment of students, including both employment by the public agency and assistance in making employment available. (34 C.F.R. § 300.107)

The standards and interpretation of how to design and provide FAPE in the LRE are continually evolving along with educational practice, legal mandates, and judicial decisions. The evolution of special education has been described. The original intent of special education was to focus on access to education, but under IDEA 2004, the intent has evolved to emphasize inclusion and academic results. As students with disabilities are required to pass the same statewide tests as their peers without disabilities, the practice of removing students with disabilities from the general education classroom to receive supports and services is increasingly under scrutiny. It is recognized that the delivery of the core curriculum and instruction occurs in the general education classroom and that special education has not demonstrated that it is able to replicate this delivery of information in separate settings. The change in expectations of the educational system and the laws ultimately increases the importance of FAPE and LRE, ensuring access to general education curriculum and access to general education content-expert teachers. Speech–language pathologists and special education teachers will also see a change in their responsibilities to create access for the students they serve. The advent of the reauthorization of ESEA and the impending reauthorization of IDEA indicate that this expectation will only increase in the future.

Landmark Court Decisions Regarding FAPE and LRE

Board of Education of Hendrick Hudson School District v. Rowley (U.S. Supreme Court, 1982)

The first special education case heard by the U.S. Supreme Court was a 1982 case out of New York: *Board of Education of Hendrick Hudson Central School District v. Rowley*,

458, U.S. 176. This case set the standard for defining an appropriate program. Amy Rowley was a student who was deaf and attending a general first-grade class, following a successful kindergarten year. School authorities provided Amy with an FM wireless assistive listening device for amplification of the teacher's voice in the classroom. She was to receive additional support from tutors and her parents. Amy's parents requested that the school also provide Amy with a sign language interpreter. The school district denied their request because a trial period with a sign language interpreter had demonstrated to the district that this service was unnecessary because Amy learned just as well without the interpreter. The Supreme Court ruling in this case held that Congress set the standard for free and appropriate public education that is still followed. In *Rowley*, the court established the following:

- A "free appropriate public education" consists of educational instruction specially designed to meet the unique needs of the handicapped child, supported by such services as are necessary to permit the child "to benefit" from the instruction. (III A)
- The requirement that a State provides specialized educational services to handicapped children generates no additional requirement that the services so provided be sufficient to maximize each child's potential "commensurate with the opportunity provided other children." (III A)
- Assuming that the [Education for All Handicapped Children Act] was designed to fill the need identified in the House Report—that is, to provide a "basic floor of opportunity" consistent with equal protection—neither the Act nor its history persuasively demonstrate that Congress thought that equal protection required anything more than equal access. Therefore, Congress' desire to provide specialized educational services, even in furtherance of "equality," cannot be read as imposing any particular substantive educational standard upon the States. (III B ii)
- Implicit in the congressional purpose of providing access to a "free appropriate public education" is the requirement that the education to which access is provided to be sufficient to confer some educational benefit upon the handicapped child. (iii)
- When the language of the Act and its legislative history are considered together, the requirements imposed by Congress become tolerably clear. Insofar as a State is required to provide a handicapped child with a "free appropriate public education," we hold that it satisfies this requirement by providing personalized instruction with sufficient support services to permit the child to benefit educationally from that instruction. Such instruction and services must be provided at public expense, must meet the State's educational standards, must approximate grade levels used in the State's regular education, and must comport with the child's IEP. In addition, the IEP, and therefore the personalized instruction, should be formulated in accordance with the requirements of the Act, and if the child is being educated in the regular classroom of the public education system, should be reasonably

calculated to enable the child to achieve passing marks and advance from grade to grade. (III C)

The *Rowley* case reinforced the importance of the IEP process in defining *appropriate education*. The standard for educational benefit, and not maximum development, has continued to be upheld by the courts in subsequent rulings. States establish their standards for FAPE. The *Rowley* interpretation of a floor, not ceiling, of opportunities is upheld in all states.

The importance of the *Rowley* decision has grown and expanded over the years. Initially, lower courts strictly applied the *Rowley* standard to other court cases. However, later courts struggled with the distinction between "some" educational benefit being more than just "trivial" benefit. Courts later moved to a less strict interpretation and extended the *Rowley* standard to that of "meaningful" educational benefit. Special educators must understand that the IEP should be designed so that it results in educational advancement or meaningful educational benefit that the student can reasonably be expected to achieve. The standards for FAPE have also changed according to the times and the new requirements under each reauthorization, specifically as related to the location of services provided to students.

While the Regular Education Initiative (REI) and the Inclusion Movement may have advocated for normalizing the setting and methods for providing services to children with disabilities (see "General and Special Education Reforms" in Chapter 1), the courts are where clarification occurred in terms of what would be acceptable settings and methods. The procedural safeguards afforded to parents allowed for either parents or school districts to request a due process hearing or mediation if there was a disagreement on any issue dealing with the identification, evaluation, educational placement, or provision of FAPE to a child, including issues arising in the IEP process. (See "Resolution Sessions, Mediation, Due Process Hearings, and State IDEA Complaints" in Chapter 8 for a full discussion.) The ruling of an administrative law judge or impartial hearing officer stands as the final decision, unless the decision is appealed. Appeals in these cases may be heard as a civil action in federal court or may be heard in a state court of competent jurisdiction. As in most other legal proceedings, complainants in due process proceedings are required to exhaust administrative remedies before filing a court action.

Following *Rowley*, court actions have defined LRE in terms of "inclusion," or placement of a child with disabilities into a general education classroom. These cases were all heard first at the level of a due process hearing and then worked their way to the court system.

Daniel R. R. v. State Board of Education (Fifth Circuit, 1989)

Daniel was an elementary school student with Down syndrome. His parents wanted him included in a regular classroom, but the school district denied the placement. Noting a strong congressional preference for mainstreaming, the Fifth Circuit Court in 1989 created a two-part inquiry for determination of placement.

First, the school must determine whether placement in the regular classroom, with supplementary services, could be achieved satisfactorily. To make that determination, the school must ask the following questions:

- Has the school taken steps to provide supplementary aids and services to modify the regular education program to suit the needs of the disabled child?
- Once modifications are made, can the child receive an educational benefit from regular education?
- What effects will the presence of the child with disabilities have on the regular classroom environment and, thus, on the education the other students are receiving?

Second, if the decision is made to remove the child from the regular classroom for all or part of the day, then the school must also ask whether the child has been mainstreamed (spending some time in the regular classroom) to the maximum extent possible.

Oberti v. Board of Education of Borough of Clementon School District (Third Circuit, 1993)

In *Oberti v. Board of Education of Borough of Clementon School District* (1993), the Third Circuit Court ruled that the school district bore the burden of proof in LRE cases and that mere token attempts at inclusion on the part of the district were not satisfactory to meet the requirement. Rafael Oberti was a student with Down syndrome placed in a developmental kindergarten class in a New Jersey school district. He was reported to show disruptive behaviors and was difficult for the teacher to manage. The findings of fact in this case chronicled that the school district did not provide enough support, or even effort, to make the placement work. The court concluded that the preference for mainstreaming was so strong that the argument in favor of the placement could be rebutted only if the school district could prove any of the following: (a) The student would receive little or no benefit from the inclusion placement, (b) the student would be so disruptive that other students' learning would be impaired, or (c) the cost of providing services in the regular classroom would have a negative effect on other students. The court found that in this case, additional teacher training might have eliminated any potential disruption to the classroom and that the necessity to modify the curriculum was not a reason for exclusion.

Sacramento City School Dist. v. Rachel H. (Ninth Circuit, 1994)

The *Sacramento City School Dist. v. Rachel H.* (1994) case involved a child with intellectual disabilities whose parents wanted her fully included in a regular classroom (see www.kidstogether.org/right-ed_files/rachel.htm). In the *Rachel H.* case, the Ninth Circuit Court established the following four-factor balancing test to consider when determining appropriate placement:

1. The educational benefits of full-time placement in a regular class
2. The nonacademic benefits of such a placement

3. The effects of the student on the teacher and other children in the class
4. The cost of a regular education placement with appropriate supplementary aids and services

In these referenced cases, the courts set forth criteria that subsequently assisted IEP teams in making decisions about placement in the least restrictive environment. School districts bear the responsibility of demonstrating that a less restrictive environment cannot work rather than arguing for a more restrictive placement without first attempting the less restrictive.

Poolaw v. Bishop (Ninth Circuit, 1995)

Poolaw v. Bishop (1995) was a Ninth Circuit Court decision that affirmed an Arizona district. In this particular case, the courts set forth criteria that subsequently assisted IEP teams in making a decision in favor of placing a 13-year-old student with significant communication needs requiring intensive instruction in American Sign Language at the state school for the deaf. Notably, the Ninth Circuit Court commented on IDEA's LRE requirement:

> In some cases, such as where the child's handicap is particularly severe, it will be impossible to provide any meaningful education to the student in a mainstream environment. In these situations, continued mainstreaming would be inappropriate and educators may recommend placing the child in a special education environment.

McWhirt by McWhirt v. Williamson County Schools (Sixth Circuit, 1994)

McWhirt by McWhirt v. Williamson County Schools (1994) is a Sixth Circuit Court inclusion decision that a fourth-grade student with multiple disabilities should be placed appropriately in a comprehensive special education class with partial mainstreaming rather than in the less restrictive resource room desired by her parents. The Sixth Circuit found that the severe nature of the student's disabilities prevented her from "functioning constructively in regular education."

Kari H. v. Franklin Special School District (Sixth Circuit, 1995)

The Sixth Circuit Court later relied on its authority in *McWhirt by McWhirt v. Williamson County Schools* in its ruling on *Kari H. v. Franklin Special School District* (1995). In that case, the inappropriate behaviors of the student in previous mainstream placements, as well as the functional gains she could realize in a special education classroom, were determined by the court to outweigh any minimal benefit she might realize from placement in the regular classroom.

A series of cases since the late 1990s have dealt with questions of what school districts were required to provide and fund under special education law. In these cases, the courts focused on how failure to follow procedural requirements can be interpreted as a denial of FAPE.

Cedar Rapids Community School District v. Garret F.
(U.S. Supreme Court, 1999)

In the *Garret F.* case, the U.S. Supreme Court was asked to consider whether a school district was required to fund necessary nursing services for a student, Garret F., who was dependent on a ventilator. The district argued that the nursing services were medical in nature and therefore should not be the responsibility of the school district to fund. The Court of Appeals disagreed, finding that these services would fall in the range of "related services" under the IDEA. In its ruling, affirming the Court of Appeals, the U.S. Supreme Court stated,

> This case is about whether meaningful access to the public schools will be assured, not the level of education that a school must finance once access is attained. It is undisputed that the services at issue must be provided if Garret is to remain in school.
>
> Under the statute, our precedent, and the purposes of the IDEA, the district must fund such "related services" in order to help guarantee that students like Garret are integrated into the public schools.

Kevin T. v. Elmhurst Community School District No. 205
(U.S. District Court for the Northern District of Illinois, 2002)

This case involved the denial of FAPE to a 19-year-old student with a learning disability, attention-deficit/hyperactivity disorder (ADHD), and bipolar disorder. Throughout Kevin's educational career, his skills declined, and he achieved failing grades. The analysis of the case involves an examination of the credibility of the witnesses, and although the teacher and case carrier were found to be credible witnesses, it was determined by the court that the school psychologist's testimony was evasive and inconsistent. Problems with the IEP included the following: (a) The goals and objectives were the same for 3 years, (b) the IEP team ignored the recommendations of an independent evaluator, (c) the district failed to review and revise the IEP, (d) the district did not address the student's reading difficulties, (e) the district did not change the IEP when the student had increasing academic problems, (f) the district did not consider whether the student needed assistive technology, (g) the district failed to appropriately address the required provisions for statewide assessment and how the student would participate, and (h) the transition plan was not appropriate. Despite all of Kevin's difficulties in school, the district decided to issue a standard diploma to him. The court found that he was inappropriately graduated and ordered compensatory education until he reached age 21 years.

M. L. by C. D. and S. L. v. Federal Way School District
(Ninth Circuit, 2003)

In this case, the school district's failure to include a general education teacher in the IEP meeting for a student who was being transferred to a special day class created a structural defect so significant that it resulted in an automatic (de facto) denial of FAPE.

Court cases may seem like they are remote and removed from the daily work of speech–language pathologists and audiologists in public schools. These cases do, however, strongly influence the direction given by administrators to IEP teams so that current rulings are reflected in decision making. Court cases provide guidance to the field (see Table 2.4) to clarify our practice. The decisions provided by court cases become known as "case law" and should be considered when districts and IEP teams are making decisions. Practice trends are often tested in the courts. Inclusion and inclusive services are more a part of the general practice in special education than it once was. (See the section in Chapter 5 on inclusion.) With a broader focus on inclusive schools and services, access to core curricula, and collaborative practice, school districts have changed the way IEP teams make decisions about placement and services. However, IEP teams do still struggle with FAPE and LRE decisions, and some of these struggles lead to legal challenges.

Zirkel (2011) reported that children with autism represented a disproportionate sample in the court decisions between 1993 and 2006. The litigation percentage for this population was 10:1 as compared to cases decided involving students with other disabling conditions. The reasons are complex, but Zirkel (2011) suggested, "As a result of the disparity between the interest groups' prescriptions and school districts' prevailing practices, with the underlying mutual motives of high costs and methodological controversy, it is not surprising that the parents of children with autism would be more prone to litigation than the parents of children with other disabilities" (p. 99). He recommended "effective communications and trust building with parents of students with autism" (p. 92) and the use of alternative dispute-resolution approaches in working with the parents of children with autism to mitigate these conflicts. In reality, these are appropriate approaches for all.

Endrew F. by Joseph F. v. Douglas County School District RE-1 (U.S. Supreme Court, 2017)

In March 2017, the Supreme Court rendered a decision in the appeal of *Endrew F. by Joseph F. v. Douglas County School District RE-1* (Case #15-827), a case out of Colorado. In this case, the parents of Endrew F. appeal decisions of the federal district court and the 10th Circuit Court of Appeals. Endrew was a student with autism who had received his education in the district special education program up to the fourth grade. His parents did not believe that he was making satisfactory progress and unilaterally placed him in a private school for children with autism. The district argued that he was making adequate progress based on the *Rowley* standard. While the district prevailed in the lower court and the 10th Circuit Court of Appeals, the Supreme Court concluded differently. The justices found that the standard did not mean that trivial benefit was enough, but rather that the LEA must offer an IEP that is "reasonably calculated to enable a child to make progress in light of the child's circumstances."

The Court rejected the parents' appeal to redefine the FAPE standard to provide opportunities substantially similar to those of nondisabled peers for academic achievement and contributions to society. The Court noted that this was not what was done in

Rowley or by Congress in subsequent reauthorizations of IDEA, so it rejected this aspect of the parents' claim.

Extending the *Rowley* standard to include the provision "in light of the child's circumstances" is now up for interpretation by other courts and IEP teams. Early interpretations of this ruling point to the provision of special considerations for students with significant disabilities to enable progress that is more than *de minimis* (i.e., trivial). In practice, this entails ensuring that assessments are comprehensive and solid and that IEP goals are written to address the specific student's needs and, importantly, that progress on goals is reported at the intervals required in the IEP. Too frequently, IEP teams carry over goals and do not make adjustments when students are not making progress. These types of procedural errors can be considered a denial of FAPE, especially under this extension of the *Rowley* standard. Table 2.4 presents the effects of case law on the practice of speech–language pathologists and audiologists.

Educational Benefit

The *Rowley* standard has long established that IEPs must confer educational benefit on the student. What is educational benefit under this standard? In general, it means that there is evidence that FAPE was provided in the LRE and resulted in educational advancement for the student because of the provision of special education and related services required to meet the student's unique educational needs. The educational benefit standard has been given increasing attention under IDEA 2004. Under the standards of *Rowley* and educational benefit, process and procedures are critical, in addition to being able to demonstrate that the student made progress in the general education curriculum and on IEP goals. The *Endrew F.* decision extends and clarifies this standard.

In IDEA 2004, the Congress established that special education must prepare students to lead productive and independent adult lives. IDEA 2004 also aligns academic demands with those of general education, increasing expectations for academic success. Both of these affect how FAPE will continue to be defined and challenged.

Application of FAPE and LRE to Speech–Language and Hearing Services

Educators feel the impact of legislative and judicial decisions on their daily work. Speech–language and hearing programs must comply with FAPE and LRE guidelines. To ensure that all children receive FAPE, the child's evaluation must be "sufficiently comprehensive to identify all of the child's special education and related services needs, whether or not commonly linked to the disability category in which the child has been classified" (34 C.F.R. § 300.304 [6]). To ensure that LRE is achieved, states are required to provide a "continuum of alternative placements to meet the unique needs of each child with a disability" (34 C.F.R. § 300.303). Speech–language pathologists and audiologists need to provide a continuum of services using several different service deliv-

(text continues on p. 55)

TABLE 2.4. A Summary of Key Court Cases and Their Effect on the Practice of Speech–Language Pathologists

Court case	Court direction	Effect on speech–language pathologists' practice
Board of Education of Hendrick Hudson Central School District v. Rowley (1982) (State of New York; U.S. Supreme Court)	The Court set standard for determination of free appropriate public education (FAPE), ruled that the goal of special education is not to maximize potential, and ruled that the goal of special education is access to educational benefit.	The ruling influences decisions for recommendations for therapy.
Daniel R. R. v. State Board of Education (1989) (State of Texas; Fifth Circuit Court of Appeals)	The court set guidelines for determination of provision of supplementary aids and services to modify the regular classroom in order for the child to receive educational benefit and considered the influence of the child with a disability on the education of other children in the class.	This decision influences the need for speech–language services to be provided either in the general education classroom or in conjunction with the work of the classroom (i.e., the curriculum).
Oberti v. Board of Education of Borough of Clementon School District (1993) (State of New Jersey; Third Circuit Court of Appeals)	The court placed the burden of proof on the school district to demonstrate that the student would receive no educational benefit from educational placement in a regular classroom, recommended teacher training to deal with potential problems, and ruled that a need to modify the curriculum was not a reason for exclusion.	The ruling influences speech–language pathologists' need to work with families and requests for services in the regular classroom; they must attempt and prove that a type of service delivery does not work.
Sacramento City Unified School Dist. v. Rachel H. (1994) (State of California; Ninth Circuit Court of Appeals)	The court established a four-factor balancing test to determine FAPE and considered educational and nonacademic benefits.	The case explains that educational and nonacademic benefit must be the basis of placement considerations.
Union School District v. B. Smith (1994) (State of California; Ninth Circuit Court of Appeals)	The court upheld the Hearing Officer's decision that the district has an obligation to make a specific offer of a FAPE, including a specific location and program, even if the parents have let it be known that they will reject the placement offer. This ruling is based on the requirements for prior written notice. The court found that the district cannot escape its obligation to make a formal placement offer.	This case finds that school districts and IEP teams must make a specific offer of placement as part of the FAPE offer in an IEP. This is true even when the parents have indicated that the offer will be declined.
Poolaw v. Bishop (1995) (State of Arizona; Ninth Circuit Court of Appeals)	The court found that in certain cases, the severity of the student's disability may require a more restrictive environment to provide the educational benefit to the child.	This ruling allows for consideration of specialized communication needs.
McWhirt by McWhirt v. Williamson County Schools (1994) (State of Tennessee; Sixth Circuit Court of Appeals) and *Kari H. v. Franklin Special School District* (1995) (State of Tennessee; Sixth Circuit Court of Appeals)	The court determined that the severe nature of a student's disability can prevent the student from receiving educational benefit in a regular classroom.	When working as part of an Individualized Education Program (IEP) team, one considers the complexities of the disability for program service decisions.

TABLE 2.4. *(continued)*

Court case	Court direction	Effect on speech–language pathologists' practice
Cypress-Fairbanks Independent School District v. Michael F. (1997) (State of Texas; No. 96-20221, Fifth Circuit Court of Appeals)	The court ruled that there are four factors that can serve as indicators of whether an IEP is reasonably calculated to provide a meaningful educational benefit under the IDEA: (a) The program is individualized on the basis of the student's assessment and performance, (b) the program is administered in the least restrictive environment, (c) the services are provided in a coordinated and collaborative manner by the key stakeholders, and (d) positive academic and nonacademic benefits are demonstrated.	IEP teams need to ensure that they follow the four indicators provided by the court to ensure that the IEP is appropriately designed to confer educational benefit to the student.
Cedar Rapids Community School District v. Garret F. (1999) (State of Iowa; 526 U.S. 66, 119 S.Ct. 992, 143 L.Ed.2d 154)	The school district was responsible for funding nursing services for a student who was ventilator dependent.	Students who have significant medical disabilities will attend public schools and will need to be provided with services and supports designed to meet their needs so they can attend school.
Kevin T. v. Elmhurst Community School District No. 205 (2002) (State of Illinois; U.S. District Court)	A 19-year-old student who had been receiving special education services since he was 6 years old demonstrated decreasing skills although he had received special education services for 12 years. The court found that the district did not appropriately assess and inappropriately graduated the student.	The court examined witness credibility, failure to review and revise goals, the student's regression of skills, and overall lack of planning as part of its consideration. IEP teams must address students' lack of progress in their IEPs, adjusting services accordingly. The consideration by the court of witness credibility is important for IEP team members to know.
Deal ex rel. Deal v. Hamilton County Board of Education (2004) (State of Tennessee; 42 IDELR 109; Sixth Circuit Court of Appeals)	A school district's predetermination of a program for a child with autism denied the parents meaningful participation in the IEP process. The district also did not consider the child's individual needs through its unofficial policy of refusing 1:1 applied behavior analysis programs.	Parent input and participation in the IEP is critical. Predetermination of placement is considered a denial of meaningful participation. School district teams can meet and confer but cannot make final decisions prior to the IEP meeting.
M. L. by C. D. and S. L. v. Federal Way School District (2003) (State of Washington; No. 02-35547, Ninth Circuit Court of Appeals)	A school district's failure to include a general education teacher in the IEP meeting created a structural defect so significant that it resulted in an automatic denial of FAPE.	The presence of a general education teacher at the IEP meeting is required to ensure the student is provided FAPE.

(continues)

TABLE 2.4. *(continued)*

Court case	Court direction	Effect on speech–language pathologists' practice
Schaffer v. Weast (2005) (State of Maryland; U.S. Supreme Court 54 U.S. 04-698)	The burden of proof in special education cases is placed on the party bringing the action (i.e., the party seeking relief).	School districts should always prepare their IEPs in a legally defensible manner, but the burden to demonstrate whether the IEP is appropriate will fall to the party (e.g., parents or school district) who made the due process request.
Doug C. v. State of Hawaii Department of Education (2013) (State of Hawaii; Ninth Circuit Court of Appeals)	The court reversed the lower court decision, finding that the student was denied a FAPE when the Department of Education held the student's IEP meeting without the parent, as the parent sought to reschedule the meeting. The court emphasized that parent participation is central to the IDEA.	In this case, the decision to hold the meeting without the parent was determined to be a denial of a FAPE. The arguments presented regarding the inconvenience to staff schedules and the impending annual review deadline were determined not as important as the parent's participation. IEP teams can hold meetings without parents only under very rare circumstances and when the parent affirmatively refuses to attend. Always seek guidance if there is difficulty securing parent participation in an IEP meeting.
I.R. by E.N. v. Los Angeles Unified School District (2015) (State of California; Ninth Circuit Court of Appeals).	The court found that waiting a year and a half to file for due process when a parent has not signed an IEP is too long and that the district should file for due process without an unreasonable delay.	The court ruling instructs districts and IEP teams that it is not permissible to let long delays to occur without seeking resolution. This does not mean that districts and parents will not continue to try to resolve differences, but speech–language pathologists should ensure that administrators know if parents are not signing IEPs.

TABLE 2.4. *(continued)*

Court case	Court direction	Effect on speech-language pathologists' practice
Endrew F. v. Douglas County School District (U.S. Supreme Court)	The Court extended and clarified the *Rowley* standard that the IEP must be designed to confer educational benefit "in light of the child's circumstances."	Minimal or trivial progress is not enough, even for students with significant disabilities. IEP goals should not be rewritten over and over, with little progress made. Speech-language pathologists and other team members must be attentive to the connections between appropriate assessment, present levels, and connecting them to goals. Reporting to parents on progress on goals and adjusting if progress is not being made are all important to implement this new standard.

ery models, which may include collaboration, coteaching, direct and pullout services, consultation, and others. A one-size-fits-all model might have been typical of service delivery in the early 1970s but is not in the spirit of FAPE and LRE.

The continuum of special education programs in schools must also be broad. This means not only that the continuum of placements will be extensive (i.e., specialized academic instruction and/or related services provided in a variety of locations, including the general education classroom, resource room, learning center, special class, special school) but also that the service delivery models of each will be varied. In working with other members of the IEP team, speech–language pathologists will need to coordinate their services with the continuum and delivery models of other service providers. These evolving applications of FAPE and LRE can provide rich rewards for students and service providers. (Chapter 5 includes further discussion of service delivery.)

Federal Laws
That Prohibit Disability Discrimination

Section 504 and the Americans With Disabilities Act

Two federal laws that are not specific to education have had an effect on school programs and facilities. Section 504 of the Rehabilitation Act of 1973 was passed to prohibit discrimination against individuals with disabilities by any program receiving federal financial assistance. The Americans With Disabilities Act (ADA) was passed in 1990 to strengthen the access requirements of Section 504 and extend them to all public domains.

ADA (1990) and Section 504 (1973) issues frequently are related. ADA deals with access to buildings, facilities, and transportation and includes the provision of auxiliary aids and services to individuals with vision or hearing impairments. Provisions under Section 504 include anything required to enable access to an instructional program, including modifications to the learning environment and materials to meet the needs of students who have identified disabilities. ADA, Section 504, and the Individuals With Disabilities Education Improvement Act of 2004 (IDEA 2004) overlap in places. (See https://doe.sd.gov/oess/documents/sped_section504_Guidelines .pdf.)

Until the 1990s, Section 504 was not commonly applied to students in schools. Because school districts receive federal assistance, however, this act applied to these agencies. Section 504 of the Rehabilitation Act of 1973 requires the following:

> No qualified handicapped person shall, on the basis of handicap, be excluded from participation in, be denied the benefits of, or otherwise be subjected to discrimination under any program or activity which receives Federal financial assistance. (Office for Civil Rights [OCR], 1999, § 104.4 [a])

Some children may receive speech–language services under Section 504 instead of special education. Speech–language pathologists and audiologists who work in schools need to know the legal and procedural bases for this provision of services, as it is quite different from that of special education. Both IDEA 2004 and Section 504 protect students' civil rights. IDEA 2004, however, provides federal funding and describes the procedural requirements required to receive this funding at state and local levels. Section 504 does not provide funding, so schools must use local resources to provide any services or facilities that help students with disabilities access school programs.

A significant difference between the laws, in relation to school-age students with disabilities, is the eligibility criteria. IDEA 2004 protects only students who, by virtue of their disabilities, require special educational services. Section 504, however, prohibits discrimination against all school-age children, regardless of whether they require special education services.

All individuals who are disabled under IDEA are also considered to be disabled, and therefore protected, under Section 504 and ADA. However, all individuals who have been determined to be disabled under Section 504 may not be disabled under IDEA 2004. With respect to most students with disabilities, many aspects of the Section 504 regulation concerning FAPE parallel the requirements of IDEA (Moore, 2013).

ADA (1990) deals with accessibility to public domains (including communication access) and prohibits discrimination against people with disabilities (USDE, 2010).

In communities and employment situations, ADA (1990) issues may become part of the work of speech–language pathologists in schools, particularly when dealing with transition to postsecondary settings. For example, a student who is deaf may need a telecommunications device for the deaf (TDD) to communicate at a work site. Recent and future advances in telecommunications can provide additional accessibility for individuals with communication impairments to be successful in the workplace, and these must be made available by employers as they become reasonable to acquire. Schools and public facilities must provide physical access for persons using wheelchairs or who have other mobility impairments (e.g., ramps and elevators), signs must be accessible to persons with visual impairments (e.g., braille), safety features must be accessible to all (e.g., flashing lights on fire alarms), and facilities, such as water fountains, sinks, toilets, and light switches, must be accessible from various heights and clearances.

Responsibilities to Students Under Section 504

Coverage under Section 504 (1973) is much broader than the eligibility criteria under IDEA 2004. An individual who is considered disabled under Section 504

- has a physical or mental impairment that substantially limits one or more major life activities, including "walking, seeing, hearing, speaking, breathing, learning, working, caring for oneself, and performing manual tasks";
- has a record of such impairment; and
- is regarded as having such impairment (USDE, 2010).

To determine whether a student is covered under Section 504, the Section 504 team uses a data-gathering process that considers information from many available sources. The individuals involved with this evaluation process compose the team and are familiar with the student and the information considered. The team then meets and determines if the student is considered disabled under the provisions of Section 504.

Section 504 requires public agencies (i.e., school districts) to provide FAPE in the least restrictive environment to any student with a disability that limits a major life function. The USDE (n.d.-b) stated,

> Section 504 requires recipients to provide to students with disabilities appropriate educational services designed to meet the individual needs of such students to the same extent as the needs of students without disabilities are met. An appropriate education for a student with a disability under the Section 504 regulations could consist of education in regular classrooms, education in regular classes with supplementary services, and/or special education and related services.

When developing a Section 504 accommodation plan and services, the 504 team should consider the following factors (USDE, 2010, p. 33):

a. Evaluation results
b. Section 504 identification determination
c. The student's unmet needs
d. Services and/or accommodations based on needs
e. Least restrictive environment for services
f. Discussion of and plan for possible staff training

As previously stated, students identified under IDEA 2004 automatically have the protections offered under Section 504. However, students who are identified as disabled using Section 504 procedures usually do not need the special education services offered under IDEA 2004 (Kaloi, n.d.). Examples of such situations would be students with attention-deficit disorder (ADD) who do not demonstrate a learning disability under IDEA 2004 or who are not found to qualify under "other health impairment" or other eligibility criteria considered in IDEA 2004. The accommodation plan would identify the necessary modifications and accommodations needed to allow the students to access their education (see Table 2.5 for examples).

If a student is found by an IEP team to be ineligible for special education, parents and teachers might advocate for the student to be identified as disabled under Section 504 with the goal of having the student receive special education and related services through Section 504.

Technically, students identified under Section 504 cannot be denied special education services. However, if a student's needs are so significant that special education services are required, then an IEP team should identify that student as a child with a disability under IDEA 2004. Accommodations and modifications such as those identified in Table 2.5 do not need to meet IDEA eligibility for implementation because they can be accomplished using general education staff and resources.

TABLE 2.5. Section 504 Examples

Identified disability	Major life activity affected	Accommodations provided
Attention-deficit disorder	Learning	• Shortened assignments • Reminder prompts • Learning center, study carrel • Timer • Reinforcers • Planning chart on desk • Reminder binder • Phone message from teacher to parent regarding homework assignments • After-school tutoring • Peer counseling
Asthma	Breathing	• Adjusted physical education requirements, per doctor's orders • Modified assignments for physical education • Health plan developed for medication needs
Spinal tumor	Working, performing manual tasks	• Extra time between classes • Peer assistant to take notes • Adjusted assignments (due to fatigue) • Teacher calls at night to discuss assignments with parents, child, or both • Homework club

Mandates under federal law across all education, civil rights, and antidiscrimination laws apply to schools and school service providers. The USDE provided an illustration (see Figure 2.1) that is helpful in distinguishing the areas covered by IDEA, Section 504, and ADA.

Table 2.6 provides a narrative comparison of these laws. This comparison will allow for an understanding of the expectations for providers and the protections for students. Further information on documentation is provided in Chapter 3.

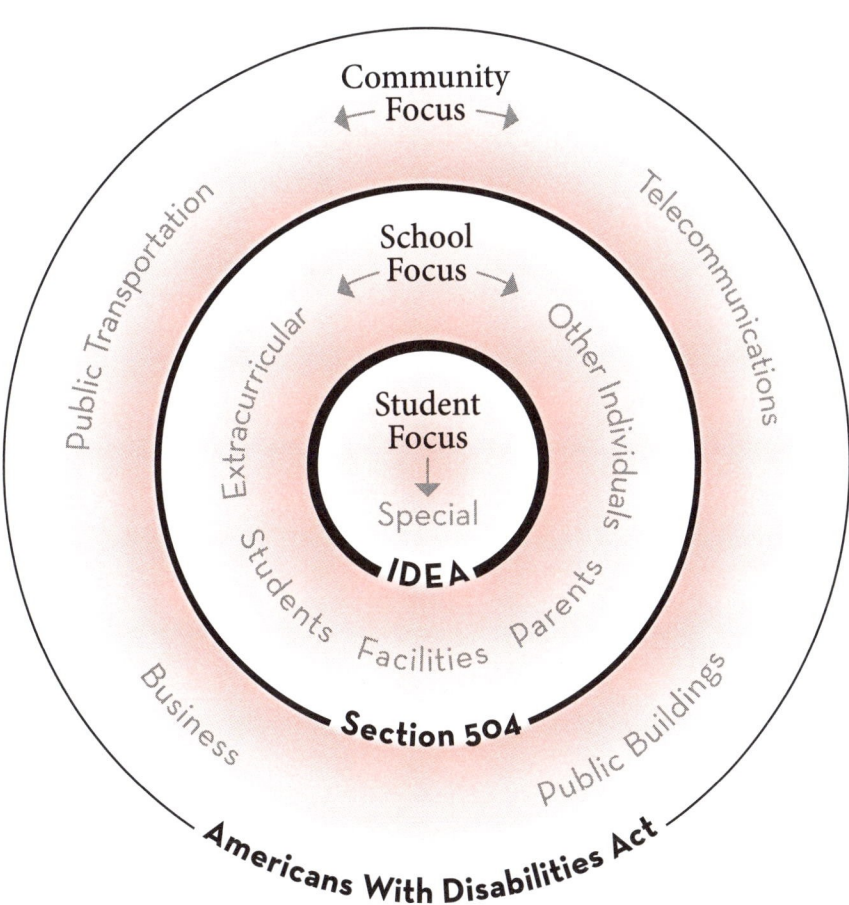

FIGURE 2.1. IDEA, Section 504, and ADA: How they relate.

Note. Adapted from "Guidelines for Educators and Administrators for Implementing Section 504 of the Rehabilitation Act of 1973—Subpart D," by U.S. Department of Education, 2010. Retrieved from https://doe.sd.gov/oess/documents/sped_section504_Guidelines.pdf.

TABLE 2.6. Summary of Federal Laws Pertaining to Documentation in Schools

Federal law	Original enactment	Most recent authorization	Legal foundations	Documentation
Individuals With Disabilities Education Improvement Act (IDEA 2004)	November 26, 1975, originally passed as P.L. 94-142, the Education for All Handicapped Children Act	December 3, 2004	IDEA 2004 requires the provision of special education and related services for students identified as children with disabilities. When students are identified as having a disability, they become members of a protected class; therefore, they secure procedural safeguards, which are realized in the procedural requirements of special education. The following are foundational concepts in special education: • Free appropriate public education • Least restrictive environment • Zero reject • Due process of law for families and children: timelines, consent, appeal procedures	**Purposes** To show that legal requirements were met, including timelines and regulations To demonstrate that parents were included in the decision making **Typical documents** • Individualized Education Program (IEP) • Assessment reports • Parent rights • Consent forms
Rehabilitation Act of 1973; Section 504	September 26, 1973	December 2008	Section 504 of the Rehabilitation Act of 1973 is a federal civil rights law that prohibits discrimination against individuals with disabilities in programs and activities that receive federal financial assistance. Section 504 is intended to prohibit discrimination on the basis of disability. All IDEA students are also covered by Section 504, but not all Section 504 students are eligible for services under IDEA. It is not necessary for IDEA-eligible students to have a Section 504 plan.	**Purpose** To ensure that the process is documented (Section 504 has regulations but not the right timelines and definitive criteria that special education has.) **Typical documents** • Section 504 accommodation plan • Reports • Consent for data collection
Family Educational Rights and Privacy Act (FERPA)	August 21, 1974, as part of the reauthorization of the Elementary and Secondary Education Act (ESEA), the Education Amendments of 1974	October 26, 2001, as part of the USA Patriot Act of 2001	FERPA provides students' parents the right to access educational records and also the right to protect transferability of records without their consent.	**Purpose** To provide regulations regarding sharing of student records to ensure the protection of privacy rights **Typical documents** School records as defined by law

TABLE 2.6. (continued)

Federal law	Original enactment	Most recent authorization	Legal foundations	Documentation
Elementary and Secondary Education Act (ESEA)/Every Child Succeeds Act (ESSA)	April 11, 1965	ESSA was the reauthorization of ESEA (e.g., Title I), signed into law December 10, 2015.	ESEA/ESSA intends to ensure that all children reach proficiency on state content standards and state assessments, to close the achievement gap between high- and low-performing students and between advantaged and disadvantaged students, and to ensure that all students are college and career ready.	**Purpose** To ensure the academic achievement of all students, including students with disabilities, English Learners, students from low socioeconomic homes, and minority students. **Typical documents** • Testing results • Data • Accountability reports
Health Insurance Portability and Accountability Act (HIPAA)	August 21, 1996	April 14, 2003	HIPAA sets forth simplified health insurance administration by establishing standards and requirements for the electronic transmission of certain health information. It specifically addresses protected health information (PHI), which includes any physical or mental health information. Education records subject to the protections of FERPA are excluded from HIPAA. The HIPAA privacy rule mandates that a "covered entity" may not use or disclose PHI except as permitted by the rule. A school district is considered the "covered entity." The PHI is germane, in most cases, to conducting evaluation and development of the IEP and/or Section 504. The intent of both HIPAA and FERPA is confidentiality. Some of the agencies (i.e., medical) that work with school districts and want records must abide by HIPAA's PHI rules, so there must be consent to exchange information.	**Purpose** Privacy of PHI **Typical documents** Most school records are covered under FERPA and excluded from HIPAA, including IEPs, evaluations, IEP meeting tapes, Medicaid reimbursement claims, student health records, and personal notes, when the personal note has become a school record (Shorter, 2004).

(continues)

TABLE 2.6. (*continued*)

Federal law	Original enactment	Most recent authorization	Legal foundations	Documentation
Americans With Disabilities Act (ADA)	July 26, 1990	September 26, 2008	ADA (1990) deals with accessibility to public domains (including communication access) and "prohibits discrimination on the basis of disability in employment, programs, and services provided by state and local governments, good and services provided by private companies, and in commercial facilities" (U.S. Department of Justice, 1999, in Moore & Montgomery, 2008).	**Purpose** Prohibits discrimination against people with disabilities; intended to give broad protections by providing physical and communication access **Typical documents** • Employment records • Facilities records • Some school records • Other records that document provision of accessibility for the public

Note. Adapted from "Documentation Issues in Speech–Language Pathology and Audiology," by B. Moore, in *Professional Issues in Speech–Language Pathology and Audiology* (4th ed.), edited by R. Lubinski & M. Hudson, 2013, Clifton Park, NY: Cengage/Delmar. Adapted with permission.

CHAPTER 3

Referral and Assessment

● *In This Chapter*

This chapter describes the process that results in a student being identified as requiring special education services. The chapter examines prereferral requirements, including the response to intervention (RTI) process and the referral and assessment process, and highlights assessment methods that are considered to be good practice for speech-language services. The importance of procedural timelines is discussed.

● *Chapter Questions*

1. Discuss the speech-language pathologist's role in assessment.
2. How does response to intervention (RTI) affect speech-language assessment in the schools?
3. What are the various types of assessment methods that may be used by speech-language pathologists or audiologists, and when would each method be appropriate?
4. Outline the requirements for assessment and eligibility determination under the Individuals With Disabilities Education Improvement Act of 2004 (IDEA 2004).

Child Find Obligations

Under the federal requirements of special education, school districts are obligated to conduct Child Find, a system to locate, evaluate, and serve children with disabilities. The *Code of Federal Regulations* (C.F.R.) requires the following:

(a) *General.* (1) The State must have in effect policies and procedures to ensure that—

(i) All children with disabilities . . . including children with disabilities who are homeless children or are wards of the state, and children with disabilities attending private schools, regardless of the severity of their disability, and who are in need of special education and related services, are identified, located, and evaluated. (34 C.F.R. § 300.111 [a])

The history of the requirements of Child Find dates back to the enabling legislation of special education, P.L. 94-142, when children with disabilities were not being consistently served in public schools. In the preamble to both Individuals With Disabilities Education Acts (IDEA Amendments of 1997 and IDEA 2004), Congress stated that public schools had realized the intent of finding and serving children with disabilities under this act but now needed to focus the law on producing results for children served under special education. With the advent of the focus on early identification and intervention, prereferral and response to intervention (RTI) processes, and universal design for learning, general education classrooms have greater responsibility for providing assistance to children who struggle in school. This shift means that processes must be in place in schools prior to referral for assessment for special education and even consideration of whether a child may have a disability. These prereferral processes are intended not to prevent or delay access to identification and services but rather to ensure that students who are struggling in school are provided intervention systematically and quickly, not made to "wait to fail," and also that children are not inappropriately identified as having disabilities. Child Find obligations work as part of a system of supports within a school, not as a separate or immediate process if a student is having difficulty. IDEA 2004 makes it clear that Child Find obligations also apply to homeless children and children in private schools, as noted previously, but that Child Find obligations also apply to

> children who are suspected of being a child with a disability . . . and in need of special education even though they are advancing from grade to grade; and (2) Highly mobile children, including migrant children. (34 C.F.R. § 300.111 [c] [1][2])

Child Find obligations are an integral part of the special education process. The avenues by which children are referred for evaluation to determine special education eligibility are sophisticated and sometimes complicated processes. Special education processes and procedures are important because failure to follow these processes may lead to a denial of the child's rights and protections under special education laws. The initial process of referring a student for assessment is linked to prereferral processes in general education and must be highly coordinated with these processes.

The Child Find activities referred to in the C.F.R. vary from state to state and from local school district to local school district but generally encompass the same basic processes, which will be defined in the rest of this section. These procedures are necessary and important to follow for many reasons, but most importantly so that children receive the assistance they need and that their rights are not violated.

Avenues to Referral

Not all children come to school having the same background and opportunities. Children come to school from homes in which English is the primary language and homes in which English is not the primary language, homes with hundreds of books and homes with no books, and homes in which bedtime stories are read every night and homes in which no one has the literacy skills to help children with homework. Regardless of these children's backgrounds, public education in the United States greets all of them and more.

Teachers and other educators are under a considerable amount of pressure to provide high-quality education to students to prepare them for living and working in the global economy. Children who do not successfully develop skills in math, language, reading, and problem solving will have great difficulty securing employment in the Digital Age. The economic reality of the widening gap between what is needed in the future work world and the potential for success for individuals who do not secure a solid education is cause for concern. Educators must face the weighty burden of dealing with each and every child who does not bring to the classroom the tools and circumstances that typically spell success. This situation is not new to schools. What is new is the intense focus on school reform, the keen societal interest in test scores and student performance, and the reality of an economic future that will not have vocational jobs for an unskilled labor force. The focus of the Common Core State Standards (www.common-corestandards.org) and 21st Century Skills (www.p21.org/our-work/p21-framework) is on skills that all students need to compete in a knowledge economy: critical thinking, communication, collaboration, and creativity. Regardless of students' abilities or background, these are the skills that educators must develop in students so that they can be competitive in their future.

How students will be referred to speech, hearing, and special education programs is undergoing a dramatic shift from what it was in the first 40 years of special education. The reason for this shift is a combination of legislative, research, and policy practices that represent a new way of thinking about what constitutes a disability and that clearly identify the responsibilities of both general and special education. Traditionally, students were referred to the special education assessment team either from a student study team (SST) or through a direct referral to a speech–language pathologist or audiologist for testing. This older model of referral reflected a fundamental belief among educators that if a child was struggling, there must be something "wrong" with the child. Student study teams and special education assessment teams then, in essence, went in search of what was "wrong" with the child, oftentimes with little consideration for the environment in which the child was being taught, the child's educational history, or the competence of the instructor. Within the focus of the Elementary and Secondary Education Act (ESEA) and IDEA 2004 underlies a belief that the system needs to adjust to learners' needs and must support learners when they struggle. The application of this belief is demonstrated in the processes now used to determine who receives and does not receive speech and language or special education services.

There are other reasons why the referral and assessment process has changed under IDEA 2004. First, early intervention can prevent eventual special education identification. Second, special education results have not been strong in terms of postsecondary academic success. Finally, the cost of special education continues to rise, with no cost–benefit realized on a grand scale in terms of academic achievement. Special education is valuable for students with disabilities. Child Find and general education processes of intervention need to be established so that systems ensure that the students are appropriately referred for assessment and ultimately served under the law, and that the students who are struggling for reasons other than disability receive the assistance they need through general education interventions.

IDEA 2004 and ESEA are meant to work together, as are general and special education. Children with educationally disabling conditions are identified for service under strict eligibility categories defined by law. The rest of this chapter discusses how students are referred and assessed to determine eligibility under IDEA 2004.

Multi-Tiered System of Supports: Response to Intervention and Early Intervening Services

Multi-Tiered System of Supports

Over the course of time since the reauthorizations of ESEA 2001 and IDEA 2004, the emphasis on interventions through general education has evolved in schools and school districts. As discussed in this chapter, a combination of factors came together in school practice that led to a change in how students came to be referred for special education. In the late 1990s, researchers and policy makers were simultaneously concerned with several interrelated factors affecting policy and practice for struggling students. These included the

1. increasing identification of students in special education;
2. increasing costs of special education;
3. results of reading research, including the National Reading Panel (2000, 2006) report, Marilyn Adams's study (Adams, 1999), and *Preventing Reading Difficulties in Young Children* (C. E. Snow, Burns, & Griffin, 1998), all of which indicated that early intervention was indicated for young children who were not learning to read; and
4. the impact of the "wait to fail" model of identification of special education eligibility.

As a result of these forces, IDEA 2004 allowed for the use of "a process which would consider a student's response to intervention" as a method to consider if a student presented with a learning disability. This was only after the student was provided instruction in the core areas of reading, as identified in ESEA, and taken from the work of the National Reading Panel and *Put Reading First* (Armbruster & Osborn, 2001). At the time, response to intervention (RTI) programs did not exist in systematic ways. However, 15 years later, as of the writing of this text, most schools throughout the country have some sort of system of interventions in place for students who are struggling academically and behaviorally. These RTI models will be discussed further, specifically as they pertain to prereferral interventions and early intervening services.

Even as schools and districts continue to develop RTI processes and programs, challenges have emerged in this evolution, leading to a new concept: Multi-Tiered System of Supports (MTSS). Early models of RTI split the interventions into academic and behavioral, and described three tiers of interventions for students who needed increasing levels of support. In these models, RTI was generally known for academic interventions, and behavioral interventions were provided through a program or approach known as *positive behavioral intervention and supports* (PBIS). The concept of MTSS brings together the efforts of RTI, PBIS, Title I, special education, English Learner services, mental health support, community support, and support for at-risk students. In this comprehensive system, all services designed to support students with academic and social–emotional and behavioral needs are coordinated. Increasingly, states are moving to this model of coordinated supports, connecting systems designed to assist students in a more cohesive manner ("A Multitiered System of Supports," 2015).

The Colorado Department of Education defined its model of MTSS in this way:

> Multi-Tiered System of Supports (MTSS) is defined as a whole-school, data-driven, prevention-based framework for improving learning outcomes for EVERY student through a layered continuum of evidence-based practices and systems. (See more at www.cde.state.co.us/mtss#sthash .fR5qwglX.dpuf.)

The Colorado Department of Education described this model thusly:

> MTSS is the idea of bringing all of our supports together within one integrated continuum of supports. Nothing we do to support our students is left out of this continuum. And it includes everyone, not just some of us. Universal supports are foundational for ALL learners. Supplemental supports we refer to as targeted supports and intensive supports are IN ADDITION TO universal supports— that's the layered continuum.

Because MTSS has become the evolution of RTI, it is considered the umbrella over systems of support, connecting "all EDs." MTSS has been identified as a broader umbrella that includes RTI, PBIS, and a continuum of services and processes ("RtI, RtI2, MTSS: Establishing Clarity," 2013; Statewide Special Education Task Force, 2015).

As MTSS and other systems of support grow and blend, the integration of special education into these systems will be realized. However, legal mandates regarding timelines and procedural protections will need to be protected. Now more than ever, special education does not live in a separate silo, and special education is a service, not a place where students go when they have difficulties in school ("Special Education: A Service, Not a Place," 2013).

Preventing Students From Needing Special Education: How We Conceptualize Disability

The movement toward early intervening services and response to intervention in IDEA 2004 represented clear congressional intent to change the way special education services were delivered in this country, beginning with the identification and eligibility phase of the process. This change represented a need for broad revision in our educational system for both general and special education. The new premise of our identification system required that students cannot be identified for special education services if they have not been instructed.

The basis of the change represented an evolution in the philosophical base of our concepts of disability, specifically learning disability, and concerns over the rising costs of special education, consequently leading to policy changes in operational procedures. In addition, since 2001, with the requirements of ESEA, schools were held accountable for the learning of every student. What all of these efforts have in common was addressing student learning needs quickly and efficiently. Old models of special education were criticized for making a struggling student "wait to fail" before providing special attention or instruction. This was widely known to not be an effective way to provide students with assistance.

Response to Intervention

Response to intervention (RTI) is a framework for problem solving and short-term intervention programs that determine how struggling students respond before assuming they must have a disability and referring them for special education assessment. RTI emphasizes a process whereby we look at how the system addresses student needs before we look at "within learner" challenges to explain why students are struggling. RTI allows for multiple attempts to provide assistance to students before identifying them as students with disabilities. RTI programs are typically operated within a tiered model of school support designed to have multiple ways to assist students. In some places, RTI and MTSS may be used interchangeably (National Center for Learning Disabilities, n.d.), but for the purpose of this discussion, *RTI* refers to general education interventions that may be used prior to referral for a special education assessment. RTI is one aspect of MTSS.

RTI programs are intended to address students' learning and behavioral needs. IDEA 2004 established that students may not be called *disabled* if they have not been instructed. This specifically applies to students with learning disabilities and speech–language disorders, which are considered "high-incidence disabilities," as they are the most frequently occurring educational disabilities. A criticism of the way the educational system previously dealt with students who had academic or behavioral issues was that they were (a) not helped early and (b) placed in special education after long periods of school failure.

The National Association of State Directors of Special Education (NASDSE) (Batsche et al., 2005) defined *RTI* as "the practice of providing high-quality instruction and intervention matched to student need, monitoring progress frequently to make decisions about changes in instruction or goals, and applying child response data to important educational decisions" (p. 3). NASDSE identified the following as the core principles of RTI:

- Effectively teach all children.
- Intervene early.
- Use a multi-tier model of service delivery.
- Use a problem-solving method to make decisions within a multi-tier model.
- Use research-based, scientifically validated interventions and instruction to the extent available.
- Monitor student progress to inform instruction.
- Use data to make decisions. A data-based decision regarding the student's response to the intervention is central to RTI practices.
- Use assessment for three different purposes:

  1. screening applied to all children to identify those who are not making academic or behavioral progress at expected rates,
  2. diagnostics to determine what children can and cannot do in important academic and behavioral domains, and
  3. progress monitoring to determine if academic or behavioral interventions are producing desired effects. (pp. 19–20)

In an updated discussion about MTSS, Batsche (2013) expanded the explanation of the problem-solving process as understood through four questions:

1. Is there a problem, and what is it? (Common Core State Standards, behavioral standards)
2. Why is this happening? (hypothesis about why they are not doing the desired behavior and assessments to verify the hypothesis)
3. What are we going to do about it? (the comprehensive, integrated intervention plan)
4. Did our intervention work? (data-based response to instruction and intervention)

Batsche (2013) commented,

> The most important step in this problem-solving process is the first one—goal identification. When the goal focuses on what we want students to know and be able to do (rather than on the problem), then problem solving and intervention focuses on building skills and behaviors, not eliminating problems. (p. 3)

Academic and behavioral goals are integrated in Step 1. The next critical step is the delivery of instruction and supports across tiers, including the intensity of instruction in both focus and time (Batsche, 2013, p. 3). In RTI and MTSS models, tiers of support are to provide increasingly intensive instruction and intervention, with Tier 2 and Tier 3 providing targeted and intense intervention. Several authors in special education and speech–language pathology have concerns about whether intensive interventions are truly being provided in these tiers, as well as within special education (Danielson & Rosenquist, 2014; Fuchs, Fuchs, & Vaughn, 2014; R. Gillam, Baker, & Williams, 2012). Fidelity to intervention is essential in RTI programs, as decisions about students are made based on their response. If the program has not been delivered with fidelity and the student does not respond, then the student may be determined to have a disability or referred for assessment to make such a determination (Danielson & Rosenquist, 2014; Fuchs et al., 2014). Table 3.1 describes considerations to be made regarding intensive intervention.

When special educators provide intervention to non-IDEA-eligible students, as part of an RTI program or model at the school, these services are known as *early intervening services*. IDEA 2004 promotes the use of special education funds for early intervening services to assist students who are not yet eligible for special education. IDEA 2004 encourages special educators to work with nonidentified students to provide interventions that may prevent the students from needing to be identified as a student with a disability.

TABLE 3.1. Considerations for Intensive Intervention

Intervention facet	Explanation
Treatment intensity and/or intense intervention	This treatment is designed to address severe and persistent learning or behavioral difficulties (Danielson & Rosenquist, 2014); examples include small-group and expanded time. The ways to increase intensity include increasing the number of sessions and pace of the session, establishing a strong routine that is learned by students, and creating activities that are highly connected to students' lives (Montgomery & Moore, 2011). This can include the number of hours, quality and quantity of services, level of participation, adult-to-student ratio, and the number of therapeutic episodes across time (Warren, Fey, & Yoder, 2007).
Dosage	*Dosage* refers to both the amount of treatment sessions and the number of teaching episodes in a single teaching session (Warren et al., 2007) and pertains to the questions "How often?" and "How much?" (Montgomery & Moore, 2011).
Fidelity	*Fidelity* refers to the accurate and consistent delivery of instruction, intervention, or assessment in a manner that is consistent with the developer's recommendations (Danielson & Rosenquist, 2014, p. 7).
Evidence-based practice	Evidence-based practice includes the integration of (a) clinical expertise, (b) current best evidence, and (c) client values to provide high-quality services reflecting the interests, values, needs, and choices of the individuals served (American Speech–Language–Hearing Association, n.d.-j).
Data-based intervention	This intervention offers a systematic method for using assessment data to determine when and how to intensify intervention in reading, math, and behavior (National Center on Intensive Intervention, 2013).
Standard intervention protocol	Standard intervention protocol is a consistent, often scripted evidence-based instructional program intended for students with similar academic or behavioral needs (Danielson & Rosenquist, 2014, p. 7).
Progress monitoring	Progress monitoring is a scientifically based practice that is used to assess students' academic performance and evaluate the effectiveness of instruction. Progress monitoring can be implemented with individual students or an entire class (National Center on Student Progress Monitoring, n.d.).

The *Code of Federal Regulations* described how special education can do this:

- An LEA [local education agency] may use up to 15 percent of its funds to develop and implement coordinated early intervening services. Agencies may blend funding to coordinate programs for students in kindergarten through grade 12 (with particular emphasis on students in kindergarten through grade 3) to provide additional academic and behavioral supports that promote success in a general education environment. (C.F.R. § 613 [f][1])
- Funds may be used for professional development for teachers and other school staff to learn scientifically-based academic instruction and behavioral interventions. Topics may include scientifically-based literacy instruction, use of adaptive and instructional software, and providing educational and behavioral evaluations, services, and supports. (C.F.R. § 613 [2])
- May coordinate IDEA-funded activities with those being carried out under ESEA. (C.F.R. § 613 [f][5])

Speech–language pathologists should be actively involved in the development of early intervening service models at their school and/or be involved in RTI at their school as part of their role in prevention (see Chapter 9).

A Tiered System of Support for All Learners

Struggling students in our educational system have traditionally had few resources available to them that could address their issues. A tiered system of supports allows learners to receive assistance when they begin to demonstrate difficulties, and they do not have to "wait to fail," as happened under the old model of special education.

Under the tiered model of supports, the intensity of interventions is heightened as students need more intervention:

- *Tier I:* General education core instruction
- *Tier II:* Strategic, targeted group instruction
- *Tier III:* Intense individual or group instruction

General education is responsible for the interventions in an RTI, PBIS, or MTSS model; however, special education staff may be involved at all levels. IDEA 2004 formalized the working of special education staff with non-IDEA-identified students who are struggling and may need assistance or intervention from staff with specialized expertise. This involvement of special education staff in providing assistance to general education struggling learners may be provided through early intervening services, which can be used at any of the tiers.

The use of scientifically based instruction, as mandated under both ESEA and IDEA 2004, begins at Tier I. When effective core instructional strategies and principles are used, it is expected that the majority of the learners in the classroom (80%–90%) will benefit. Students who struggle in the general education classroom (10%–20%) may need to be moved to Tier II for targeted assistance. Within Tier II, it is expected that 80% to 85% of the students will benefit from that program, leading to either returning the student to Tier I or perhaps providing additional assistance through Tier II. A much smaller number of students, then, will continue to struggle and require intensive assistance through Tier III. Each of these tiers involves interventions provided through general education resources, including Title I or other categorical programs. Special education staff may provide early intervening services for students in any of the tiers, but it is most likely that intense services are provided at Tier III. See Table 3.2 for the instructional characteristics and methods that may be used at each tier.

Critical to the implementation of a tiered model of instructional supports is an *instructional support team* (IST). (See the later section "Instructional Support Team, Instructional Consultation Team, and Problem-Solving Team" for more information.) Under the IST, instructional consultation team (ICT), or problem-solving team model, the team is charged with looking at factors external to the student rather than at deficits within the student. Importantly, the first step to assistance is not special education.

Working within a tiered system provides opportunities for all students to learn, benefits English Learners and other students in need of intense language experiences due to linguistic deficits that are not due to a disability, and allows for progress monitoring to determine students' response to intervention.

Under this type of system, speech–language pathologists and other special educators will be working "inside" and "outside" of special education. The philosophy of this approach is to allow students access to specialists so that we might prevent students from becoming identified for special education.

TABLE 3.2. Instructional Characteristics and Methods of a Tiered System

Tier	Instructional characteristics	Methods
I	• Methodologies enhance the likelihood of learner success for all learners. • Progress is monitored for all students.	• Universal instruction • Universal design differentiated instruction • Universal screening
II	• Methodologies are targeted to address learner needs and enhance the likelihood of learner success. • Intervention is provided for a specified period of time. • Progress is monitored to determine the learner's response to intervention.	• Targeted instruction • Selected interventions using scientifically based instructional strategies that may not be available through general education • Increased intensity • Smaller group size
III	• Methodologies are specialized to address learner needs and enhance the likelihood of learner success. • Intervention is provided for a specified period of time. • Progress is monitored to determine the learner's response to intervention.	• May use programs and strategies previously reserved for special education • May be provided by special educators as early intervening services • May be small-group or individualized instruction

Speech–language pathologists, as members of the school team, have a good deal to contribute to RTI programs at their school. Several authors in the field have addressed these roles (Ehren, 2009; Rudebusch, 2008; Rudebusch & Wiechmann, 2011; Wallach, 2008). (See further discussion of RTI as a service delivery model in Chapter 5.) The early work of Troia (2005) still applies when outlining these different roles in each of the tiers:

Tier I: Assist in Providing Professional Development to Teachers
- Provide strategies for teaching literacy-based skills, such as alphabetic principle, strategies for decoding and spelling, and how to deliver instruction.
- Provide instruction in later vocabulary development, roots and prefixes, and how to select scientifically validated materials.
- Consult on how to deliver effective universal instruction, set up screening, and monitor progress.
- Monitor and assist school teams.

Tier II: Be a Consultant for Teams Delivering Targeted Instruction and Interventions
- Provide directed instruction for diagnostic and therapeutic instructional purposes.
- Make recommendations for interventions that prevent long-term problems. (If the student does not respond to the interventions, then a comprehensive assessment may be indicated.)

Tier III: Provide Direct and/or Indirect Intervention
- Provide specialized treatments for poor readers with language deficits who have not responded to universal instruction and targeted interventions.
- Consult with special educators to help them make their services maximally beneficial.

Early Intervening Services

Continuous school improvement in the era of accountability has changed practice in schools to intervene early with struggling students. Districts may use IDEA 2004 funds to develop policies and procedures to help students who are not currently identified for special education but may be in need of additional academic assistance. Early intervening services can be developed for use at all levels, but the law encourages emphasis on students in kindergarten through Grade 3 who need additional academic or behavioral supports (IDEA 2004, § 613 [f][1]). Early intervening services may be either professional development activities or evaluation services and supports, including scientifically based literacy instruction (IDEA 2004, § 613 [f][2]).

Speech–language pathologists will recognize that early intervening services, along with appropriate identification and intervention procedures and the use of evidence-based practice and a workload analysis approach, will shape their model for service in a positive way. As early intervening service models continue to develop throughout the country, they will likely be based on RTI models that have proved successful, as well as the integration of RTI and workload analysis (Montgomery & Moore-Brown, 2005; Rudebusch & Wiechmann, 2011). Many states and local districts have established models that have been successful. Some examples are a model using a 9-week intense literacy instruction program cotaught by resource specialists and speech–language pathologists (Moore-Brown, Montgomery, Bielinski, & Shubin, 2005), an expanded screening model for providing articulation intervention prior to identification, and a clinical reading model where the speech–language pathologist instructs first and second graders in phonemic awareness for 20 minutes three times a week, for 3 months. All of these models have proved successful in preventing students from ultimately requiring special education (Montgomery & Moore-Brown, 2005; Rudebusch, 2008).

School districts are required under IDEA 2004 to document their early intervening services and report how many students avoided special education. Speech–language pathologists will need to communicate with administrators when developing these programs, to be sure of the documentation necessary and to provide appropriate notice to parents.

Early intervening services have both funding and practice implications. These are discussed in Chapter 9 but are featured here as well. Early intervening services are not limited to speech–language intervention. Audiologists may also be able to consult or provide interventions in auditory training, acoustic modifications, or consultation services for students with hearing issues.

Funding Implications

IDEA 2004 includes a provision for the use of up to 15% of Part B funds for early intervening services. Part B is the portion of IDEA that requires special education services for identified students aged 3 to 22 years. Early intervening services allow for the use of these funds for programs and services to nonidentified students who are struggling academically and/or behaviorally and who could benefit from the resources normally reserved for students in special education. Permissive use of funds for prereferral activities was allowed under IDEA Amendments of 1997. The specific provisions for early intervening services in IDEA 2004 make it very clear that Congress intends for special education to be engaged in activities that will prevent students from ultimately needing special education identification.

The early intervening services provision addresses concerns about the much-criticized "wait to fail" model of special education identification, specifically in the area of learning disabilities. Through the use of early intervening services and adoption of RTI models, struggling students can receive academic and behavioral supports prior to being eligible for special education. The intent of this provision is to prevent ultimate special education identification by supporting and helping these students early.

The section of the *Code of Federal Regulations* (C.F.R. § 300.226 [b]) that outlines early intervening services indicates that these services may include the following:

(1) Professional development, which may be provided by entities other than local education agencies (LEAs) for teachers and other school staff to enable them to deliver scientifically based academic instruction and behavioral interventions, including scientifically based literacy instruction and, when appropriate, instruction on the use of adaptive and instructional software; and

(2) Providing educational and behavioral evaluations, services, and supports, including scientifically based literacy instruction.

Commentary by the U.S. Department of Education (USDE) to the C.F.R. clarifies the following about early intervening services:

- Not to delay an evaluation of a student suspected of having a disability
- Recipients do not have the rights and protections of special education
- Intended for students in Grades K–12
- Emphasis on K–3
- Cannot be used for preschool
- May be used to purchase instructional materials to support these efforts
- May include related services personnel in the development and delivery of educational and behavioral evaluations, services, and supports

The following comment was made by the USDE in relation to the funds and the rationale for allocating special education funds in this way:

> The authority to use some Part B funds for early intervening services has the potential to benefit special education, as well as the education of other children, by reducing academic and behavioral problems in the regular education environment and reducing the number of referrals to special education interventions. Therefore, we believe the use of Part B funds for early intervening services should be encouraged, rather than restricted. (C.F.R. Commentary, pp. 46626–46627)

School districts with significant disproportionality of students in special education based on race and ethnicity will be required to use 15% of their Part B funds for early intervening services to serve children in the local education agency particularly, but not exclusively, and children in those groups who were significantly overidentified.

States will be required to identify the specifics of how early intervening services will be provided, including who will be involved. The C.F.R. commentary provided by the USDE stated, "Nothing in this Act or regulations prevents States and LEAs from including related services personnel in the development and delivery of educational and behavioral evaluations, services, and supports for teachers and other school staff to enable them to deliver coordinated early intervening services" (C.F.R. Commentary, pp. 46627–46628).

Early Intervening Services and Speech-Language Pathologists

Using special education funds to provide early intervening services to nonidentified, but struggling, students is an example of funding flexibility. Special education personnel have historically limited their work exclusively to students with identified disabilities in most situations. With the early intervening services provisions under IDEA 2004, special education resources, including personnel time, can and should be spent in part on attempting to prevent struggling students from needing special education identification.

Through this avenue, speech–language pathologists have a unique opportunity to engage in prevention activities, including collaboration and consultation, professional development for teachers, and direct and indirect services through RTI programs for struggling students.

Because this is a shift in how speech–language pathologists' time is spent, coordination at the school and district levels will be needed. Reporting requirements include tracking which students receive early intervening services, so the process for referral and the types of services provided must be clearly identified.

Practice Implications

The clear intent of Congress is to use the expertise of special education professionals, including speech–language pathologists, to work with students who are struggling academically to prevent such students from becoming IDEA 2004 eligible. In doing so, caseload counts should decrease. However, although this concept is readily understood by those in both general and special education, a shift in practice will be required. Speech–language pathologists and other special educators who engage in early intervening services must account for their time so that it is recognized as part of the 15% (early intervening services) Part B funding. In addition, general and special education staff must look at their current model of referral and supports for students to ensure that old methods that are not consistent with this intent are updated.

Some speech–language pathologists are concerned about requirements or trends to work with nonidentified students for the following reasons: (a) They imagine that this work will be in addition to already demanding workloads, and (b) the funding formula in their state counts identified students, which may result in a decrease in funds for the school district.

Some specialists are also concerned that if they reduce their caseloads, positions will be cut or eliminated. Again, because requirements encourage the use of special education funds to serve nonidentified students, this concern should not be realized. However, it is important for all parties, particularly administrators and business staff, to understand that the funding of positions should not be established on caseload counts. Maintenance of effort requirements for special education also prevent such reductions in staffing when reduction in caseload counts is realized.

Some educators are excited when they hear about "the 15%" of funds that can be allocated to early intervening services. It is important to remember that this is 15% of the Part B funds, not a new pot of money. Accessing and tracking these funds is important. By providing early intervening services, speech–language pathologists can not only positively affect performance for all students but also begin to implement work-load management efforts. Speech–language pathologists in schools are encouraged to be a part of local planning and implementation.

Screening Procedures

In some school districts, speech–language pathologists engage in individual or mass screenings annually or periodically to identify students with communication difficulties who may not be referred by teachers, other professionals, or parents. *Screening* refers to a rapid pass–fail procedure used by speech–language pathologists to record the communicative behaviors of all students of a particular grade level, category, or class and identify candidates for formal evaluation. In the past, the speech–language pathologist could, for example, screen all kindergartners, all third graders, all new students, all children at risk, or all children in the first quartile of reading achievement. This practice was part of the Child Find system.

While still evident in some school districts, this practice has generally been eliminated in most systems for a variety of reasons, primarily because this practice is contrary to the belief systems of Multi-Tiered System of Supports or response to intervention (RTI). In other words, when children have difficulties, whether in speech or language development, the first question is whether there are interventions that could assist through general education. Screening methods that operate separate from the RTI or MTSS model not only remove students from the intervention model and philosophy of RTI and MTSS but also cause speech–language pathologists to operate outside of the system. Finally, the change in consideration of disability suggests that a snapshot of a student can potentially overidentify. (See the Appendix, "To Screen or Not to Screen . . . That is the Question.")

Screening for communication impairments based on a direct referral to the speech–language pathologist is discouraged under current practice, although screening is still included in the ASHA Preferred Practice Patterns in assessment. The key is distinguishing between screening, assessment, and observation. If the purpose of the screening is to determine whether a student has a disability, then the screening can be construed as an assessment and therefore would need parental consent. A good rule of thumb is that anything that is done for an individual student versus the whole group of students (e.g., classroom) likely would need parental consent, even for an observation or screening.

Screening usually employs a short face-to-face interview with the child, but screening may also include a teacher interview. The speech–language pathologist engages a child in a series of questions, a conversation, or both to decide whether more in-depth observation or assessment is necessary. If the speech–language pathologist conducts a screening program, his or her responsibilities are as follows:

- Select screening measures with technical adequacy
- Administer and/or interpret a speech–language screening
- Administer and/or interpret a hearing screening in accordance with state and local policy, procedures, and staffing patterns (ASHA, 2004e)

The main reasons that screening is not indicated as a preferred practice in the public schools are that students must be considered in the instructional environment in which they are achieving or not achieving, and that all areas of suspected disability must be considered if a child is having difficulty in school. Under the tiered model of interventions, screening of a different kind occurs. This screening is known as *universal screening* and applies to all children in the general education classroom. Through universal screening, the progress of all children in the educational system is monitored and considered closely. This type of screening is the responsibility not of special education personnel but of general educational personnel. When students are not progressing in the manner in which they should, appropriate interventions should be applied. However, this does not mean that these children will require special education, only that they may require intense instruction in their areas of need.

The *Code of Federal Regulations* does clarify that screening for instructional purposes is not evaluation:

> The screening of a student by a teacher or specialist to determine appropriate instructional strategies for curriculum implementation shall not be considered to be an evaluation for eligibility for special education and related services. (34 C.F.R. § 300.302)

Instruction and Interventions in a School Improvement Environment

Schools across the United States are concerned with student learning in ways that are unprecedented. Throughout this book, speech–language pathologists who work in schools are encouraged to understand and participate in these efforts. Understanding the issues and pressures of public education will help in adjusting to the demands placed on the educational system.

To address the requirements of ESEA and meet the mandates demanding high achievement, many schools have embarked on initiatives to strengthen the teaching–learning connection. As discussed, schools are establishing systems that support student learning needs and are now addressing these needs systematically and routinely as part of their school operations. Professional learning communities (PLCs) (DuFour, Dufour, Eaker, & Karhanek, 2004) represent one way that schools are attempting to work collaboratively to create a school system that is designed specifically to address student learning needs. PLC schools focus on learning—not teaching—and create a positive environment for both learners and teachers (DuFour et al., 2004). A community of learners ensures that the whole school has a culture of wanting to help, and provides established interventions. For many years in education, students who struggled had few opportunities for extra or specialized instruction outside of special education or Title I programs. In the current educational environment, and within the context of accountability, school programs are now being designed to support learners who struggle.

Most efforts to improve student achievement in our schools involve examining how the processes in our schools are designed to address student learning needs for all students. As seen in the discussion on MTSS, the goal of these efforts is to design an educational system that will focus on learning and provide supports and processes for those learners who struggle. These processes may involve special education personnel but will not necessarily mean that all students will be identified as special education eligible.

The first step in creating schools that effectively meet the needs of all students is to begin with instruction in the general education classroom. Under the framework of the tiered approach, this is Tier I but should also be considered "Job One" for all educators. In the era of accountability, schools are responsible for the learning of all students, so systems need to be in place that can address each student's learning needs. This is far different from sending a student somewhere other than the general education classroom for assistance if the student is not mastering the curriculum in the classroom. Manthey (2007) pointed out that students are sent out for "intervention" but that "instruction" occurs in the classroom. In addition, there is increasing concern about the importance of ensuring that students with disabilities continue to have access to the common core standards and core curriculum as delivered by the general education teacher, the curriculum expert.

At the heart of this approach is defining what educators believe about students' learning struggles, and also the educational system's capability to respond to these struggles. The focus on improving student achievement ties together several initiatives including the mandates of ESEA and IDEA 2004 to use scientifically based research practices, also known as evidence-based practice. Strong, powerful, proven instructional strategies are at the center of what general education needs to provide to all students, but educators also need to believe that all students can learn, and then act accordingly.

Research in school-based speech–language pathology has directed the field to curriculum, reading, and collaboration for over 20 years. The requirements for identification and accountability mean that speech–language pathologists working in schools must be well versed in standards and curriculum. The value-added feature that speech–language pathologists bring to the school environment lies in using their expertise in considering how the language demands of the curriculum create challenges for learners. The speech–language pathologist brings expertise to the team and can help others understand this disconnect and generate solutions for struggling learners.

The Prereferral Prevention-Intervention Process

Long before a speech–language pathologist becomes involved with a student for consultation or service, a teacher typically encounters the student in his or her classroom. Observant general education teachers immediately help students if they begin to struggle with classroom demands. Such assistance may include providing individualized instruction, assigning the student an adult to help support the student (e.g., an instructional aide or other adult support), changing or modifying the materials or mode of presentation, using peer or cross-age tutoring, changing the student's seating position in the classroom, or making a variety of other adjustments to the classroom instructional program. All of these approaches constitute good teaching and are usually appropriate and effective, though such strategies may need to be reviewed and revised throughout the year, depending on the student's success. Students receiving such support are not likely to need outside assistance. However, if left unassisted, these students may continue to struggle and eventually be referred to the special education system.

Prior to IDEA 2004, speech–language pathologists in public schools generally dealt only with identification of and remediation for students with communication disorders. Today, however, speech–language pathologists are also engaged in prevention and prereferral activities.

Instructional Support Team, Instructional Consultation Team, and Problem-Solving Team

Nearly all schools have some type of formalized process to support students who are struggling, which is critical to the implementation of a tiered model. In the past, many schools used a student study team (SST) model. The name of this team varied in different parts of the country (e.g., student success team, child study team, student assistance team). Typically, these teams would analyze a student's strengths and needs, make recommendations, and follow up. As a whole, the SST model was not proven successful for students and was often criticized as being just a delay or precursor to special education. With the shift in focus from referring struggling learners for special education to providing more timely assistance within the realm of general education, this model has been replaced by instructional support teams (ISTs) or instructional consultation teams (ICTs). In this text, reference to a *problem-solving team* may be used interchangeably with IST or ICT; however, there may be some operational differences in these teams. Using this approach, the team looks first at possible external factors, such as lack of instruction, rather than deficits within the student. In other words, the first step to assistance is not special education but providing assistance to the student, as determined by the team. The IST provides help to any student in the school who is having difficulties in the classroom, as well as his or her teachers and family, by using a problem-solving process to examine the instructional environment and how it is or is not assisting the student. The team usually consists of general education teachers from different grade levels, an administrator or counselor, a special education representative, and possibly the school psychologist or speech–language pathologist. The parents, and student, if appropriate, are invited to the instructional support meeting. Under this model, the team facilitator leads the team in a problem-solving discussion about the student, following a familiar two-part process.

1. Gathering Known Information
   - What are the student's strengths?
   - What do we know about the student?

- What are the concerns?
- What intervention strategies (i.e., accommodations and modifications) have been attempted?
- What were the results?

2. Troubleshooting
   - Brainstorm ideas for assistance.
   - Select what to try next and assign responsibility.
   - Schedule when to meet again to report on progress.

Strengthening general education programs to be able to address all students' learning needs is central to improving all aspects of the overall educational system. Batsche (2013) stated, "The two critical elements in an MTSS are (1) the use of a databased problem-solving process and (2) the delivery of instruction/intervention in varying levels of intensity across multiple tiers" (p. 3). Central to this process is consistency in practice and procedures, as well as the concept that both students and teachers need to be learning all the time. This problem-solving approach allows a collaborative team to consult regarding students' learning needs and then learn new ways to address the students' difficulties. Critical to the problem-solving approach is the use of data to inform decision making.

To increase student achievement toward the goal of producing learners and thinkers, we must in some way enhance teacher learning and thinking. In this context, resolving problems regarding a student's difficulty in learning basic math processes implies that learners be able to learn and think about math processes in different ways. The bottom line is that looking for deficits within a student benefits neither the teacher nor the student in reaching the ultimate goal. To create learners and thinkers means that teachers need the support and resources to move themselves and their students toward this target. Again, a fundamental concept within this type of model is to first consider how the learning environment can be adjusted to address student learning needs versus first assuming or searching for needs within the student.

Professional learning communities (PLCs) operate according to three critical questions that drive how teachers, parents, and administrators work together to ensure that all students succeed (DuFour et al., 2004):

1. Exactly what is it we want all students to learn?
2. How will we know when each student has acquired the essential knowledge and skills?
3. What happens in our school when a student does not learn?

According to the National Association of State Directors of Special Education (NASDSE) (Batsche et al., 2005, p. 21), implementation of RTI requires three essential components:

1. Multiple tiers of intervention service delivery
2. A problem-solving method
3. An integrated data-collection and assessment system to inform decisions at each tier of service delivery

According to the National Center on Response to Intervention (2010), required components are as follows:

- Data-based decision making
- Screening
- Progress monitoring
- Multilevel prevention system

The problem-solving process is recommended at every level or tier and consists of the following steps:

- Define the problem (What is the problem and why is it happening?).
- Develop a plan (What are we going to do?).
- Implement the plan (Carry out the intervention).
- Evaluate (Did our plan work?) (Batsche, 2013; Batsche et al., 2005).

As models evolve to incorporate these premises and operations, old practices will improve or be abandoned. An instructional support team (IST) is necessary, to focus on individual student learning needs. However, these teams will have new and expanded obligations, including helping develop interventions within the tiers (e.g., pyramid of interventions), monitoring the effectiveness of the general education instructional program, and recreating a special education program that better meets the needs of individual students. The problem-solving team and/or IST may be one team in a school, or there may be multiple teams to deal with student needs. The important part is to have a team of people who are evaluating student need based on data and identifying resources and environmental supports for students, not searching for a place to send the students.

The Speech–Language Pathologist's Role in the IST and in RTI

The speech–language pathologist can contribute in several ways to the prevention–intervention process, including in-service training, consultation with parents and teachers, ideas for prereferral interventions, and screenings (ASHA, 2010a, 2010b). Being an active member of the intervention team may also serve to prevent inappropriate referrals for speech–language services but also allows the speech–language pathologist to contribute to the overall school program. Participation on this team can have the collateral benefit of marketing the skills of speech–language pathologists, as they demonstrate their knowledge and expertise to parents, teachers, and administrators.

Speech–language pathologists should function as regular members of a prereferral–referral committee, if this committee is separate from the problem-solving team, RTI program, or IST. Decisions are made within this committee that directly affect their caseload, but more importantly, if speech–language pathologists are to be seen as vital members of the school community, they need to be involved when decisions are being made about student achievement. Speech–language pathologists are uniquely qualified to assist the IST members in their functions. In the document "Responsiveness to Intervention: New Roles for Speech–Language Pathologists" (Ehren, Montgomery, Rudebusch, & Whitmire, 2006), the authors suggested the following:

> As a schoolwide prevention approach, RTI includes changing instruction for struggling students to help them improve performance and achieve academic progress. To meet the needs of all students, the educational system must use its collective resources to intervene early and provide appropriate intervention and support to prevent learning and behavioral problems from becoming larger issues.
>
> Speech–language pathologists can play a number of important roles in using RTI to identify children with disabilities and provide needed instruction to struggling students in both general education and special education settings. But these roles will require some fundamental changes in the way speech–language pathologists engage in assessment and intervention activities. (p. 1)

Mills (2005, pp. 98–102) outlined the following implications for speech–language pathologists on problem-solving teams, in RTI programs, and in ISTs:

- Recognizes the speech–language pathologist as having a role in early intervening services
- Gives the opportunity for speech–language pathologists to intervene with children and youths early, without having to go through the special education process
- Provides speech–language pathologists with increased opportunities to work collaboratively with classroom teachers
- Provides an opportunity for some speech–language pathologists to be employed under the 15% funding for intervening services
- Challenges speech–language pathologists to consider their role in the elusive and not-so-well-defined area of prevention
- Increases opportunities for speech–language pathologists to become more accepted as a member of the school team responsible for student achievement
- Has potential for reducing paperwork associated with referrals to and eligibility determination for special education
- Provides speech–language pathologists with opportunities to coteach students with general education teachers, allowing the speech–language pathologist to model good "language of instruction" for the teacher and to learn from the teacher as well
- Provides speech–language pathologists with opportunities to help teachers become more knowledgeable about listening, speaking, reading, and writing
- Provides speech–language pathologists with the opportunity to become increasingly familiar with the state's standard course of study/learning standards
- Expects speech–language pathologists to conduct authentic/classroom-based assessments, reducing reliance on and the need for standardized testing

- Gives speech–language pathologists an opportunity to learn more about behavior management and positive behavior supports
- Provides opportunities for the speech–language pathologist to help classroom teachers learn how to "language load" their instruction
- Needs to be included in the curriculum of the communication science and disorders preservice program at institutions of higher education

Children with perceived "speech only" problems, such as articulation, fluency, or voice disorders, may be referred directly to the speech–language pathologist, bypassing the IST process. The benefit of using the IST process, instead of going directly to referral for assessment, is to ensure that other academic or social issues are not also affecting the student. Whether the need is speech or language, concern about academic impact must be considered. For example, as the impact of phonemic awareness on literacy development has become more evident, the team should consider a student with an articulation disorder in terms of reading skills. Using the IST guarantees that the team reviews the student's progress in all learning areas. As a result of the speech–language pathologist's participation on the IST, other team members will develop awareness about the relationship of speech–language skills to academic performance. Some speech–language pathologists have developed specific referral systems for "speech improvement" programs, which are operated as an RTI model through general education for single-sound disorders in their districts. While this may be an efficient and effective system, there must be a connection to the IST model of the school, ensuring that the speech–sound disorders are truly the only issue present for the student.

The Referral Process

Most referrals for speech and language evaluations will come from within the school setting, from either teachers or the IST; however, some other outside professionals who work with children may also refer a child with a suspected disability to the school district. These professionals include physicians, nurses, teachers at state or county residential facilities, psychologists, social workers, probation officers, and administrators of social agencies. Before making the referral, the professional must inform the parent that the referral will be made. The referral must be in writing and must include the reason(s) why the child is believed to have a disability. Parents will also request evaluations, which require a specific response within certain timelines. Classroom behaviors that may be indications of possible communication problems and lead to referral include the following:

- Difficulty with reading
- Difficulty with spelling and writing
- Difficulty being understood when speaking in class
- Vague or evasive answers

- Frequent absences or avoidance of school
- Inability to attend or stay focused
- Rubbing ears or complaining of pain in ears
- Unusual vocal quality or recurrent hoarseness
- Avoiding making eye contact with teachers or others (not culturally based)
- Unwillingness to speak in front of the class
- Social skills difficulties

Speech–language pathologists often find it useful to conduct in-service training for teachers regarding communication behaviors and learning patterns that might be indicators of a communication disorder. As has been mentioned, the best way for teachers to understand the work of speech–language pathologists is to work together on specific cases, consult in the classroom, and work together on problem-solving teams. These opportunities will create natural situations where teachers and speech–language pathologists have an opportunity to learn from each other for students' benefit.

Referrals for assessment may come from many sources: parents, teachers, school psychologists, physicians, and students themselves. If parents ask the school to assess their child, the speech–language pathologist or audiologist, as members of the team, must address this request immediately. Referral by a teacher or a parent should still be processed through the IST process in most states and will generally require general education interventions before a formal assessment is undertaken. The reason that the parent's request should be addressed by an IST is that the team can discuss the parent's concerns in order to better understand what led to the parent's request for an assessment. In other words, foundational to a special education assessment is the suspicion of a disability. If a parent, rather than school personnel, is the one requesting the assessment, then the team needs to understand what concerns the parent (or other) has so that an assessment plan is appropriately developed to assess in all areas of suspected disability. On occasion, the discussion at the IST may lead to a determination that an assessment is not warranted and that other interventions can be implemented to address the parent's concerns. If parents agree to withdraw their request for assessment in order to allow for interventions through RTI to occur, this withdrawal must be in writing. If an assessment is agreed to, written permission from parents is necessary to continue in the formal assessment process for determination of special education eligibility (i.e., informed consent). (See the following section, "Assessment for Speech, Language, and Hearing Disabilities.")

In a model of MTSS that uses a problem-solving team or IST to consider student needs and identify interventions, all students who have challenges should be involved in this process. As mentioned earlier, in many schools and districts, speech–language pathologists have developed RTI-type models of intervention specifically for speech–sound disorders (see Chapter 5). In these cases, the referral may go directly to the speech–language pathologist and not through the IST. Speech–language pathologists should be wary of having systems separate from the general problem-solving team or IST. If the system of referral and intervention is run separately, the student's needs and the work of the speech–language pathologist will be unknown to the rest of the school team, which works contrary to the intent of MTSS. A connection to the team is important.

Assessment for Speech, Language, and Hearing Disabilities

Backward Planning: What Does the Law Require?

In a school system, students must qualify as having a disability in order to receive special education, including speech–language services. A great deal of emphasis is currently being placed legislatively and operationally on trying to provide assistance to students who are struggling, in order to prevent them from requiring special education services. However, some students who participate in interventions through the RTI process and receive assistance in various programs, and who subsequently fail to respond to these interventions, will ultimately be referred for special education assessment. Because the law requires a multidisciplinary assessment team (MDAT), the speech–language pathologist will not be working in isolation when a referral is received (34 C.F.R. § 300.308).

Assessment in schools is for the following purposes:

- Determining eligibility
- Identifying strengths and areas of need
- Identifying how the student's disability affects his or her ability to succeed in the general education curriculum
- Identifying how the student performs compared to his or her nondisabled peers
- Generating recommendations for goals, programs, and services

As has been indicated in the first part of this chapter, prereferral activities are part of the process that will need to be considered should a student be referred for an assessment due to lack of response to interventions (RTIs) provided. Figure 3.1 illustrates the various activities within the prereferral, referral, and assessment processes.

The terms *assessment* and *evaluation* are often used interchangeably (Shipley & McAfee, 2009), although *assessment* mostly refers to the process of gathering diagnostic information, whereas *evaluation* refers to the decision-making process involved in determining the diagnosis or eligibility for services. To distinguish these processes, think of standardization, reliability, validity, and using different assessments for different purposes as describing assessment, or the process of gathering information. Evaluation, on the other hand, refers to the process of using information to make decisions (Hosp, 2006). Furthermore, assessment includes the use of multiple measures to gather data, including standardized and nonstandardized measures and procedures that will be used to establish how the student is performing, while evaluation includes "inte-

Prereferral ➜ Referral ➜ Assessment ➜ Eligibility Determination

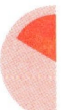

Prereferral

Problem-solving team, instructional support team

Response to intervention

Tiers of intervention

Early intervening services

Not intended to be a delay in referring to special education

Referral for Aesment

May come from the instructional support team

May come from the parent

Need to demonstrate that general education interventions cannot meet needs prior to referral

Need to have a clear understanding of the areas of suspected disability

Be careful about those trying to refer so the student will "get in" through speech and language.

Assessment

Must assess in all areas of suspected disability

Can use standardized and nonstandardized measures

Need to understand the assessment questions

Need to coordinate with members of the multidisciplinary assessment team

Assessment results will be used to make eligibility determination and for the development of the Individualized Education Program, if the student qualifies.

FIGURE 3.1. Prereferral, referral, and assessment processes.

grating, interpreting, and summarizing the comprehensive assessment data, including indirect and preexisting sources" (National Joint Committee on Learning Disabilities, 2010, p. 1).

Section 300.315 Evaluation

Evaluation means procedures used in accordance with Sections 300.304 through 300.311 to determine whether a child has a disability and the nature and extent of the special education and related services that the child needs.

Source. 20 U.S.C. § 1414(a)–(c).

In schools, there are several types of assessments, including classroom assessments, statewide or high-stakes assessments, school or district assessments, program assessments, chapter assessments, and common assessments. For the purposes of special education eligibility, assessments are individual assessments, which also need to include information on the other types of assessments completed by the school in other arenas.

Initial Evaluation

The processes mandated for initial evaluations are set out in C.F.R. § 300.301 and require the following:

(a) The public agency must conduct a full and individual evaluation in accordance with § 300.305 and § 300.306, before the initial provision of special education and related services.

(b) A parent or a public agency may initiate a request for an initial evaluation to determine if a child is a child with a disability.

Child With a Disability (§ 300.8)

(a) General.

(1) Child with a disability means a child evaluated in accordance with § 300.304 through § 300.311 as having mental retardation, a hearing impairment (including deafness), a speech or language impairment, a visual impairment (including blindness), a serious emotional disturbance (referred to in this part as "emotional disturbance"), an orthopedic impairment, autism, traumatic brain injury, another health impairment, a specific learning disability, deaf-blindness, or multiple disabilities, and who, by reason thereof, needs special education and related services.

(2) (i) Subject to paragraph (a)(2)(ii) of this section, if it is determined, through an appropriate evaluation under § 300.304 through § 300.311, that a child has one of the disabilities identified in paragraph (a)(1) of this section, but only needs a related service and not special education, the child is not a child with a disability under this part.

(ii) If, consistent with § 300.39 (a)(2), the related service required by the child is considered special education rather than a related service under State standards, the child would be determined to be a child with a disability under paragraph (a)(1) of this section.

(b) Children aged three through nine experiencing developmental delays. Child with a disability for children aged three through nine (or any subset of that age range, including ages three through five), may, subject to the conditions described in § 300.111 (b), including a child—

(1) Who is experiencing developmental delays, as defined by the State and as measured by appropriate diagnostic instruments and procedures, in one or more of the following areas: Physical development, cognitive development, communication development, social or emotional development, or adaptive development; and

(2) Who, by reason thereof, needs special education and related services.

(c) Definitions of disability terms. The terms used in this definition of a child with a disability are defined as follows:

(1) (i)   Autism means a developmental disability significantly affecting verbal and nonverbal communication and social interaction, generally evident before age three, that adversely affects a child's educational performance. Other characteristics often associated with autism are engagement in repetitive activities and stereotyped movements, resistance to environmental change or change in daily routines, and unusual responses to sensory experiences.

   (ii)   Autism does not apply if a child's educational performance is adversely affected primarily because the child has an emotional disturbance, as defined in paragraph (c)(4) of this section.

   (iii) A child who manifests the characteristics of autism after age three could be identified as having autism if the criteria in paragraph (c)(1)(i) of this section are satisfied.

(2) Deaf-blindness means concomitant hearing and visual impairments, the combination of which causes such severe communication and other developmental and educational needs that they cannot be accommodated in special education programs solely for children with deafness or children with blindness.

(3) Deafness means a hearing impairment that is so severe that the child is impaired in processing linguistic information through hearing, with or without amplification that adversely affects a child's educational performance.

(4) (i)   Emotional disturbance means a condition exhibiting one or more of the following characteristics over a long period of time and to a marked degree that adversely affects a child's educational performance:

      (A) An inability to learn that cannot be explained by intellectual, sensory, or health factors.

      (B) An inability to build or maintain satisfactory interpersonal relationships with peers and teachers.

      (C) Inappropriate types of behavior or feelings under normal circumstances.

      (D) A general pervasive mood of unhappiness or depression.

      (E) A tendency to develop physical symptoms or fears associated with personal or school problems.

   (ii)   Emotional disturbance includes schizophrenia. The term does not apply to children who are socially maladjusted, unless it is determined that they have an emotional disturbance under paragraph (c)(4)(i) of this section.

(5) Hearing impairment means an impairment in hearing, whether permanent or fluctuating, that adversely affects a child's educational performance but that is not included under the definition of deafness in this section.

(6) Intellectual Disability means significantly subaverage general intellectual functioning, existing concurrently with deficits in adaptive behavior and manifested during the developmental period, that adversely affects a child's educational performance.

(7) Multiple disabilities means concomitant impairments (such as mental retardation-blindness or mental retardation-orthopedic impairment), the combination of which causes such severe educational needs that they cannot be accommodated in special education programs solely for one of the impairments. Multiple disabilities does not include deaf-blindness.

(8) Orthopedic impairment means a severe orthopedic impairment that adversely affects a child's educational performance. The term includes impairments caused by a congenital anomaly, impairments caused by disease (e.g., poliomyelitis, bone tuberculosis), and impairments from other causes (e.g., cerebral palsy, amputations, and fractures or burns that cause contractures).

(9) Other health impairment means having limited strength, vitality, or alertness, including a heightened alertness to environmental stimuli, that results in limited alertness with respect to the educational environment, that—

    (i) Is due to chronic or acute health problems such as asthma, attention deficit disorder or attention deficit hyperactivity disorder, diabetes, epilepsy, a heart condition, hemophilia, lead poisoning, leukemia, nephritis, rheumatic fever, sickle cell anemia, and Tourette syndrome; and

    (ii) Adversely affects a child's educational performance.

(10) Specific learning disability

    (i) General. Specific learning disability means a disorder in one or more of the basic psychological processes involved in understanding or in using language, spoken or written, that may manifest itself in the imperfect ability to listen, think, speak, read, write, spell, or to do mathematical calculations, including conditions such as perceptual disabilities, brain injury, minimal brain dysfunction, dyslexia, and developmental aphasia.

    (ii) Disorders not included. Specific learning disability does not include learning problems that are primarily the result of visual, hearing, or motor disabilities, of mental retardation, of emotional disturbance, or of environmental, cultural, or economic disadvantage.

(11) Speech or language impairment means a communication disorder, such as stuttering, impaired articulation, a language impairment, or a voice impairment, that adversely affects a child's educational performance.

(12) Traumatic brain injury means an acquired injury to the brain caused by an external physical force, resulting in total or partial functional disability or

psychosocial impairment, or both, that adversely affects a child's educational performance. Traumatic brain injury applies to open or closed head injuries resulting in impairments in one or more areas, such as cognition; language; memory; attention; reasoning; abstract thinking; judgment; problem-solving; sensory, perceptual, and motor abilities; psychosocial behavior; physical functions; information processing; and speech. Traumatic brain injury does not apply to brain injuries that are congenital or degenerative, or to brain injuries induced by birth trauma.

(13) Visual impairment including blindness means an impairment in vision that, even with correction, adversely affects a child's educational performance. The term includes both partial sight and blindness.

Source. 20 U.S.C. § 1401 (3); § 1401 (30).

Procedures for Initial Evaluation

The initial evaluation

(1)(i) Must be conducted within 60 days of receiving parental consent for the evaluation; or

(ii) If a state establishes a timeline within which the evaluation must be conducted, within that timeframe; and

(2) Must consist of procedures—

(i) To determine if the child is a child with a disability under § 300.8, and

(ii) To determine the educational needs of the child.

Speech–language pathologists should be familiar with the requirements for conducting evaluations as identified in the C.F.R. § 300.304. This section identifies the procedures the public agency must follow:

(b)(1) Use a variety of assessment tools and strategies to gather relevant functional, developmental, and academic information about the child, including information provided by the parent that may assist in determining:

(i) Whether the child is a child with a disability under § 300.8, and

(ii) The contents of the child's IEP, including information related to enabling the child to be involved in and progress in the general education curriculum (or for preschool child, to participate in appropriate activities).

(2) Not use any single measure or assessment as the sole criterion for determining whether a child is a child with a disability and for determining an appropriate educational program for the child, and

(3) Use technically sound instruments that may assess the relative contribution of cognitive and behavioral factors, in addition to physical or developmental factors.

In addition, the law requires that the following must occur during the course of an evaluation:

(c)(1) Assessments and other evaluation materials need to assess a child under this part—

    (i)   Are selected and administered so as not to be discriminatory on a racial or cultural basis;

    (ii)   Are provided and administered in the child's native language or other mode of communication and in the form most likely to yield accurate information on what the child knows and can do academically, developmentally, and functionally, unless it is clearly not feasible to so provide or administer;

    (iii)   Are used for the purposes for which the assessments or measures are valid or reliable;

    (iv)   Are administered by trained and knowledgeable personnel; and

    (v)   Are administered in accordance with any instructions provided by the producer of the assessments.

Both initial evaluations and reevaluations (e.g., triennial evaluations, requested evaluations) must include the following components:

(a) As part of an initial evaluation (if appropriate) and as a part of any reevaluation ... the IEP team or a team of other qualified professionals, as appropriate, must—

    (1) Review existing evaluation data on the child, including:

        (i)   Evaluations and information provided by the parents of the child;

        (ii)   Current classroom-based, local, or State assessments, and classroom-based observations; and

        (iii)   Observations by teachers and related services providers; and

    (2) On the basis of that review, and input from the child's parents, identify what additional data, if any, are needed. (34 C.F.R. § 300.305)

Becoming familiar with the requirements of the law in terms of evaluations is necessary in order to plan what needs to be done as part of the evaluation process. Another section of the law that is critical is § 300.306, which outlines the special rule for eligibility determination, or what needs to happen in the instructional area prior to referral for initial assessment. The following requirements are critical for planning in the IST process:

§ 300.306 (b) Special Rule for Eligibility Determination. A child must not be determined to be a child with a disability under this part—

    (1) If the determinant factor for that determination is—

        (i)   Lack of appropriate instruction in reading, including the essential components of reading instruction (as defined in § 1208 [3] of the ESEA);

(ii) Lack of appropriate instruction in math; or

(iii) Limited English proficiency.

(2) If the child does not otherwise meet the eligibility criteria under § 300.8 (a);

§ 300.306 (c) Procedures for determining eligibility and educational need.

(1) In interpreting evaluation data for the purpose of determining if a child is a child with a disability under § 300.8, and the educational needs of the child, each public agency must—

(i) Draw upon information from a variety of sources, including aptitude and achievement tests, parent input, and teacher recommendations, as well as information about the child's physical condition social or cultural background, and adaptive behavior; and

(ii) Ensure that information obtained from all of these sources is documented and carefully considered.

The eligibility determination process allowed under IDEA 2004 in the area of specific learning disability (SLD) changed the way that school districts operate in eligibility determination. The impact of requiring specific instruction and intervention prior to eligibility determination has been widespread and applied to all other disability conditions. In terms of instruction needed prior to referral for special education assessment, the *Code of Federal Regulations* outlines the following procedures for identifying students with specific learning disabilities. These procedures lay the foundation for RTI:

§ 300.307 (a)(2) Must permit the use of a process based on the child's response to scientific, research-based intervention.

The multidisciplinary assessment team may determine the existence of a specific learning disability if the following occur:

§ 300.309 (a)(1) The child does not achieve adequately for the child's age or to meet State-approved grade-level standards in one or more of the following areas, when provided with learning experiences and instruction appropriate for the child's age or State-approved grade-level standards:

(i) Oral expression.

(ii) Listening comprehension.

(iii) Written expression.

(iv) Basic reading skill.

(v) Reading fluency skills.

(vi) Reading comprehension.

(vii) Mathematics calculation.

(viii) Mathematics problem solving.

§ 300.309 (a)(2)(i) The child does not make sufficient progress to meet age- or State-approved grade-level standards in one or more of the areas identified in paragraph (a)(1) of this section when using a process based on the child's response to scientific, research-based intervention; or

(b)(1) Data that demonstrate that prior to, or as part of the referral process, the child was provided appropriate instruction in regular education settings, delivered by qualified personnel;

(2) Data-based documentation of repeated assessments of achievement at reasonable intervals, reflecting formal assessment of student progress during instruction, which was provided to the child's parents.

In addition, the *Code of Federal Regulations* lays out requirements for conducting observation as part of the evaluation process:

§ 300.310 (a) The public agency must ensure that the child is observed in the child's learning environment (including the regular classroom setting) to document the child's academic performance and behavior in the areas of difficulty.

Reevaluation

The requirements for conducting reevaluations are as follows: (a) Must be conducted at least every 3 years (known as the 3-year or triennial evaluation), or (b) parent, teacher, or IEP team may request a reevaluation (34 C.F.R. § 300.300). The procedure for the reevaluation is the same as for the initial evaluation, with these exceptions: (a) The multidisciplinary assessment team (MDAT) reviews existing data and determines that additional assessment is not needed; the team decides whether or not the child continues to need special education and related services based on this existing data, or (b) the MDAT reviews the existing data and determines that additional data are needed, which may not include formal or standardized testing. Checking on the local procedures for implementation is important, but this provision allows for a more meaningful process to gather data about what the child needs as opposed to conducting testing and evaluation using measures that might not be as meaningful (34 C.F.R. § 300.305).

If the IEP team, parent, or student's teacher requests a reevaluation for the purpose of changing the student's eligibility, then a full evaluation must be completed (34 C.F.R. § 300.3052 [e]).

Conducting and Completing the Assessment Process

Once a referral is received, the speech–language pathologist gathers information from the referring source, consults with the parents, observes the student according to outlined procedures, and then decides what diagnostic testing is necessary. Written parent permission is generally required before the formal evaluation process begins. This is always true of an initial evaluation. In some states, parent consent for a triennial reevaluation may not be necessary. (See the section "Parental Consent" later in this chapter.) In some instances, parents will need reassurance. Parents should always understand what areas of need are being evaluated. The speech–language pathologist will need to coordinate with other members of the multidisciplinary assessment team. Psychologists may need corroborating data for a diagnosis that includes a communication component. General educators may be unaware of the academic impact of a hearing loss or auditory processing deficit and will need guidance during this information-collection stage.

A child may be referred for a speech–language or hearing evaluation in a variety of ways. Most typically, the student will be referred from either the IST or the child's parents. Referrals may also come directly from classroom teachers, mass-screening coordinators, and medical or mental health professionals. Some school districts have received referrals from judges who order assessments to be completed in child custody cases, juvenile justice courts, or other types of situations. If a referral of this nature is received, special education administration should be consulted by the team or individual receiving the referral. Districts and states may choose a variety of ways to respond to such a referral. Although the majority of referrals for assessment will come through the IST, the speech–language pathologist and other educators should never ignore any request for assessment. These professionals must have a complete understanding of the process and procedures for dealing with any referral.

No child may be provided special education and related services until an evaluation is completed (34 C.F.R. § 300.301). This is a critical part of the law. "Comprehensive assessment (data collection) and evaluation (interpretation of that data) enable the speech–language pathologist to identify students with significant communication disorders that are educationally relevant" (ASHA, 1999, p. 32). Any information about RTI interventions will be part of the assessment process and may be used in eligibility determination. The requirements regarding instruction prior to assessment further reinforce the need for speech–language pathologists in schools to know about and understand curriculum and instruction.

Conducting an evaluation before providing services is a logical course of events. The potential difficulty for a speech–language pathologist may arise if a parent, teacher, or administrator tries to pressure the speech–language pathologist by saying, "Just put Johnny in speech class. He only needs a little bit of help with his speech." Regardless of whether a student is involved in a tiered intervention that is being provided by the speech–language pathologist or the student is involved in an assessment, there is always a process involved that must not be violated. Students must be evaluated and then determined eligible because they meet eligibility criteria and require special education services. Any attempt to circumvent this process is considered a violation of the student's due process rights. In addition, evaluation allows for a thorough assessment of the student's learning strengths and needs, which will lead to the decisions regarding eligibility, need, and goals before services can be considered.

The importance of an accurate and thorough evaluation cannot be overstated. The evaluation is the key to detecting the existence of a student's disability or disabilities, and it sets the parameters for the course of special education and related services that will follow if the student is determined to be eligible. Knowing the legal requirements will help both the IST and the MDAT know what needs to be done before and during a formal assessment process. These processes and whether they were followed are also potential areas for challenge in a legal dispute (see Chapter 8, "Resolution Sessions, Mediation, Due Process Hearings, and State IDEA Complaints"). Table 3.3 provides a summary of the requirements for evaluations and eligibility determinations under IDEA 2004.

TABLE 3.3. IDEA 2004 Evaluation and Eligibility Determination

Law

- If a parent refuses to consent for an initial evaluation, districts may file for a due process hearing. If the parent refuses services following an initial evaluation, the district may not file for due process and is not responsible for providing FAPE. (§ 614 [a][1][D][ii])
- Parents and districts may agree that a three-year reevaluation is unnecessary. (§ 614 [a][2][A][ii])
- Districts are required to use a variety of assessment tools and strategies to gather relevant functional, developmental, and academic information, including information provided by the parent. (§ 614 [b][2][A])
- Districts must coordinate with the previous school districts when students transfer during an evaluation. (§ 614 [b][3][D])
- A child may not be determined eligible for special education if the determining factor is lack of appropriate instruction in reading, including the essential components of reading instruction as defined in NCLB. (§ 614 [b][5][A])
- IEP Teams determining whether a child has a specific learning disability are not required to consider a severe discrepancy between achievement and intellectual ability in several performance areas. (§ 614 [b][6][A])
- IEP Teams determining whether a child has a specific learning disability may use a process that determines if the child responds to scientific, research-based interventions. (§ 614 [b][6][B])
- As part of initial and reevaluations, the IEP Team and others shall review existing evaluation data including local and state assessments. (§ 614 [c][1][A][ii])
- Eligibility determination and determinations of whether the child continues to have a disability must include consideration of the educational needs of the child. (§ 614 [c][1][B][i])
- Eligibility determination and determinations of present levels of performance must include academic achievement and related developmental needs. (§ 614 [c][1][B][ii])
- LEAs are not required to conduct an evaluation if the reason for termination in service is due to graduation or aging out of the program. (§ 614 [c][5][B][i])
- Upon graduation or aging out of the program, LEAs shall provide to the parent and/or child a summary of performance of the child's academic achievement and functional performance, including recommendations on how to assist the child in meeting post-secondary goals. (§ 614 [c][5][B][ii])

Implications for speech–language pathologists

Speech–language pathologists should note the emphasis on both academic achievement and functional performance when conducting evaluations and making eligibility determinations. Also notable is the change in the criteria for *specific learning disability*, which removes the requirement for a discrepancy between academic achievement and intellectual ability and allows for the use of a response to the intervention process as part of the eligibility determination for specific learning disability. Review requirements for evaluations carefully and follow district and state guidance on reporting.

Note. From Individuals With Disabilities Education Improvement Act of 2004, 20 U.S.C. § 1400 *et seq.* (2004). FAPE = free appropriate public education; IEP = Individualized Education Program; LEA = local education agency.

Team Approach

Assessments to determine eligibility must be conducted by trained and knowledgeable personnel (34 C.F.R. § 300.304 [b][3][c][iv]). Speech–language pathologists will work as members of a multidisciplinary assessment team. No one person determines whether a child has a disability. Children must be assessed in all areas of suspected disability (34 C.F.R. § 300.304 [4]), and the assessment must be "sufficiently comprehensive to identify all of the child's special education and related services needs, whether or not commonly linked to the disability category in which the child has been classified" (34 C.F.R. § 300.304 [c][6]).

Working together as assessment team members means that all personnel must have knowledge of each other's areas of expertise and evaluation, in addition to being familiar with the assessment instruments and processes that each professional discipline will use.

The *Code of Federal Regulations* gives guidance as to who should be a part of the MDAT when considering a child as potentially having a specific learning disability. The C.F.R. indicates the team should consist of the child's parents and a team of qualified professionals, including the child's teacher and "at least one person qualified to conduct individual diagnostic examinations of children, such as a school psychologist, speech–language pathologist, or remedial reading teacher" (34 C.F.R. § 300.308 [3][b]). The commentary to the C.F.R. by the U.S. Department of Education (USDE) indicates that in all assessments for the purposes of determining eligibility, flexibility is granted so that the teams can use the people whose expertise is needed for each different type of assessment in any disability area.

Consultation with other team members is essential when conducting assessments and determining eligibility. The synergy that is created when professionals of various disciplines work together is important to the inquiry process of evaluation. Individual team members should not work in isolation but should collaborate to ensure that all aspects of the student's functioning is examined and considered.

Speech–language pathologists need to learn, know, and understand the skills and competencies of their fellow team members. When planning to conduct an evaluation, team members will find it helpful to share information about which assessment instruments will be used during an assessment. Some team members may also choose to conduct their assessments simultaneously, as in an arena assessment, which is common with infant and toddler assessments but may also be useful for other types of assessments. Another valuable process is to have one member of the assessment team observe while another conducts testing or other assessment processes (Moore-Brown, Huerta, Uranga-Hernandez, & Peña, 2006). Most importantly, each professional member of the assessment team must be respectful of the knowledge and skills that other team members bring to the process. Each team member has a different perspective, and it is the combination of each of these perspectives that will complement and complete the picture of the student's learning needs (see also Table 4.1, "School Team Members," and the section "Teaming on Goals" in Chapter 6).

Parental Consent

Parental participation is one of the cornerstones of special education. Informed parent consent is one of the most important procedural safeguards afforded to parents, ensuring their involvement in the process and that they have been informed that their child is suspected of having a disability. (Chapter 8 provides a full discussion of procedural safeguards in "Parental Notification and Involvement.")

According to 34 C.F.R. § 300.9, consent means the following:

(a) The parent has been fully informed of all information relevant to the activity for which his or her consent is sought, in his or her native language, or other mode of communication;

(b) The parent understands and agrees in writing to the carrying out of the activity for which his or her consent is sought, and the consent describes that activity and lists the records (if any) that will be released and to whom; and

(c) (1) The parent understands that granting of consent is voluntary on the part of the parent and may be revoked at any time.

    (2) If a parent revokes consent, that revocation is not retroactive (i.e., it does not negate an action that has occurred after the consent was given and before the consent was revoked).

Under the requirements of 34 C.F.R. § 300.504 (a)(1), a copy of the procedural safeguards notice must be given to parents upon the initial referral or parent request for evaluation. Districts are also required to provide written notice to parents when the district does the following (C.F.R. § 300.503):

(a) (1) Proposes to initiate or change the identification, evaluation or educational placement of the child or the provision of FAPE [free appropriate public education] to the child; or

    (2) Refuses to initiate or change the identification, evaluation, or educational placement of the child or the provision of FAPE to the child.

These provisions are included in what is known as *prior written notice* (PWN). All members of the IEP team, including administrators and speech–language pathologists, must be aware of the requirements of PWN. Failure to provide PWN in the format that is required by law can lead to legal challenges and findings that districts have not afforded parents due process. Consent forms for evaluations and meeting notices generally are written in a manner that meets the PWN requirements. In other instances, such as when a district is denying a parent's request for services, a formal PWN letter must be written. This type of a letter generally will come from the district office, but site personnel may need to provide input. (See Figure 3.2 for a model of a PWN letter.) In light of this requirement, teams must be vigilant as to whether parent requests need a PWN response if the IEP team or district is intending to deny the parent's request. Just saying "no" in the IEP isn't enough: A PWN may be needed. In these situations, it is always necessary to contact the special education administrator.

Prior Written Notice

Under 34 C.F.R. §300.503(a), the school district must give a written notice (information received in writing), whenever the school district: (1) Proposes to begin or change the identification, evaluation, or educational placement of [a] child or the provision of a free appropriate public education (FAPE) to [a] child; or (2) Refuses to begin or change the identification, evaluation, or educational placement of [a] child or the provision of FAPE to [a] child. The required content under 34 C.F.R. §300.503(b) is listed below in this model form. The school district must provide the notice in understandable language (34 C.F.R. §300.503[c]).

This model form provides a format that States and/or school districts may choose to adopt to construct the form that they will use to provide that notice. The school district will need to insert the required child- and situation-specific information, and must inform parents, as part of the notice, that they have protection under the procedural safeguards of Part B of IDEA.

Prior Written Notice Under Part B of IDEA

Description of the action that the school district proposes or refuses to take:

Explanation of why the school district is proposing or refusing to take that action:

Description of each evaluation procedure, assessment, record, or report the school district used in deciding to propose or refuse the action:

Description of any other choices that the Individualized Education Program (IEP) team considered and the reasons why those choices were rejected:

Description of other reasons why the school district proposed or refused the action:

Resources for the parents to contact for help in understanding Part B of IDEA:

If this notice is not an initial referral for evaluation, how the parent can obtain a copy of a description of the procedural safeguards:

FIGURE 3.2. Part B prior written notice.

Note. Adapted from "Prior Written Notice," by U.S. Department of Education, n.d.-a. Retrieved from http://idea.ed.gov/download/modelform2_Prior_Written_Notice.pdf.

An initial assessment must not begin until a parent returns a consent form. Informed parent consent must be obtained before conducting an initial evaluation (34 C.F.R. § 300.300 [a][1][i]) or reevaluation (34 C.F.R. § 300.300 [a][4][c][i]). Consent to an initial evaluation cannot be construed as consent to provide special education and related services to the child with a disability (34 C.F.R. § 300.300 [a][ii]).

The speech–language pathologist may know the child through membership on the IST or because of serving the student in an RTI model. When the consent form is sent to a parent or guardian, notification of procedural safeguards or parent and child rights must be sent as well. As stated, the parent must agree in writing to the assessment. During the assessment, parents should be interviewed by the speech–language pathologist, as IDEA 2004 requires parent input in the assessment process. Teacher interviews are also necessary in order to get a complete picture of how the student's needs are affecting the potential for his or her classroom success. Interviews provide essential information for the diagnostic process (Haynes & Pindzola, 2012).

The initial assessment is the first of several times that parents must be informed of their procedural rights. Members of the multidisciplinary assessment team must make sure that parents and students understand their rights. The speech–language pathologist is often responsible for providing a copy of the rights to parents, and it is important to document that the parents received a copy of the procedural safeguards that contain a description of the parent rights. (See Chapter 8 for a further discussion of parent and child rights.)

Parents sometimes refuse to give their consent for assessment. If school district personnel believe that a child has a disability, the school district may need to request mediation or a due process hearing on the right to assess (34 C.F.R. § 300.506 [b]), depending on state law. In California, for example, state law requires that school districts file for (i.e., request) a due process hearing if the parent's actions do not afford the child access to FAPE. The C.F.R. also directs school districts that "a public agency may not use a parent's refusal to consent to one service or activity . . . to deny the parent or child any other service, benefit, or activity of the public agency" (C.F.R. § 300.300 [c][3]). However, parents cannot just agree to one service and decline another, as the FAPE offer includes all aspects of the offer. Generally, school districts are not allowed to simply agree to or ignore a refusal of consent because of legal and educational ramifications. Speech–language pathologists should always consult a special education administrator when these questions or issues arise.

The majority of the time, parents do consent to the proposed assessment. The case manager should always note on the assessment plan the date that the signed plan was returned to school. Sometimes parents forget to return the paper. If this should happen, a phone call or note home is generally enough of a reminder. E-mail has become a common method of communication between school staff and parents. Be careful not to rely on e-mail only to communicate with parents about informed consent. An e-mail approval does not substitute for a parent's signature on an assessment plan. These are legal documents and need to be signed with a live signature on the form. Ultimately, copies of the consent will need to be placed in the district's special education file, as this is a student record.

Timelines

Once the assessment plan is received, the MDAT has a certain period of time in which to complete the assessment. IDEA 2004 requires that the district complete the evaluation and make services available within 60 days of receiving the parental consent for assessment (34 C.F.R. § 300.301 [c][1][i]). Specific timelines can vary from state to state, but no state can have a timeline that exceeds 60 days to complete an assessment. The only exceptions to this timeline are if a child moves or if the parent refuses to make the child available for the evaluation (34 C.F.R. § 300.301). If the parent is not making the student available for assessment or if the child is ill and unable to attend school, a special education administrator should be contacted for guidance.

Diagnostic testing may take upward of 6 hours, a scheduling challenge for many busy speech–language pathologists. Timelines for the assessment process, such as the sample in Table 3.4, are designed by many states and school districts to aid special educators in meeting the IDEA 2004 requirements. Note that the speech–language pathologist must respond to the parents within 15 days when an assessment is requested and have the results of the assessment within 60 days after the date of permission to assess is received. In some school districts, one or more speech–language pathologists rotate from school to school to help with testing so that timelines can be maintained. It is important for the speech–language pathologist to notify a supervisor if help is needed, as violations of timelines are considered serious problems, with repercussions at local, district, and state levels.

If parents request an assessment, the school team may choose to meet with them in an IST meeting to further discuss the parents' concerns that led to the request for assessment. When parents make a request for assessment, it means that they suspect that their child has a disability. If the request comes from the parent and not the school team, there may be a difference of opinion regarding how the student is functioning. To develop an assessment plan to assess in all areas of suspected disability, parents and

TABLE 3.4. Evaluation Action Timelines

Action	Timelines	Notes
Request for assessment received	The team has 10–15 days to present the parent with an assessment plan.	If the parent does not return the assessment plan signed, follow-up is needed.
Signed assessment plan received	The team has specified days (30–60) to complete the assessment.	All days indicated are calendar days.
Individualized Education Program meeting held	The meeting notice is sent 1–15 days prior to the meeting date. Providing parents as much advance notice as possible of the proposed meeting is recommended to be respectful of their time and other commitments.	The team presents the completed reports.

school staff, including the child's teacher, need to meet to discuss presenting student needs. If a school district determines that an assessment is not warranted, then a PWN letter needs to be written. However, the risk of refusing an assessment is that the family may then secure a private assessment and expect the school district to pay for it.

State-imposed timelines refers to the number of calendar days (not school days or workdays) the MDAT has between the time the family returns the assessment plan and when an IEP meeting is convened.

The regulations, timelines, documentation, and procedures of special education are all tightly regulated and extremely important. Although timelines may seem to be just another rule, it is important to remember that these timelines are part of the procedural safeguards provided to the family. Violations of timelines can be construed as a denial of the child's FAPE if services were delayed in being implemented. Timelines are critical.

Timelines and Diversity

Families who are from cultures other than that of mainstream America or who are struggling with issues of daily living may not always be responsive to the important timelines and deadlines in special education. Some speech–language pathologists have experienced working with refugee families who are fearful of authority because of the oppression in the countries they fled. In other situations, cultural parameters value oral, not written, communication, so meeting notices go unheeded, but visits to the home are welcomed. Individuals may also operate on a different value system regarding time. The team may find that the family arrives for a meeting (sometimes with many family members) either several hours early or several hours late. Transportation issues may also prevent families from coming to a meeting; for example, a family may not have the resources to access transportation services that might be available to them.

Sometimes, issues arising as a result of cultural differences become the responsibility of the IEP team. Helping families with these issues, and respecting their challenges, will help the students in the long run. Speech–language pathologists must use their own judgment to know when paperwork and compliance with the legal parameters of the special education process are overwhelming or outside of the purview of the student's family. In these situations, assistance of a very different nature may be necessary (see also ASHA, n.d.-c; Torres, 2013).

Selecting the Appropriate Speech–Language Assessment Processes and Measurement Instruments

Selecting appropriate assessment tools is the next step in the assessment process. Speech and language assessment involves determining what procedures and processes need to be completed to gather the information needed in the assessment. Tests alone do not make up an assessment.

Speech–language functioning may be assessed using many different methods or a combination of methods. There are basically three methods for assessing students: standardized tests; performance-based measures, including curriculum-based measures; and dynamic protocols. Each method helps speech–language pathologists gather information in a different way. Speech–language pathologists need to be familiar with each method and the appropriate tools for that method, and know when to use them.

ASHA's (2004c, pp. 10–12) "Preferred Practice Patterns" described the clinical process for a comprehensive speech–language assessment:

> Assessment may be static (i.e., using procedures designed to describe structures, functions, and environmental demands and supports in relevant domains at a given point in time) and/or dynamic (i.e., using hypothesis testing procedures to identify potential for change and elements of successful interventions and supports).

A thorough assessment may include the following:

- Relevant case history, including medical status, education, vocation, and socio-economic, cultural, and linguistic backgrounds
- Review of auditory, visual, motor, and cognitive status
- Patient or client and family interview
- Standardized and/or nonstandardized measures of specific aspects of speech, spoken and nonspoken language, cognitive-communication, and swallowing function
- Analysis of associated medical, behavioral, environmental, educational, vocational, social, and emotional factors
- Identification of potential for effective intervention strategies and compensations
- Selection of standardized measures for speech, language, cognitive-communication, and/or swallowing assessment with consideration for documented ecological validity
- Follow-up services to monitor communication and swallowing status and ensure appropriate intervention and support for individuals with identified speech, language, cognitive-communication, and/or swallowing disorders

As the speech–language pathologist and the multidisciplinary assessment team consider how to assess the student, consideration must be given to IDEA 2004 requirements for assessment conducted by the local education agency. Read this section of the law carefully to ensure that the process used meets the legal requirements set forth.

Sec. 300.304 Evaluation Procedures

(a) Notice. The public agency must provide notice to the parents of a child with a disability, in accordance with Sec. 300.503, that describes any evaluation procedures the agency proposes to conduct.

(b) Conduct of evaluation. In conducting the evaluation, the public agency must—

(1) Use a variety of assessment tools and strategies to gather relevant functional, developmental, and academic information about the child, including information provided by the parent, that may assist in determining—

   (i) Whether the child is a child with a disability under Sec. 300.8; and

   (ii) The content of the child's IEP, including information related to enabling the child to be involved in and progress in the general education curriculum (or for a preschool child, to participate in appropriate activities);

(2) Not use any single measure or assessment as the sole criterion for determining whether a child is a child with a disability and for determining an appropriate educational program for the child; and

(3) Use technically sound instruments that may assess the relative contribution of cognitive and behavioral factors, in addition to physical or developmental factors.

(c)   Other evaluation procedures. Each public agency must ensure that—

(1) Assessments and other evaluation materials used to assess a child under this part—

   (i) Are selected and administered so as not to be discriminatory on a racial or cultural basis;

   (ii) Are provided and administered in the child's native language or other mode of communication and in the form most likely to yield accurate information on what the child knows and can do academically, developmentally, and functionally, unless it is clearly not feasible to so provide or administer;

   (iii) Are used for the purposes for which the assessments or measures are valid and reliable;

   (iv) Are administered by trained and knowledgeable personnel; and

   (v) Are administered in accordance with any instructions provided by the producer of the assessments.

(2) Assessments and other evaluation materials include those tailored to assess specific areas of educational need and not merely those that are designed to provide a single general intelligence quotient.

(3) Assessments are selected and administered so as best to ensure that if an assessment is administered to a child with impaired sensory, manual, or speaking skills, the assessment results accurately reflect the child's aptitude or achievement level or whatever other factors the test purports to measure, rather than reflecting the child's impaired sensory, manual, or speaking skills (unless those skills are the factors that the test purports to measure).

(4) The child is assessed in all areas related to the suspected disability, including, if appropriate, health, vision, hearing, social and emotional status, general intelligence, academic performance, communicative status, and motor abilities;

(5) Assessments of children with disabilities who transfer from one public agency to another public agency in the same school year are coordinated with those children's prior and subsequent schools, as necessary and as expeditiously as possible, consistent with Sec. 300.301(d)(2) and (e), to ensure prompt completion of full evaluations.

(6) In evaluating each child with a disability under Sec. 300.304 through Sec. 300.306, the evaluation is sufficiently comprehensive to identify all of the child's special education and related services needs, whether or not commonly linked to the disability category in which the child has been classified.

(7) Assessment tools and strategies that provide relevant information that directly assists persons in determining the educational needs of the child are provided.

Source. 20 U.S.C. § 1414(b)(1)–(3), 1412(a)(6)(B).

The other consideration when planning an assessment is how eligibility determination is different with RTI, as RTI data will need to be included in the evaluation report. Since the passage of IDEA 2004 and the increase of RTI practice, the development of formal procedures to include RTI information as part of eligibility determination has occurred in many states (Arizona, 2012; California, 2009; Illinois, 2012; New York, 2010; Virginia, 2009). Initial guidance regarding the use of RTI as part of eligibility determination came from the National Association of State Directors of Special Education (NASDSE) (Batsche et al., 2005), who recommended that in-depth assessment was not required unless there is a "likelihood that serious impairment in a specific domain is a significant factor in the student's poor achievement, behavior, or both" (p. 28). Instead, in RTI, eligibility determination for special education services occurs when a student's response to both core instructional and supplemental interventions does not result in movement toward achieving benchmarks and peer performance level.

Eligibility determination can be made using the convergence of data from multiple sources to document each of the following four eligibility criteria (Batsche et al., 2005, p. 28):

- Level difference, such as large performance differences compared to peers and benchmark expectations in relevant domains of behavior
- Rate of learning difference, such as large differences in rate of learning compared to peers and trajectories toward benchmarks when provided with high-quality interventions implemented over a significant period
- Documented adverse impact on education and need for special education
- Exclusion factors: (a) rule out sensory impairments and absence of instructional opportunities, and (b) depending on the state education agency's (SEA's)

disability categories, rule out [intellectual disability], emotional behavioral disorders and speech, language, and other disabilities as the primary cause of the
significant achievement deficiency

This initial NASDSE (Batsche et al., 2005) framework is seen as foundational to
the subsequent state guidelines that were developed. For example, California (2009)
guidelines specifically mentioned the role of the speech–language pathologist in RTI
and eligibility determination. School personnel should always check their state guidelines for guidance.

As school districts have developed and expanded the use of RTI as a method of prevention and intervention in order to first assist students and also to prevent unnecessary
identification for special education, methods as assessment are also being developed
that match with this philosophy. In the late 1990s, curriculum-based measurement/
curriculum-based assessment (CBM/CBA) processes were developed, which more
closely aligned with the teaching and learning that was occurring in classrooms. These
processes and other more authentic processes are encouraged in the assessment, evaluation, and eligibility determination processes. An increasingly popular method for use
when considering RTI data for eligibility determination, especially in the area of specific learning disabilities, is consideration of patterns of strengths and weaknesses. The
federal guidelines for specific learning disability identification include language to all
for the use of a patterns of strengths and weaknesses process; however, just like RTI, the
processes for the use of patterns of strengths and weaknesses are still emerging (Lichtenstein & Klotz, 2007). However, some states, such as Oregon, have well-established
 processes for patterns of strengths and weaknesses (see www.ode.state.or.us/
offices/slp/sld_ttsd_understanding_eligibility.doc). This approach may gain
more specificity and usability in the future.

Guidelines for assessment can be found in professional documents, graduate school
textbooks, and state departments of education regulations. The National Joint Committee on Learning Disabilities (NJCLD, 2010) (ASHA is a member of this organization)
document "Comprehensive Assessment and Evaluation of Students With Learning Disabilities" provided clear guidance for multidisciplinary assessment teams about appropriate procedures to use during assessment. This document is highly recommended by
the authors for an in-depth discussion on these issues. IDEA 2004 defined each eligible
disability category, including a speech–language disability (see the section "Federal Eligibility Criteria for Special Education" in Chapter 4). Speech–language pathologists are
reminded that assessment is for the purpose of determining eligibility and identifying
needs that will be used to develop goals and services needed to implement the goals.
Students who are eligible for special education because of disabling conditions other
than speech and language may still have needs in the area of communication. The information given earlier on assessment that uses RTI data and patterns of strengths and
weaknesses may not apply to students with more severe disabilities that include complex communication needs. In these situations, the assessment and determination of

need will often include measures that are authentic, nonstandardized, and performance based. The National Joint Committee for the Communication Needs of Persons With Severe Disabilities (2002) (ASHA is a member) provides guidance as to considerations for eligibility for services in a position statement and technical report that are recommended when making these determinations.

This section discusses what constitutes *good practice* in communication assessment and gives guidance in identifying a speech–language disability. States may specify what instruments to use, and local school districts may also specify particular approaches and tools for the speech–language pathologist. When embarking on an assessment, the speech–language pathologist must keep in mind what the diagnostic questions are that need to be answered during the assessment and use these questions to approach the assessment and determine what approaches would be appropriate to find the answers to the questions (see Table 3.5).

Table 3.6 provides examples of methods of assessment that are commonly used in school settings.

Standardized Measures

Norm-referenced tests are produced by commercial publishers and are standardized on large populations of students. Such tests divide language and speech into components that are probed with a series of questions or tasks. Examiners must administer the tests in a standardized format and readminister a test only in the prescribed manner. The

TABLE 3.5. Types of Assessment Methods

Type of assessment	Description	Clinical question
Norm-referenced assessment	• Standardized measures • Compare performance to peers • Static; right–wrong answer	Does the child have a specific language impairment?
Criterion-referenced assessment	• Performance compared to a prespecified standard or skill • Documents ability at a particular point in time; static	How can this child perform this particular communicative or academic task?
Dynamic assessment	• Nonstatic approach • Identify the skills that a child possesses and learning potential • "Fluid and responsive" • Observes how child modifies his or her language after demonstration • Effectively distinguishes between language difference and disorder	Given exposure and opportunity, can this child perform a particular language or academic task?

Note. Adapted from *Language Disorders in Children: Fundamental Concepts of Assessment and Intervention*, by J. N. Kaderavek, 2010, Upper Saddle River, NJ: Pearson. Adapted with permission.

TABLE 3.6. Methods of Assessment Commonly Used in School Settings

Standardized tests for each ability area	
• Articulation, phonology • Language • Voice • Fluency • Reading and writing skills	• Vocabulary • Memory • Word retrieval • Auditory processing • Social skills, pragmatics

Performance-based measures, including curriculum-based measures
• Videotaping, audiotaping • Physiological functioning: vital capacity, oral motor examinations • Checklists and scales of learning • Local proficiency tests • Unit tests • Fine motor skills • Self-help skills • Social-emotional skills

Dynamic measures
• Cognitive tasks in nonstandardized format • Checklist with levels of support

Additional methods of assessment	
Screening results • Statewide assessment results • Hearing **Interviews** • Parents • Teachers • Student • Other educators	**Observations** • Classroom • Playground • Home • Peer activities **Review of student products** • Oral • Written • Technology based

student's correct answers are tallied, and this raw score is converted to a score on a statistical scale yielding a standard score, which can be compared to the table of norms or average scores for other children of the same age. If the student's score is significantly lower than comparison expectations, he or she is determined to have a deficit in that area. Standardized tests are static measures. They are administered in a prescribed way using one set of criteria and take a "snapshot" of the student at one point in time.

Speech–language pathologists use standardized tests primarily to identify speech impairments, language disorders, auditory perceptual deficits, and academic achievement. There is a norm, or expected performance, for each tested skill at different ages. Students' abilities can be compared to those of other students of the same age across the country. In other related areas, such as psychological testing, standardized tests are also used.

Standardized tests are constructed to account for the amount of growth expected within a year for a typically developing student, reflected in the scaled or standard score. After administration of a standardized test, retesting a year later is likely to show approximately the same or lower standard score. If a student made 1 year's growth in 1 year, the standard score would stay the same. If the student made less than 1 year's growth—common for many students with disabilities who learn at a slower rate—the standard score would be lower than it was at the initial testing because the standard score compares growth with the expected growth for that period of time for students in the sample.

This statistical representation of growth is the reason that many thoughtful speech–language pathologists do not use standardized tests to measure change. If a student is making month-for-month progress, there will be no apparent improvement in the score. If a student makes less than 1 year's progress in 1 year, his or her skills will appear to decline because of the lower score. A student's standard score will increase only if he or she makes exceptionally fast progress and surpasses the rate of growth in the norming sample. Therefore, standardized tests are the most useful the first time they are given, especially for identification and initial assessment purposes, and they become less useful each time they are given thereafter. In some cases, students will show improvement on a standardized test, but the next two types of assessment procedures discussed are more reliable for this purpose. In addition, as students move into middle school and high school, standard score comparison may be misleading or confusing to parents and teachers. Understanding how to describe and use these indicators is important. This also means it is important to understand what to report. Grade- and age-level metrics are not statistically meaningful measures or reliable indicators, yet they are often reported. Great caution should be used when reporting results from standardized measures. In addition, all reports should connect the information to the classroom expectations and show how the results will inform how the student will be able to access the core curriculum.

Items on standardized tests are assumed to be appropriate for all children, though they are often normed on a population sample that does not reflect the cultural and linguistic diversity found in today's schools. Many of these tools are biased toward children in the economic, cultural, and linguistic mainstream. They assume that all students have the same experiences, language opportunities, and styles of learning. For this reason, such tests must be selected and interpreted with care.

A standardized test should always be given in its entirety. Using subtests, or parts of tests, invalidates standard scores, and therefore these scores cannot be reported. Subtest tasks are viewed as performance indicators, not test scores. A few standardized tests are actually a battery of tests, and those subtests may be given independently. Speech–language pathologists need to be completely familiar with the administration and technical manuals of the standardized tests they use. It is unwise to use standardized tests in nonstandardized ways at any time. Doing so prevents speech–language pathologists from administering a valid test at a later date, because the student's performance would be affected by familiarity with the items.

Reading the test manual must be standard practice before administering a standardized assessment to any student in order to ensure that the test is appropriate for the student's age and cultural and linguistic background and that the test will help answer the diagnostic questions of the assessment. Using standardized measures on populations that do not meet the norming sample (e.g., using a preschool test to evaluate an adolescent who is developmentally disabled with limited language skills) is an inappropriate practice. An excellent resource for professional behavior in assessment is the *Code of Fair Testing Practices in Education* (ASHA, 2004b).

In the environment of RTI, it has been mentioned that standardized, in-depth assessments will not be necessary to determine eligibility or even baseline functioning. Standardized instruments will likely always have a place in the assessment battery of speech–language pathologists in schools, as well as in other disciplines. In the past, there was a heavy reliance on these instruments. ASHA (2014a) offered the following regarding the role of standardized tests in the assessment process:

> Results of standardized tests provide the speech–language pathologist with valuable information regarding the communication abilities in specific areas. However, ASHA recognizes that standardized tests are only one component of a comprehensive assessment process. Nonstandardized or informal assessment procedures, including behavioral and pragmatic observations in natural contexts and spontaneous and structured language sampling, provide valuable information that standardized tests alone may not.

Wiig and Secord (2006), the authors of several standardized measures, explained the balance that is necessary between standardized measures and other approaches and said, "A test provides a lens for examiners to observe behavioral segments of language and communication within a narrow, wide-angle, or panoramic view. A test lens is not intended to provide a picture of the world of language and communication in its complexity." They indicated that new information in our field has expanded what we, as a field, believe about the functions of standardized measures. Knowledge about brain–behavior relationships and the necessity to include contextualized information from the student's social–behavior and academic performance has broadened the lens of examiners so that in our evaluations, "performance and assessments should serve to verify one another."

Just as speech–language pathologists need to ensure that the assessment results from standardized testing match the actual communication performance of a student, psychologists and teachers need to ensure that standardized test results match a student's skills and abilities. One concern about standardized assessments in these areas is that they may be culturally or linguistically biased, as in the case of intelligence testing, which may result in lower scores. Another concern is that the academic tests do not match the curriculum that is taught in the classroom. Speech–language pathologists in particular should become familiar with the instruments that their allied professional colleagues use so that a profile of the student's skills, abilities, strengths, and deficits can be accurately described.

Performance-Based Assessments

Performance-based assessments, another form of static testing, require students to demonstrate knowledge and skills in either artificially created or authentic situations. Speech–language pathologists may engage students in conversation to assess, for example, topic maintenance, focus, vocabulary, fluency, or degree of dysarthria. Students may be asked to write, draw, explain, persuade, summarize, read a passage in a book, or retell a story. The process of collecting and analyzing a language sample is an example of performance-based assessment. The tasks are in real time and reveal the actual performance of the student.

Student products, rather than student behavior, may also be analyzed in performance-based testing. Speech–language pathologists may look at journal writing, artwork, term papers, homework, or school projects. Increasingly, teachers and schools have developed matrices to measure student performance on standards. These may be useful in analyzing student progress on real classroom tasks. Students may be observed participating in class or communicating with peers. Some speech–language pathologists use video- or audiotape to record the performance of a student for later, often team, analysis.

Recording physiological functioning—vital capacity, oral peripheral examinations, hearing acuity tests, monitoring of throat clearing—is another example of a performance-based assessment familiar to speech–language pathologists. Assessing a person with highly dysarthric speech, swallowing problems, a hearing loss, or English as a second language requires a speech–language pathologist to interact with the individual rather than make determinations based on a standardized test (Kaderavek, 2011). Augmentative and alternative communication (AAC) users should be assessed on performance-based measures, because speech–language pathologists are interested in how well the AAC users communicate their ideas and how they physically and linguistically create and transmit their messages. Speech–language pathologists often want to determine whether a student initiates and responds to communication in a natural setting, or they might want to measure communicative intent. Roles and responsibilities for assessing in the area of AAC are outlined in an ASHA position statement (ASHA, 2005c).

Performance-based measures are not typically prepared commercially, although speech–language pathologists may be familiar with some tools that require students to make, create, or do something that is suggested on a checklist. Generally, performance-based assessments are portfolios, performances, or projects. The examiner is instructed to watch the child perform the activity and record how a problem is solved, an object is described, or a barrier is surmounted. Speech–language pathologists commonly use protocols to record the performance when instrumentation is used (e.g., audiometers, nasometers, digital recorders). Speech–language pathologists may begin or end an assessment with performance-based tasks, making notes on students' syntax, fluency, word choice, or eye contact without the restrictions of standardized questions, time limits, or uniform administration of items.

Performance-based testing is not informal assessment, although it is conducted in a nonstandardized manner. This manner of assessment is based on what students do in various situations, not on how they respond to an examiner's topic through standardized questioning, and is more reflective of how students' communication skills affect progress toward learning and mastering curricular goals. A student's skills are not compared to other students' skills or found superior, average, deficient, or lacking. Rather, student performance is described, recorded, analyzed, and evaluated as a way of understanding what a student has learned and how he or she communicates.

Curriculum-based evaluations (CBEs) (may be called *curriculum-based assessments* [CBAs] or *curriculum-based measurements* [CBMs]) are a common type of performance assessment used in schools that are directly linked to the student's curriculum. They can be helpful in identifying where the student is compared to classroom expectations and peers. Performance-based or authentic assessments are used for two main reasons: (a) Because communication skills are highly influenced by context and vary across situations, performance-based assessment allows the assessor to document the student's communication performance across settings; and (b) standardized results are not useful in planning treatment (Justice, 2006b).

Requirements for Initial Evaluations

Evaluation materials are selected and administered so as not to be discriminatory on a racial or cultural basis.

Evaluation materials are in the child's native language or mode of communication as much as feasible.

Materials and procedures minimize the effect of English-language skills for students with limited English proficiency.

A variety of tools and strategies gather relevant functional and developmental information.

Information from parents must be included.

Information must be included related to enabling the child to be involved in and progress in the general curriculum or appropriate preschool activities.

Information must assist in determining whether this is a child with a disability and what the contents of the IEP should be.

Standardized tests are valid for the purpose and administered by trained and knowledgeable personnel according to directions.

Any nonstandard uses of tests are reported.

Evaluation materials include those tailored to assess specific areas of educational need, not just a single general intelligence quotient.

Tests are selected and administered to minimize effects of impaired sensory, manual, or speaking skills.

No single procedure is used as the sole criterion for determining if this is a child with a disability or determining an appropriate program.

The child is assessed in all areas related to the suspected disability, including, if appropriate, health, vision, hearing, social and emotional status, general intelligence, academic performance, communicative status, and motor abilities.

Comprehensive assessment identifies all special education and related service needs, whether or not these are commonly linked with the disability area identified with the child.

Technically sound instruments are used which may assess the relative contribution of cognitive and behavioral factors, in addition to physical or developmental factors.

Source. 34 C.F.R. § 300.304.

Dynamic Measures

Dynamic testing is the observation of language or learning during the mediation or learning process (ASHA, n.d.-l; Gutiérrez-Clellen & Peña, 2001; Lidz & Peña, 1996). Dynamic testing is not a static method of assessment. Rather than taking a snapshot of performance (as standardized tests do) or analyzing a student's behavior, work, or functioning (as performance-based assessments do), dynamic testing looks for a description of behavior under varying conditions. The examiner is actively engaged in the task with the student, using a process-oriented approach that looks at the child as a learner (Justice, 2006b). Dynamic assessment has been recognized as appropriate for use with culturally and linguistically diverse (CLD) students, specifically because these are non-biased assessments, and also they have been shown to be excellent at distinguishing between a language difference and a language disorder.

Dynamic testing uses a test–teach–retest approach. A task is presented to the student, who is then supported by the speech–language pathologist, in all manner of ways, to accomplish the task. In this way, the speech–language pathologist can ascertain what type and degree of assistance is needed for the student to be successful. The examiner continues to provide assistance to the student until the student can perform. The examiner's role is interactive, not passive, as it is in static testing. Dynamic assessments emphasize the learning process the child is using, not the products of past learning.

Known as *process-oriented testing*, dynamic assessment is based on the work of Vygotsky (1978), who demonstrated that children achieved more when their teachers varied the learning tasks in deliberate ways. He considered intellectual development as a socially created phenomenon that could be manipulated by the adults in a child's world. Dynamic testing is used as the method to find out what types and amounts of manipulation are helpful to student learning. This assessment information leads directly to intervention planning. Student success is measured by how much less mediation is needed to get the same result after intervention. Dynamic approaches are a valuable tool in an RTI environment (Lidz & Peña, 2009; Rosa-Lugo, Rivera, & Rierson, 2010).

Dynamic testing does not result in scores. Instead, this method requires speech–language pathologists to record the student's level of performance, along with the type and degree of assistance that was most helpful as a starting point for the intervention process. *Modifiability* is the term used to describe the degree of assistance the student needs to be successful (Gutiérrez-Clellen & Peña, 2001; Peña, 2000). Dynamic protocols can be used for assessing reading difficulties, articulatory behaviors, voice abnormalities, pragmatics, and stuttering. Determining a student's specific phoneme stimulability is a dynamic assessment technique. There are no set items or materials needed to conduct the assessment, and any conducive environment may be used. Dynamic assessment is particularly useful in an RTI environment.

Successful applications of dynamic assessment have included the assessment of preschool children, children who are culturally and linguistically diverse (Moore-Brown et al., 2006), and students with severe disabilities. Speech–language pathologists in some school districts with culturally diverse populations have been taught to use dynamic assessment methods.

Criterion-Referenced Measures

Criterion-referenced tests examine a student's mastery of particular skills or information according to absolute standards. The individual's performance is judged against a set standard or criterion. Justice (2006b) indicated there are three important qualities that define criterion-referenced testing:

1. Clear standard of performance (p. 124)
2. Design of specific tasks that reliably document individual performance against the standard (p. 125)
3. Clear guidance for interpreting performance and determining whether an individual has achieved the standard (p. 125)

Because the criterion-referenced test gives detailed information about how the student is performing, and consequently how the student is learning, the results of this testing may be more useful to parents, teachers, and students. In the area of speech–language–hearing assessment, criterion measures may be used to determine hearing levels, swallowing skills, and rate of dysfluencies. Criterion-referenced instruments are also often used in academic settings to measure mastery of early cognitive concepts and mastery of academic standards.

The Assessment Report

The speech–language assessment should give an overall picture of the child as a communicator in the school setting. Framing statements about the child as a student in his or her class is very important. If terms like *pragmatics*, *syntax*, or *lexicon* are used, the speech–language pathologist should give curriculum-related examples so that educators and family members can comprehend the impact of problems in these areas.

Assessment of the students is conducted during the school day, through arrangements with the teacher for suitable periods of time that the student may leave class. The student needs to be assessed in the areas identified by the referral. Testing, observation, checklists, and other forms of assessment can take many hours to complete, depending on the child's age and attention and skill levels. Discussions with parents, teachers, or caregivers and use of communication development checklists may provide more information for diagnosis than actual interactions with the child, especially if the child is unknown to the speech–language pathologist (and vice versa).

The speech–language pathologist should meet with other team members to compare and validate findings. The report should describe the presenting problem; describe the nature of the assessment, including the purpose and results of the tests; and include recommendations for intervention or support services. In some districts, the team will write one comprehensive report with each member contributing rather than have several separate reports from each assessor. Predetermining placement and services is a violation of the procedural safeguards under IDEA 2004; however, professional staff should be prepared to make recommendations and know in advance whether there is going to be disagreement among team members at the IEP. Most importantly, the staff should know whether another assessor has information salient to the findings and the recommendations being made.

Speech–language pathologists should use good judgment when interpreting behaviors or interactions and have sufficient documentation for conclusions. The report should be concise, cover all required areas, and be available at the meeting to all team members. IDEA requires that "the public agency provides a copy of the evaluation report and the documentation of determination of eligibility at no cost to the parent" (34 C.F.R. § 300.306 [2]). Parents may request to see the report before the IEP meeting. This is generally a good idea and good practice, especially if the parents are concerned. Providing parents a copy of the report ahead of the meeting allows for greater parent participation and involvement in the discussion at the IEP meeting. School-based speech–language pathologists need to become skilled at writing succinct but complete reports, using descriptions understood by team members representing other disciplines. Speech–language pathologists may need to write a longer, more comprehensive report if there are extenuating circumstances, such as a due process situation or a complicated case.

Speech–language pathologists may be able to use a template to present all the information about a student's assessment and functioning level. Using one format is particularly helpful for students with complex medical needs or developmental disabilities for which large amounts of evidence and observational information must be conveyed to the team. This approach is also meaningful for recording observations and comments to use as an assessment report. The profile form can streamline the efforts of all team members when students have complicated behaviors.

An assessment is not just standardized testing but a comprehensive analysis of the student. Assessments must comply with the education code. An assessment may include review of records, standardized testing, nonstandardized testing, classroom observations, observations in other relevant areas, and parent, teacher, and student interviews. Speech–language pathologists must be sure the report includes

- a pertinent background, a discussion of assessment results, and an explanation of the choice of assessment instruments;
- documentation on suspected areas of need and explanation of student needs;

- justification for needed services;
- connection to other reports and assessments; and
- information on interviews with parents and teachers.

Reports should be written in a professional manner, using professional terminology, but written so parents understand (Moore, 2014b).

Assessment Report Format

- Reason for assessment
- Background information
- Assessment and testing
  - Standardized assessments or tests
  - Observation in natural setting
  - Nonstandardized assessment or methods
  - Activities within natural setting
- Behaviors observed during assessment
- Information on progress in academic or curricular areas
- Information on classroom assessments and statewide assessments
- Information from others (parents, teachers, aide, other MDAT members)
- Input from the student
- Impressions
- Summary and conclusions
- Recommendations

As the speech–language pathologist works with a group of educators over time, team members are likely to learn speech–language or audiology terminology, diagnoses, and corresponding interventions. In schools, unlike health-care or private practice settings, the speech–language pathologist is often the only person in the building who is a professional in this field. Speech–language pathologists should consider how to increase the knowledge base of all the other team members each time they assess a student, write a report, or work with an educator or family.

Assessment is a critical aspect of working in the school setting. Unlike intervention, which may be carried out by teachers, aides, family members, assistants, bus drivers, and others under the supervision or direction of the speech–language pathologist, assessment is carried out solely by the speech–language pathologist. Finding a baseline of student abilities, recognizing the value and limitations of standardized tests, and determining present levels of communication performance allow the educational team to make the best decisions about the student's eligibility for services. A well-crafted report is vital to the family, student, team, and school district.

Assessment reports provide the legal documentation that the school district and family need regarding completion of the requirements. Clearly documenting the processes and procedures followed, results, and conclusions provides the district with a legally defendable report that will allow everyone to follow what happened during the assessment process should there be a challenge to the decisions. The importance of accuracy and timeliness of the assessment report cannot be overstated.

Independent Educational Evaluation

From time to time, parents may disagree with the school team's findings and feel that an outside evaluator would arrive at different conclusions or recommendations. Often when this happens, parents are seeking a conclusion that includes an intervention program at school that is different from the one that is desired or recommended by the school IEP team or MDAT members.

If parents do not agree with an evaluation completed by school district personnel, they have the right to request an independent educational evaluation (IEE) conducted by a qualified examiner at public expense. In these situations, the school district has the option to fund the requested independent evaluation or file for due process to defend its evaluation. If the district chooses to fund the independent evaluation, the parents will generally be provided with a list of two or three choices of qualified evaluators. Parents choose from this list, and the district is responsible for the cost, as well as for reconvening an IEP meeting to consider the results of the independent assessment. Increasingly, parents may seek to choose an assessor who is not from the list. The district is not obligated to adopt all the recommendations of the independent evaluation, but if it has funded the evaluation, it is difficult not to accept the results and recommendations. School districts are highly advised to have policies on IEEs, including what they determine to be reasonable fees for such evaluations.

In situations where parents seek or present the school district with an independent evaluation that they obtained at their own expense, the school district must consider the results of the evaluation (34 C.F.R. § 300.502 [c]). Parents who seek reimbursement for an evaluation obtained at their own expense should be referred to the administrator in charge of the special education program, as this would not be determined by the speech–language pathologist. Immediate attention to such requests is required, however, so the speech–language pathologist should contact the special education administrator immediately upon receiving such a request. Never ignore a report from an outside provider. Action is necessary, and a meeting to consider the information must be convened.

If a situation arises where parents disagree with the findings of an assessment and/or seek an outside assessment, the speech–language pathologist should understand that this does not necessarily reflect on his or her skills and abilities but may be a function of other issues in the case. If the state's eligibility criteria are adhered to, and the speech–language pathologist's assessment is complete and well administered, the school district should be on solid ground. Judges and hearing offices will, however, consider reports with great attention and specifically consider the professionalism of the report, including compliance with the procedures outlined in this chapter. School-based speech–language pathologists must know and agree to work within the federal, state, and local parameters of a speech, language, or hearing disability, as defined by IDEA 2004, rather than the broader definitions that might be available within other work settings. Working with legal and procedural safeguards, setting and maintaining timelines, and making team decisions are all part of the daily experience of a speech–language pathologist or audiologist and can require great flexibility. Working closely with one's mentors and supervisors in the schools is advisable should any conflicts arise. (See also the section "Independent Educational Evaluation" in Chapter 8.) The following describes Section 300.502, Independent Educational Evaluation:

(a) General.

(1) The parents of a child with a disability have the right under this part to obtain an independent educational evaluation of the child, subject to paragraphs (b) through (e) of this section.

(2) Each public agency must provide to parents, upon request for an independent educational evaluation, information about where an independent educational evaluation may be obtained, and the agency criteria applicable for independent educational evaluations as set forth in paragraph (e) of this section.

(3) For the purposes of this subpart—

(i)   Independent educational evaluation means an evaluation conducted by a qualified examiner who is not employed by the public agency responsible for the education of the child in question; and

(ii) Public expense means that the public agency either pays for the full cost of the evaluation or ensures that the evaluation is otherwise provided at no cost to the parent, consistent with Sec. 300.103.

(b) Parent right to evaluation at public expense.

(1) A parent has the right to an independent educational evaluation at public expense if the parent disagrees with an evaluation obtained by the public agency, subject to the conditions in paragraphs (b)(2) through (4) of this section.

(2) If a parent requests an independent educational evaluation at public expense, the public agency must, without unnecessary delay, either—

(i)   File a due process complaint to request a hearing to show that its evaluation is appropriate; or

(ii) Ensure that an independent educational evaluation is provided at public expense, unless the agency demonstrates in a hearing pursuant to Sec. § 300.507 through 300.513 that the evaluation obtained by the parent did not meet agency criteria.

(3) If the public agency files a due process complaint notice to request a hearing and the final decision is that the agency's evaluation is appropri-

ate, the parent still has the right to an independent educational evaluation, but not at public expense.

(4) If a parent requests an independent educational evaluation, the public agency may ask for the parent's reason why he or she objects to the public evaluation. However, the public agency may not require the parent to provide an explanation and may not unreasonably delay either providing the independent educational evaluation at public expense or filing a due process complaint to request a due process hearing to defend the public evaluation.

(5) A parent is entitled to only one independent educational evaluation at public expense each time the public agency conducts an evaluation with which the parent disagrees.

(c)   Parent-initiated evaluations. If the parent obtains an independent educational evaluation at public expense or shares with the public agency an evaluation obtained at private expense, the results of the evaluation—

(1) Must be considered by the public agency, if it meets agency criteria, in any decision made with respect to the provision of FAPE to the child; and

(2) May be presented by any party as evidence at a hearing on a due process complaint under subpart E of this part regarding that child.

(d)   Requests for evaluations by hearing officers. If a hearing officer requests an independent educational evaluation as part of a hearing on a due process complaint, the cost of the evaluation must be at public expense.

(e)   Agency criteria.

(1) If an independent educational evaluation is at public expense, the criteria under which the evaluation is obtained, including the location of the evaluation and the qualifications of the examiner, must be the same as the criteria that the public agency uses when it initiates an evaluation, to the extent those criteria are consistent with the parent's right to an independent educational evaluation.

(2) Except for the criteria described in paragraph (e)(1) of this section, a public agency may not impose conditions or timelines related to obtaining an independent educational evaluation at public expense.

Source. 20 U.S.C. § 1415(b)(1) and (d)(2)(A).

Additional Resources

For further discussion on the screening process, see "To Screen or Not to Screen" in the Appendix.

CHAPTER 4

The IEP Process and Procedures

In This Chapter

This chapter explains the who, when, and what of the Individualized Education Program (IEP) process, including federal and state criteria for speech–language eligibility and services in schools. This chapter traces the procedures for determining a student's need for services through the procedures for determining when a student is no longer in need of services. This approach ensures that legal requirements are met, as well as provides accountability and assists families. This chapter discusses the IEP meeting process required by the Individuals With Disabilities Education Improvement Act of 2004 (IDEA 2004), not to be confused with the methodologies involved in speech–language assessments described in Chapter 3 or the delivery of services described in the ensuing chapters.

Chapter Questions

1. Examine a textbook from any core subject, and consider the information about universal design for learning (UDL). Does this text lend itself to the precepts of universal design? How could you adapt this text for students identified as having speech or language impairments?

2. What is the difference between *eligibility* and *placement*? Why is this distinction important?

3. Discuss the importance of the requirement that general education teachers attend IEP meetings. What are some of the challenges in ensuring their participation, and how can the speech–language pathologist help in overcoming these challenges?

4. Explain how educational relevance would pertain to the impact of a communication disorder and why the federal government requires that "adverse educational affect" must be documented in eligibility determination.

5. Discuss why you think that definitions and criteria for speech–language impairment (SLI) and speech and language services vary so much from state to state. Is this an advantage or a disadvantage? Explain your answer.

6. Examine Common Core State Standards. Select areas that could be used as benchmarks or objectives for students with communication disorders.

7. Describe the precautions you must take in documentation and recordkeeping.
8. What is the purpose of triennial assessment?
9. When should a speech-language pathologist decide on dismissal criteria? Why?
10. Contact a speech-language pathologist in your area or study your own caseload. How many students are culturally and linguistically diverse (CLD)? What percentage of the entire caseload is CLD? Is there a disproportionate representation of students from particular groups on this caseload? Why did it occur? Is it justifiable? Why or why not? What can be done about this?

The IEP Meeting Process

The language that describes Individualized Education Programs (IEPs) is sometimes confusing because of the acronyms and dual meanings for some of the terminology used. An *IEP* may refer to "a written statement for a child with a disability that is developed, reviewed, and revised" (34 C.F.R. § 300.22). Common vernacular also uses *IEP* to refer to the process of the meeting or to the meeting itself.

For children 2 years 11 months of age and younger, an Individualized Family Service Plan (IFSP) is developed in place of an IEP as the written document resulting from the IEP meeting. For children 3–5 years old, the Individuals With Disabilities Education Improvement Act (IDEA 2004) permits states to use an IFSP to meet IEP requirements if using that plan is agreed to by the local education agency (LEA) and the parents (34 C.F.R. § 300.323 [b][ii]). (See Chapter 6 for further discussion of preschool-age children.)

IEP forms include all the required components of the IEP. These components are more than just lines on a page or an intent to create burdensome paperwork. Each of these areas relates to a specific requirement of the federal or state special education law. With the computerization of IEPs, the information put into the IEP document is frequently processed directly into the LEA's management information system, which then generates state and federal reports. The forms guide the IEP team through the steps of the IEP meeting process. The sections that follow describe this process.

Who Composes the IEP Team?

The *Code of Federal Regulations* (34 C.F.R. § 300.321 [a]) specifies that the members of the IEP team include the following:

(1) The parents of the child;
(2) Not less than one regular education teacher of the child (if the child is, or may be, participating in the regular education environment);
(3) Not less than one special education teacher of the child, or where appropriate, not less than one special education provider of the child;

(4) A representative of the public agency who—

   (i) Is qualified to provide, or supervise the provision of, specially designed instruction to meet the unique needs of children with disabilities;

   (ii) Is knowledgeable about the general curriculum; and

   (iii) Is knowledgeable about the availability of resources of the public agency;

(5) An individual who can interpret the instructional implications of evaluation results, who may be another member of the team described in paragraphs (a)(2) through (a)(6) of this section;

(6) At the discretion of the parent or the agency, other individuals who have knowledge or special expertise regarding the child, including related services personnel as appropriate; and

(7) Whenever appropriate, the child with a disability.

Others may also attend the IEP meeting. Parents or the district may bring anyone to an IEP meeting who they determine has knowledge or special expertise regarding the child. Often a friend or relative can give parents some support for the meeting. A notable exception is if a parent intends to bring an attorney or educational advocate to the IEP meeting. (See "Impartial Due Process Hearings" in Chapter 8.) School district participants may only be individuals who have a legitimate educational interest in the purpose of the IEP meeting. The requirements of confidentiality apply to such meetings and all information shared in the meeting. (See "Recordkeeping and Documentation" later in this chapter for a discussion on confidentiality.) Individuals such as union representatives or secretaries may not attend IEP meetings if their purpose for being there is not related to the development of the IEP for the child. Individuals attending IEP meetings must possess the required "knowledge or special expertise" about the child. Under this provision, the party who invites the individual with "knowledge or special expertise" is responsible for that determination (34 C.F.R. § 300.321 [a][6]).

The expectations of the regular education teacher's participation in the development of the child's IEP, specifically with regard to positive behavioral supports and supplementary aids and services, program modifications, and support for school personnel, are set forth in the law. The section in the IEP that identifies support for school personnel is intended to be directed so that the child can advance toward his or her IEP goals, be involved in the general education curriculum, and be able to participate in the regular class and activities like children without disabilities (34 C.F.R. § 300.324 [a][3]).

Note that the members of the multidisciplinary assessment team (MDAT) may also be members of the IEP team. Certain MDAT members, such as a psychologist, may not be able to attend all IEP meetings. Table 4.1 compares the types of teams and potential members of each. Team responsibilities are an important part of the speech–language pathologist's role in schools.

Parent participation in IEP meetings was given increased emphasis under IDEA 2004. Perceived lack of parent interest and the inconvenience of scheduling IEP meetings are common frustrations for school personnel. School-based professionals need

TABLE 4.1. School Team Members

Instructional support team	Multidisciplinary assessment team (MDAT)	Individualized Education Program team
• General education teacher • Special education teacher • School administrator • Counselor • Parent • Student (if appropriate) • Psychologist[a] • Speech-language pathologist[a] • Education specialist[a] • School counselor (middle school, high school) • Nurse (if necessary)	• Speech-language pathologist • Psychologist • Nurse • General education teacher • Special education teacher • Parent • Occupational therapist[a] • Physical therapist[a] • Teacher of hearing impaired[a] • Teacher of visually impaired[a] • Behavior specialist[a]	• Parent • Local education agency representative (administrator) • General education teacher • Special education teacher • Members of the MDAT (if reviewing assessment results) • Student (if appropriate) • Individuals invited by parent or school district

[a]Specialists who potentially might be team members.

to give particular attention to the requirements for involving families, including the requirements for documenting attempts at scheduling the IEP meeting at a mutually agreed-on time and place (34 C.F.R. § 300.322 [a][2]), which may be a conference call if attendance is not possible (34 C.F.R. § 300.322 [c]). Holding meetings before or after the speech–language pathologist's identified work hours may have legal, safety, and union ramifications. These considerations can be arranged with the administrator and require flexibility on everyone's part. IEP meeting attendance is a necessary and important part of the professional responsibilities of speech–language pathologists and all educators. Generally, school districts have not been required to hold meetings outside of normal working hours, even though this may exceed contracted hours.

Parent Participation in IEPs

(a) Public agency responsibility—general. Each public agency shall take steps to ensure that one or both of the parents of a child with a disability are present at each IEP meeting or are afforded the opportunity to participate, including—

(1) Notifying parents of the meeting early enough to ensure that they will have an opportunity to attend; and

(2) Scheduling the meeting at a mutually agreed on time and place.

(b) Information provided to parents.

(1) The notice required under paragraph (a)(1) of this section must—

(i) Indicate the purpose, time, and location of the meeting and who will be in attendance; and

      (ii) Inform the parents of the provisions in Sec. 300.344 (a)(6) and (c) (relating to the participation of other individuals on the IEP team who have knowledge or special expertise about the child).

  (2) For a student with a disability beginning at age 14, or younger, if appropriate, the notice must also—

      (i)   Indicate that a purpose of the meeting will be the development of a statement of the transition services needs of the student required in Sec. 300.347 (b)(1); and

      (ii) Indicate that the agency will invite the student.

  (3) For a student with a disability beginning at age 16, or younger, if appropriate, the notice must—

      (i)   Indicate that a purpose of the meeting is the consideration of needed transition services for the student required in Sec. 300.347 (b)(2);

      (ii) Indicate that the agency will invite the student; and

      (iii) Identify any other agency that will be invited to send a representative.

(c)   Other methods to ensure parent participation. If neither parent can attend, the public agency shall use other methods to ensure parent participation, including individual or conference telephone calls.

(d)   Conducting an IEP meeting without a parent in attendance. A meeting may be conducted without a parent in attendance if the public agency is unable to convince the parents that they should attend. In this case the public agency must have a record of its attempts to arrange a mutually agreed on time and place, such as—

  (1) Detailed records of telephone calls made or attempted and the results of those calls;

  (2) Copies of correspondence sent to the parents and any responses received; and

  (3) Detailed records of visits made to the parent's home or place of employment and the results of those visits.

(e)   Use of interpreters or other action, as appropriate. The public agency shall take whatever action is necessary to ensure that the parent understands the proceedings at the IEP meeting, including arranging for an interpreter for parents with deafness or whose native language is other than English.

(f)   Parent copy of child's IEP. The public agency shall give the parent a copy of the child's IEP at no cost to the parent.

Source. 34 C.F.R. § 300.322.

The requirements for parent participation in meetings are set forth in 34 C.F.R. § 300.501:

(b)(1) The parent of a child with a disability must be afforded an opportunity to participate in meetings to inspect and review all educational records to—

(i)　The identification, evaluation, and educational placement of the child; and

(ii) The provision of FAPE to the child.

IDEA 2004 contains provisions regarding meeting attendance and excusal of team members. These provisions must be utilized with caution, as the purpose of the IEP meeting is to ensure that the whole team is aware of the child's needs and programs. However, Congress recognized that sometimes there is a need to have a meeting and some team members may not be able to be in attendance.

(e)　IEP Team attendance.

(1) A member of the IEP Team described in paragraphs (a)(2) through (a)(5) of this section is not required to attend an IEP Team meeting, in whole or in part, if the parent of a child with a disability and the public agency agree, in writing, that the attendance of the member is not necessary because the member's areas of the curriculum or related services is not being modified or discussed in the meeting.

(2) A member of the IEP Team described in paragraph (e)(1) of this section may be excused from attending an IEP Team meeting, in whole or in part, when the meeting involves a modification to or discussion of the member's area of the curriculum or related services, if—

(i)　The parent, in writing, and the public agency consent to the excusal; and

(ii)　The member submits, in writing to the parent and the IEP Team, input into the development of the IEP prior to the meeting. (34 C.F.R. § 300.320)

The U.S. Department of Education (USDE) cautions school districts to use this provision with reserve. The intent is to provide school districts with flexibility but not to deny participation of the team members or to deny parents access to these members.

> An LEA may not routinely or unilaterally excuse IEP Team members from attending IEP Team meetings as parent agreement or consent is required in each instance. We encourage LEAs to carefully consider, based on the individual needs of the child and the issues that need to be addressed at the IEP Team meeting whether it makes sense to offer to hold the IEP Team meeting without a particular IEP Team member in attendance or whether it would be better to reschedule the meeting so that person could attend and participate in the discussion. . . . An LEA that routinely excuses IEP Team members from attending IEP Team meetings would not be in compliance under the Act. (71 Fed. Reg. 46674)

The excusal provision must be used cautiously, in light of the provision of free appropriate public education (FAPE). Several due process cases and court decisions have held that the absence of certain teachers constituted a de facto (e.g., automatic) denial of FAPE for the child (see Chapter 8).

Team members are allowed to meet and confer outside of an IEP regarding students without parents being present. Such a meeting does not include informal or unscheduled conversations involving public agency personnel and conversations on issues such as teaching methodology, lesson plans, or coordination of service provision. Such a meeting may include preparatory activities that public agency personnel engage in to develop a proposal or response to a parent proposal that will be discussed at a later meeting. The IEP team members may not meet and predetermine placement or recommendations, but they are allowed to plan and prepare for the IEP.

When Are IEP Meetings Held?

An IEP meeting must be held at least once each year (known as an annual review) and when a reevaluation is completed. Reevaluations can be completed for different reasons: because it is time for a triennial reevaluation (also known as a 3-year evaluation) as required by IDEA 2004, because of requests from the student's parents or teachers, or because the school district determined reevaluation was warranted (34 C.F.R. § 300.305). (See the section "Annual and Triennial Assessments" later in this chapter and "Reevaluation" in Chapter 3 for more details.) IDEA 2004 requires that an IEP meeting be held within 30 days of an initial determination that a student needs special education and related services (34 C.F.R. § 300.323 [c][1]). In some states, the processes for the initial determination of eligibility and the development of the IEP are separate processes. In other states, this process occurs sequentially by the same team.

An IEP meeting should also be held any time new factors that affect the student's program occur. Such examples include the following: (a) The student is not making anticipated progress on goals, (b) the student is having difficulties in school (e.g., behavior problems or failing a class), (c) a new service is being considered, or (d) any member of the IEP team, including the parent or teacher, requests a meeting. At the IEP meeting, the team develops the student's IEP, which constitutes the basics of the student's specially designed program. Additional meetings held during the year to revise the IEP may be held as an addendum to the existing program. Local practice dictates how this process is handled.

Who Is Responsible for Sending the IEP Meeting Notice?

The responsibility for sending the notice of an IEP meeting to the parent and other members of the IEP team varies from district to district and may depend on the nature of the meeting. Generally, a case manager is responsible for sending the IEP meeting notice, because he or she coordinates the special education program for the student. Most often, the case manager is the person who is the student's primary service provider. If the speech–language pathologist is the only service provider, then he or she is likely to be the one responsible for sending out the meeting notice. Federal regulations require that parents be notified of the meeting early enough to ensure that they will have an opportunity to attend and that the meeting will be held in a mutually agreeable time and place (34 C.F.R. § 300.322 [a][1][2]). States and local education agencies vary in terms of accepted practice for the amount of time to notify a parent of a meeting. Generally, a week to 10 days is acceptable.

What Must Be Considered at an IEP Meeting?

In developing each child's IEP, the IEP team shall consider the following:

(i)   The strengths of the child;

(ii) The concerns of the parents for enhancing the education of their child;

(iii) The results of the initial evaluation or most recent evaluation of the child; and

(iv) The academic, developmental, and functional needs of the child. (34 C.F.R. § 300.324 [a])

The same section of the code (34 C.F.R. § 300.324 [2]) specifies that the IEP team must also consider special factors, such as the following:

- The need for positive behavioral supports for the child whose behavior is impeding his or her learning or the learning of others
- Language needs for a child with limited English proficiency
- Instruction in braille and the use of braille for a child who is blind or visually impaired, as well as the need for appropriate reading and writing media
- The communication needs and academic instructional needs of a child who is deaf or hard of hearing
- Assistive technology (AT) devices and services (including an intervention, accommodation, or other program modification needed by the student to learn or use the device or service)

During the assessment and identification process (see Chapter 3) and in the development of the IEP, the language needs of children identified as being *limited English proficient* (LEP) are considered. The processes must ensure that students are not identified as having a disability due to a language difference and also that the IEP developed for identified students addresses English-language development. Speech–language pathologists may be called on to differentiate between a language difference and a language disorder. Speech–language pathologists have knowledge of and expertise in the normal developmental process for second-language acquisition, because some of these processes may present like a language disorder. The American Speech–Language–Hearing Association (ASHA) indicated that all speech–language pathologists should be culturally competent when providing services to individuals who are culturally and linguistically diverse (CLD) (ASHA, n.d.-c.).

Federal and state laws for special education specifically deny eligibility if the reasons for the child's learning difficulties are due to "environmental or economic disadvantage; or limited English proficiency" (34 C.F.R. § 300.309 [a][3][v]–[vi]). The demands of a student population that is increasingly diverse necessitate that speech–language pathologists be culturally competent and aware of the social issues outside of school that affect students, including mobility, poverty, literacy, access to education, access to health care, variability of language or cultural upbringing, and parental participation in the child's education.

What Are the Steps in the IEP Meeting Process?

IEP forms should guide the IEP team through the procedural requirements of the IEP. When developing an IEP, following a particular process is very important. The recommended process will not only guarantee that the requirements of IDEA 2004 are followed but also ensure that each member of the team can follow along and assist in building a program for the child that will provide a free appropriate public education.

When developing an IEP, think of the process and resulting document as a road map to the student's education. The IEP meeting process has three parts: (a) determination of present levels of academic achievement; (b) development of goals and short-term objectives or benchmarks; and (c) determination of program, placement, and services. Following this three-step process at every IEP meeting will allow for information to be shared and the resulting decisions to be made based on the requisite information. (Table 4.2 highlights important IEP requirements under IDEA 2004 and their implications for speech–language pathologists.)

Determination of Present Levels of Academic Achievement and Functional Performance

The first step in the IEP meeting process is determining present levels of academic achievement and functional performance. Depending on the type of meeting being held, present levels of academic achievement are considered by any and all of the following methods:

- Reviewing assessments, including statewide, school-wide, or classroom, as well as specialist or psychoeducational assessments
- Reviewing classroom work
- Reviewing grade reports
- Reviewing teacher or specialist reports (oral or written)
- Considering parent and student information and interests
- Reviewing the previous year's goals and the progress made
- Considering new information brought forth by any member of the team
- Reporting on student progress and behavior by service providers
- Reviewing discipline and behavioral information
- Considering statewide assessment results

TABLE 4.2. IDEA 2004 Individualized Education Program Processes and Procedures

Law

- Present levels of performance statements include the child's present levels of academic achievement and functional performance. (§ 614 [d][A][i][I])
- For students who take alternate assessments, include benchmarks or short-term objectives aligned to alternate achievement standards on the IEP. (§ 614 [d][A][I][cc])
- IEPs must include statements of measurable annual academic and functional goals designed to meet the child's needs that result from the child's disability. Goals must support the child's progress in the general education curriculum and meet each of the child's other educational needs resulting from the child's disability. (§ 614 [d][B][II][aa][bb])
- Periodic reports of the child's progress toward the annual goals are to be provided concurrent with report cards. (§ 614 [d][A][i][III])
- To the extent practicable, statements of special education, related services, and supplementary services will be based on peer-reviewed research. (§ 614 [d][1][A][i][IV])
- Special education, related services, modifications, and supports will be planned to help the child advance toward attaining annual goals, be involved in and make progress in the general education curriculum, participate in extra-curricular and other nonacademic activities, and participate with other children with and without disabilities. (§ 614 [d][1][A](i)[IV])
- The IEP must include a statement of accommodations necessary on State and districtwide assessments. (§ 614 [d][1][A](i)[VI][aa])
- Transition goals and services must be included in the IEP by the time the child is age 16. (§ 614 [d][A][VIII])
- Language regarding IEP Team members notes that "not less than one" general education teacher and "not less than one" special education teacher or service provider are to be included in the composition of the IEP Team. The representative of the LEA must be knowledgeable in the general education curriculum. (§ 614 [d][B])
- Attendance at the IEP meeting is not necessary for a member of the IEP Team whose area of curriculum or related service is not being modified or discussed at the meeting, and if the parents and LEA agree that person does not need to be in attendance. (§ 614 [d][1][C][i])
- Attendance at the IEP meeting is not necessary for a member of the IEP Team if that area of curriculum or related service is being modified or discussed when the parent and LEA agree to the excusal and the member submits input to the IEP Team in writing prior to the meeting. (§ 614 [d][1][C][ii])
- Parent consent to excusal of IEP Team members must be in writing. (§ 614 [1][d][C][iii])
- In addition to considering the strengths of the child, the concerns of the parent for enhancing the education of their child, and the results of initial evaluation or reevaluation of the child, the IEP Team must also consider the academic, developmental, and functional needs of the child. (§ 614 [d][3][A])
- After the annual IEP meeting, parents and LEAs may make agreements not to reconvene an IEP meeting to amend or modify the child's current IEP. Instead they may develop a written document to agree on the amendment(s). (§ 614 [d][3][D])
- Upon request, parents will receive a revised copy of the IEP with the amendments incorporated. (§ 614 [d][3][F])
- LEAs are encouraged to consolidate reevaluation meetings and other team meetings. (§ 614 [d][3][E])]]

TABLE 4.2. (*continued*)

Implications for speech–language pathologists
IEP development and meetings emphasize consideration of the child's academic achievement and functional performance. This underscores the need for speech–language pathologists to have goals that are curriculum related and to understand and address how the child's communication disorder affects the child's ability to both access and meet the goals of the general education classroom. This also includes considering adaptive or functional skills that interfere with academic performance. Note that the former language, "at least one" general education teacher and "at least one" special education teacher or service provider, has changed to "not less than one." Allowances for IEP amendments and excusal of certain participants from IEP meetings should be reviewed carefully. Guidance should be sought at the local level on these requirements. Make sure parent agreement is documented in writing. Now, even more than before, speech–language pathologists should develop and maintain strong, compassionate, and professional relationships with parents. These relationships can result in important contributions from parents during the evaluation and IEP planning processes.

Note. From Individuals With Disabilities Education Improvement Act of 2004, 20 U.S.C. § 1400 *et seq.* (2004). LEA = local education agency.

TABLE 4.3. Writing Positive Statements of Present Levels of Academic Achievement

Negative	Positive
Cannot understand speech	Able to produce five single words intelligibly
Does not use words	Uses gestures to communicate intent
Does not know alphabet	Able to distinguish between letters and numbers
Has not mastered sound–symbol relationships	Identifies words that begin with the same sound 60% of the time
	Present levels should be stated in terms of what the student is able to do. When describing present levels of academic achievement and functional performance, discuss the student's strengths and state needs in positive terms.

When writing present levels of achievement, evaluators should use positive rather than negative statements (see Table 4.3). IDEA 2004 regulations require that all IEPs include the following:

(a)(1) A statement of the child's present levels of academic achievement and functional performance, including—

(i) How the child's disability affects the child's involvement and progress in the general curriculum; or

(ii) For preschool children, as appropriate, how the disability affects the child's participation in appropriate activities. (34 C.F.R. § 300.320)

Speech–language pathologists in public schools must be able to integrate knowledge of communication disorders with knowledge of the scope and developmental sequence of curricula. Classroom curricula are built on taxonomies that reflect the developmental levels of children in each grade. Curricula are reflective of the Common Core State Standards (CCSS) in most states. Children with disabilities may face challenges with the curriculum of the classroom, but that does not mean they cannot master it with appropriate supports and instruction. To help the child in his or her interaction with the curriculum and to develop the IEP with standards in mind, speech–language pathologists must know what the expectations are for students in each grade. This means going beyond sharing the results of standardized or nonstandardized assessments of communication skills and interpreting how those results are related to what happens in the classroom, to design interventions to meet curriculum-based goals or outcomes.

Application to Students With Disabilities

The Common Core State Standards articulate rigorous grade-level expectations in the areas of mathematics and English language arts. These standards identify the knowledge and skills students need in order to be successful in college and careers.

Students with disabilities—students eligible under the Individuals With Disabilities Education Act (IDEA)—must be challenged to excel within the general curriculum and be prepared for success in their post-school lives, including college and/or careers. These common standards provide an historic opportunity to improve access to rigorous academic content standards for students with disabilities. The continued development of understanding about research-based instructional practices and a focus on their effective implementation will help improve access to mathematics and English language arts (ELA) standards for all students, including those with disabilities.

Students with disabilities are a heterogeneous group with one common characteristic: the presence of disabling conditions that significantly hinder their abilities to benefit from general education (IDEA, 34 C.F.R. Section 300.39, 2004). Therefore, *how* these high standards are taught and assessed is of the utmost importance regarding this diverse group of students.

Source. Common Core State Standards, n.d.-a (www.corestandards.org/assets/application-to-students-with-disabilities.pdf).

The present-level requirements reflect the connection between the Elementary and Secondary Education Act (ESEA)/Every Student Succeeding Act (2015) and IDEA 2004, in addition to the IDEA 2004 emphasis on postschool outcomes. The IEP is the document that ties together the goals of both laws: including children with disabilities in the accountability system while still ensuring attention to a student's individual learning needs.

The mandate to make a statement about the student's academic achievement and have a discussion about how the disability affects the student's ability to succeed in the general education curriculum again directs the IEP team and service providers to the curriculum and the general education program. Furthermore, IDEA 2004 requires that the LEA representative on the IEP team be knowledgeable about the general curriculum (34 C.F.R. § 300.321 [a][4][ii]) to direct the linkage between the special education pro gram and the general education curriculum and setting. To ensure access to the general education curriculum, IDEA 2004 suggests the use of universal design principles during instruction.

Universal design for learning (UDL) is a framework for curriculum design that creates access for all learners. The term *universal design for learning* means a scientifically valid framework for guiding educational practice that

> provides flexibility in the ways information is presented (recognition), in the ways students respond or demonstrate knowledge and skills (action and expression), and in the ways students are engaged (engagement); and reduces barriers in instruction, provides appropriate accommodations, supports, and challenges, and maintains high achievement expectations for all students, including students with disabilities and students who are English Language Learners. (Higher Education Opportunity Act of 2008)

The CCSS are grounded in the use of UDL. Speech–language pathologists will find ample opportunity to collaborate with teachers on UDL application in order to provide access to students by using the framework of recognition, action and expression, and engagement.

Federal Eligibility Criteria for Special Education

If the purpose of the IEP meeting is to review initial assessments (see Chapter 3 for a discussion of the initial assessment process), then present levels of academic achievement and functional performance will be determined when eligibility is considered. If the IEP meeting is part of a triennial reevaluation (see the section "Annual and Triennial Assessments" later in this chapter), continuing eligibility will be considered.

In either case, a child may not be determined to be eligible if the following:

(b)(1) The determinant factor for that eligibility determination is—
  (i) Lack of appropriate instruction in reading, including the essential components of reading instruction (as defined in section 1208 [3] of the ESEA);
  (ii) Lack of appropriate instruction in math; or
  (iii) Limited English proficiency; and
  (2) The child does not otherwise meet the eligibility criteria under Sec. 300.8. (34 C.F.R. § 300.306)

If it is determined that a child is not eligible for special education, the next two steps in the IEP meeting process—development of goals and short-term objectives or benchmarks and determination of program, placement, and services—do not occur. The IEP team may instead do any of the following: (a) make some general recommendations to the classroom teacher for assisting student in the classroom, (b) refer the student back to the IST or a tiered RTI program, or (c) refer the student to the 504 team for eligibility determination under Section 504. (See the section "Section 504 and the Americans With Disabilities Act" in Chapter 2.) In these situations, IEP teams should ensure that some form of assistance is provided so that the child does not continue to struggle and fail in school.

If a child is determined to be eligible for special education, the next two steps in the IEP process do take place. The MDAT can determine that a student is eligible if the student has one or more disabilities that require special education and related services because of the disability or disabilities. The 13 eligibility categories identified under IDEA 2004 appear in the following box.

Federal Eligibility Categories for Special Education

Autism
Deaf-blind
Developmental delay (state option)
Emotional disturbance
Hearing impairment
Intellectual disability
Specific learning disability

Multiple disabilities
Other health impairment
Orthopedic impairment
Speech or language impairment
Traumatic brain injury
Visual impairment

States may also authorize school districts to include the condition of "developmental delay" for children aged 3 through 9 years or a subset of this age group.

Source. 34 C.F.R. § 300.7 (a)(1).

Impairment refers to the existence of an abnormality of the structure or function of the student's communication at an organic level (e.g., vocal nodules, a tongue thrust, a distorted /r/ phoneme, hearing loss, repetition of the initial phoneme in words, cognitive limitations). The presence of impairment can be ascertained with the traditional instruments and standardized tests that are common to the field. These tools will help determine whether the person's communication deviates from the norms for age and ability. Traditional diagnostic measures can and should be used to determine impairment in any setting the student is seen for assessment. Impairment can be determined by comparing the child's standard score with age-appropriate norms (i.e., percentiles or similar measures from a nondisabled population).

Disability refers to the functional consequence of the known impairment. Speech–language pathologists must use functional status measures to determine the communication problems that impede the student's daily life activities. In school, the broadest educational environment is used to determine functional status: class grades, class participation, self-esteem, oral and written work, school leadership, parents' concerns, peers' reactions, and so on. There are almost no functional status tests in common use for speech and language, so speech–language pathologists must rely on reports from teachers, parents, peers, the student, and a review of class performance, including grades. If functional status does not appear to be affected by the identified impairment, the student is not educationally disabled and therefore not eligible for speech–language services under IDEA 2004. A preliminary set of functional status measures were made available by ASHA (1998b). (See the section "Functional Outcomes and the School-Based Speech–Language Pathologist" in Chapter 5 for samples of these statements.)

Handicap refers to society's perception of what an individual can or cannot do based on what people without disabilities believe is possible. There may be many genuine social consequences of a disability: joblessness, isolation, fewer friends, fewer educational opportunities, and other limitations on how one communicates with others. Although impairment causes a disability, it is the failure to ameliorate that disability that leads to a handicap. Because communication is such a vital activity of daily living, a communication impairment is usually disabling, but when an impairment is remediated or modified to no longer limit a student's ability to learn or interact successfully, it may not be a handicap.

In determining eligibility and placement, IDEA 2004 directs the IEP team to do the following:

(i) Draw upon information from a variety of sources, including aptitude and achievement tests, parent input, and teacher recommendations, as well as information about the child's physical condition, social or cultural background, and adaptive behavior; and

(ii) Ensure that information obtained from all of these sources is documented and carefully considered. (34 C.F.R. § 300.306 [c])

There is a distinct and important difference between *eligibility* and *placement*. Eligibility refers specifically to considering the student's assessment results as they compare to the outlined eligibility criteria to determine whether the student has a disability and, because of that disability, requires special education and related services.

Any of the 13 listed eligibility categories for special education may have speech–language issues involved with the presenting exceptionality. For example, when the IEP team determines that a student qualifies as a child with autism or traumatic brain injury (TBI), the student will likely present with speech or language issues as well. The IEP team should identify speech and language as an area of need and subsequently discuss goals and services to address this need as part of the student's special education program.

Speech–language services in schools are part of special education and must meet the requirements of IDEA 2004. Students are determined to be in need of such services by following a two-step process. First, the student is assessed using the procedures described in Chapter 3. If the student scores significantly below expected levels, speech–language pathologists must go to the second step, which is determining whether these identified communication deficits impede the student's educational performance. IDEA 2004 regulations stated, "Speech or language impairment means a communication disorder, such as stuttering, impaired articulation, a language impairment, or a voice impairment, that adversely affects a child's educational performance" (34 C.F.R. § 300.8 [c][11]). The key to this definition is the requirement that the impairment "adversely affects a child's educational performance." Speech–language pathologists may identify, for example, that a student has a myofunctional disorder resulting in a reverse swallow (e.g., tongue thrust) without a frontal lisp. Such a student is not considered eligible under IDEA 2004 because there is no adverse educational impact.

ASHA sought guidance from the Office of Special Education Programs (OSEP) regarding the limitations, if any, to the requirements on adverse effect, as well as other items. In response to ASHA's query, a letter from the office's director (Posny, 2007) clarified "that the determination of whether or not a child is a child with a disability is not limited to academic performance" (p. 1).

Under IDEA 2004, speech–language services (and all special education services) may be provided to students in school only if both conditions are satisfied; that is, a disability exists and it adversely affects the child's educational performance. The adverse effect may be shown in one or more areas: academic, social, or vocational. This second step is a distinct departure from similar services in health care and private practice.

This two-step process is frequently misunderstood. Nonschool agencies and parents may not understand the restriction that the educational system has in terms of providing special education services. Speech–language pathologists in school systems must abide by the eligibility criteria set forth in state and federal laws. Students with mild impairments may not qualify to receive services in schools. Although services may help the student, it is not the responsibility of the education system to assume the cost of such services because there is no adverse educational effect. Federal regulations require that parents receive a copy of the team's evaluation report and documentation of the eligibility determination (34 C.F.R. § 300.306 [a][2]).

Increasingly, some milder speech–language impairments may be treated under a response to intervention (RTI) model and never require an IEP. As this model of service delivery is expanding, speech–language pathologists in schools are discovering a way to provide assistance to these students in addition to students who are IDEA eligible. (See Chapter 5 for more information on RTI as a service delivery.)

State Eligibility Criteria for Speech–Language Services

The definition of a speech or language impairment is interpreted by each of the states in its own special education laws. The combination of tests needed for a valid assessment, the number and types of tests, and the "cutoff" points on standardized tests are determined by each state. Consequently, a student could have an educationally related communication disorder identified in one state but not in another. This does not happen often, but it is possible.

Issues in determining eligibility for language disorder are complicated by several factors, including what constitutes a significant level of language disability, as well as regulations imposed by government agencies and local school districts. Since the inception of IDEA in the mid-1970s (then known as the Education for All Handicapped Children Act [EAHCA]), language disability has been a confusing entity for states and regulatory agencies to define. Defining language and language disorder has also evolved in the field. Over the years, notions of child language have grown from a simpler one of expressive and receptive vocabulary development to a sophisticated one portraying the interplay of phonology, morphology, syntax, semantics, and pragmatics. The constructs of content, form, and use are employed in some states. Students with literacy difficulties may also be in need of language intervention. (See Chapter 6 for a discussion of how language now also encompasses reading and writing as the functional outcomes of language intervention that are related to academic success [ASHA, 2000b].)

States determine which children with language impairments (and a corresponding adverse educational effect) are eligible for services. Many states include some component of RTI in their documentation, but many are still evolving in this area.

Two of the more widely used approaches to determining eligibility are normative reference points and severity ratings. These approaches are discussed in the sections that follow.

Normative Reference Points

Several normative reference points for expected language development have been used by states to determine eligibility. Two are most common: mental age (MA) and chronological age (CA). If language performance matches MA, some states declare the child ineligible for speech–language services. (This approach is referred to as *cognitive referencing*.) In other states, if language performance matches MA but still falls below CA expectations, the child may still be eligible for speech–language services. A speech–language pathologist needs to know the issues involved in MA referencing versus CA referencing (i.e., cognitive referencing) and what his or her state requires. ASHA has a comprehensive site dedicated to this topic:

> Cognitive Referencing is the practice of comparing IQ scores and language scores as a factor for determining eligibility for speech–language intervention. Cognitive referencing is based on the assumption that language functioning cannot surpass cognitive levels. However, according to research, some language abilities may in fact surpass cognitive levels. Therefore, ASHA does not support the use of cognitive referencing. (ASHA, n.d.-b)

The relationship between language and cognition is complex. Some educators try to separate the two; others believe there is a causal relationship between language and intelligence. Arguments in support of cognitive referencing contend that language skills can never exceed a student's intellectual capability; therefore, language intervention is not warranted if performance on language tests is equivalent to performance on intellectual measures. Determining intellectual capability is problematic, however, because most intelligence tests rely on students' verbal skills. In addition, cognitive referencing emphasizes scores on static norm-referenced assessments and tends to overlook the potential of intervention to improve functional outcomes. Cognitive referencing is not a recommended practice (ASHA, 1991, 2005b). Guidance for the speech–language pathologist can be found on the ASHA cognitive referencing page. Speech–language pathologists are advised to follow the dictates of his or her state department of education, while at the same time remaining vigilant about professional options and developments in the field.

Severity Ratings

State severity ratings are used by some state education agencies (SEAs) to manage the potentially large number of children who could qualify for services. There is considerable variation in the types of severity ratings used, and states may alter their eligibility criteria or coding process to some degree at some point in time. States may use scales with one to six levels and/or the terms *mild*, *moderate*, and *severe*. According to Ireland, Hall-Mills, and Millikin (2013), "The intended purpose of severity rating scales varies widely throughout the nation." Among the various uses for severity rating scales are creating consistency between providers for describing speech and language concerns, determining adverse effect, or determining eligibility and the amount of services indicated. Speech–language pathologists are required to follow federal and state regulations, as well as local guidance, when evaluating students to determine whether they meet eligibility criteria and/or are in need of speech–language services (Ireland et al., 2013).

Once a child is found to meet eligibility criteria, *goals and short-term objectives or benchmarks* are established in the identified areas of need. Following eligibility determination and establishment of goals in the areas of need, consideration is given to program placement and services (e.g., speech–language services). Placement may be thought of as the description of the program that meets the student's individual educational needs. After reviewing the student's present levels of academic achievement and functional performance and making an eligibility determination (if necessary), the next consideration is which skills and abilities the student needs to develop.

Special Considerations in Eligibility Determination

Severe Disabilities and Complex Communication Needs

Anecdotal and government reports have indicated a dramatic increase in the numbers of children with severe or significant disabilities, which also means an increase in the intensity of their needs and requisite services. Students identified in the eligibility categories of intellectual disability, multiple disabilities, and autism are generally considered individuals with severe disabilities. Compilation of data takes time, so while the information appears dated, it is from the most current reports and reflects current trends. These are individuals who "require ongoing extensive support in more than one major life activity in order to participate in integrated community settings and enjoy the quality of life available to people with fewer or no disabilities. They frequently have additional disabilities including movement difficulties, sensory losses, and behavior problems" (National Dissemination Center for Children With Disabilities, 2004). Characteristics of these individuals include limited speech or communication, difficulty in basic physical mobility, the tendency to forget skills through misuse, trouble generalizing skills from one situation to another, and a need for support in major life activities. Data reported by the Centers for Disease Control (CDC) come from the findings of Boyle et al. (2011) regarding trends in the prevalence of developmental disabilities (DDs) in children in the United States from 1997–2008. The data also mirror what is reported by the U.S. Department of Education in its 35th Annual Report to the Congress (USDE, 2014). In addition, the CDC reported an increase in the number of children identified as having autism (see Figure 4.1).

The study showed that DDs are common: About 1 in 6 children in the United States had a DD in 2006–2008. These data also showed that the prevalence of parent-reported DDs increased 17.1% from 1997 to 2008. This study underscored the increasing need for health, education, and social services and more specialized health services for people with DDs (Centers for Disease Control and Prevention, 2016).

Identified Prevalence of Autism Spectrum Disorder, Autism and Developmental Disabilities Monitoring Network, 2000–2010, Combining Data From All Sites				
Surveillance year	Birth year	Number of ADDM sites reporting	Prevalence per 1,000 children (range)	This is about 1 in X children
2000	1992	6	6.7 (4.3–9.9)	1 in 150
2002	1994	14	6.6 (3.3–10.8)	1 in 150
2004	1996	8	8.0 (4.8–9.8)	1 in 125
2006	1998	11	9.0 (4.1–12.1)	1 in 110
2008	2000	14	11.3 (4.8–21.2)	1 in 88
2010	2002	11	14.7 (14.3–15.1)	1 in 68

FIGURE 4.1. Identified prevalence of autism spectrum disorder.

Note. From "Autism Spectrum Disorder (ASD) Data and Statistics," by Centers for Disease Control and Prevention, n.d. Retrieved from http://www.cdc.gov/ncbddd/autism/data.html.

Table 4.4 illustrates the percentages of students served in various disability categories in fall 2011 (USDE, 2014).

Examining the eligibility categories shows that students with disabilities that would be considered severe (intellectual disabilities = 9.9%, multiple disabilities = 2.2%, autism = 2.0%) represent a relatively small percentage of the total number of students served in special education (5,789,884 students ages 6–21 years served under IDEA 2004 reported in 2011) (USDE, 2014). However, these students often manifest multiple and intense needs requiring multiple services. Because of the nature of these disabilities, these students may be identified as having complex communication needs. Justice (2006b) indicated, "Complex communication needs result from significant speech, language, motor and/or cognitive impairments that prevent individuals from communicating in conventional ways" (p. 501).

When speech–language pathologists are part of assessment teams for students with severe disabilities, the question is typically not whether the student will meet eligibility criteria for special education but whether the student has needs in the areas of speech, language, or hearing that will require speech and language or audiological support services. The advent of assistive technology (AT) and advanced augmentative and alternative communication (AAC) systems has improved access for students with complex communication needs (CCN). Guidance from the National Joint Committee for Persons With Severe Disabilities is offered through ASHA, but speech–language pathologists must be cautious to follow the protocols of IDEA and of the field. Assessments should identify communication needs, opportunities, vision and motor skills, communication partners, and environments (Justice, 2006b) in addition to opportunities for access. The focus of intervention should be on developing a functional communication system and attaining socially effective communication repertoires. However, students with significant disabilities and complex communication needs should also be involved in academic instruction related to the Common Core State Standards (CCSS), and therefore, assessment and intervention should consider this focus as well (Moore, 2014a; Sturm, 2012).

To determine the need for services, how and when services occur, and the nature of the services to students with complex communication needs, goals will first need to be established indicating how to develop communication competence for each individual (Furr, Motteler, & Heiling, 2009; Justice, 2006b). Old methods of using cognitive refer-

TABLE 4.4. Categories of Severe Disabilities

Fall 2011	Intellectual disability	Emotional disturbance	Multiple disabilities	Autism	Traumatic brain injury
Ages 6–21 years	580,375	480,187	130,443	118,092	21,384
Ages 6–21 years	9.9%[a]	8.1%[a]	2.2%[a]	2.0%[a]	0.4%[a]

Note. From "New Accountability Framework Raises the Bar for State Special Education Programs," by U.S. Department of Education, 2014, Washington DC: The Education Trust.

[a]Reflects disability distribution for students served in this age group under IDEA 2004.

encing as an approach to determine whether a student with a severe disability would be entitled to speech and language services are not appropriate for any student. A statement from the National Joint Committee for the Communication Needs of Persons With Severe Disabilities (2002) provided specific guidance regarding historical practices that denied individuals with severe disabilities access to services because of the utilization of criteria that were not appropriate for making such determinations (see the following box). Speech–language pathologists in schools need to be familiar with these position statements and why older methods of determining who may and may not be eligible for service (e.g., cognitive referencing) are not appropriate for students, although these methods may have previously been perceived to be a method of caseload management.

> ## National Joint Committee for the Communication Needs of Persons With Severe Disabilities' Position on Eligibility for Communication Services and Supports
>
> It is the position of the National Joint Committee for the Communication Needs of Persons With Severe Disabilities that eligibility for communication services and supports should be based on individual communication needs. Communication services and supports should be evaluated, planned, and provided by an interdisciplinary team with expertise in communication and language form, content, and function, as well as in augmentative and alternative communication (AAC). Decisions regarding team composition; types, amounts, and duration of services provided; intervention setting; and service delivery models should be based on the individual's communication needs and preferences. Eligibility determinations based on a priori criteria violate recommended practice principles by precluding consideration of individual needs. These a priori criteria include but are not limited to (a) discrepancies between cognitive and communication functioning; (b) chronological age; (c) diagnosis; (d) absence of cognitive or other skills purported to be prerequisites; (e) failure to benefit from previous communication services and supports; (f) restrictive interpretations of educational, vocational, and/or medical necessity; (g) lack of appropriately trained personnel; and (h) lack of adequate funds or other resources. (National Joint Committee for the Communication Needs of Persons With Severe Disabilities, 2002)

Disproportionality

Concerns about the overrepresentation of minority students have been an issue since the inception of special education (Fergus, 2010a; Harry & Klingner, 2007; National Education Association, 2007, 2008). In the reauthorization of IDEA 2004, Congress identified this problem as one of the most important issues to be addressed in the implementation of the law.

The National Education Association (2008) called disproportionate representation of culturally and linguistically diverse (CLD) students in special education one of the most complex issues in the field of special education, pointing out that this has been an issue for over four decades. Reference to disproportionality includes both the overrepresentation and the underrepresentation of a particular demographic group in special education as compared to that group's representation in the general student population. The Equity Alliance (Fergus, 2010a) reported the following representative data: "In 2008, the school enrollment of Blacks (15.5%) differed greatly from their representation in special education (20.4%) and among students with an Emotional Disturbance classification (29.1%); while enrollment of Whites (55.5%) was mirrored in special education (55.9%) and among students with an ED classification (56.9%)" (p. 3).

The national data do not find disproportionality in disability categories that are more obvious, such as hearing, vision, or orthopedic impairments. In these categories, students from ethnic minority groups are represented in proportion to their representation in the general population. The areas of disproportionality appear in the categories considered "judgmental" or "those areas usually identified after a child starts school and by school personnel rather than by a medical professional" (Gamm, 2007, p. 4) (see Table 4.5).

These numbers reflect overall percentage comparisons and not a comparison of specific eligibility categories, but it can be seen that Black/African American students are increasingly identified under Part B for school-age children.

Disproportionality is a concern for several reasons, according to the National Education Association and National Association of School Psychologists (National Education Association, 2007):

> Labeling students as disabled when they really are not leads to unwarranted services and supports. Misidentified students are likely to encounter limited access to a rigorous curriculum and diminished expectations. And, more important, mislabeling students creates a false impression of the child's intelligence and academic potential. Here's why:
>
> - Once students are receiving special education, they tend to stay in special education classes (Harry & Klingner, 2006).
> - Students are likely to encounter a limited, less rigorous curriculum (Harry & Klingner, 2006).
> - Lower expectations can lead to diminished academic and postsecondary opportunities (Harry & Klingner, 2006; National Research Council, 2002).
> - Students in special education programs can have less access to academically able peers (Donavan & Cross, 2002).
> - Disproportionality can contribute to significant racial separation (Harry & Klingner, 2006; Losen & Orfield, 2002, p. 2).

Solving the problems of overidentification and disproportionality is a complex process at best, beginning with how deficits are viewed (Harry & Klingner, 2007; National Education Association, 2007). To begin to address the issue, the *Code of Federal Regulations* requires each state to collect data with regard to the identification, placement,

TABLE 4.5. U.S. Department of Education Report on IDEA 2004

Program	Ethnic group	Risk ratio	Likelihood to be served compared to children in other racial or ethnic groups
IDEA Part C (birth through 2 years)	White	1.2	Slightly more likely
	Native Hawaiian/Other Pacific Islander	1.1	Slightly more likely
	American Indian or Alaska Native	0.9	Slightly less likely
	Hispanic/Latino	0.8	Slightly less likely
	Asian	0.6	Slightly less likely
	Black or African American	1.0	As likely
IDEA Part B (3–5 years)	White	1.2	More likely
	Native Hawaiian/Other Pacific Islander	1.5	More likely
	American Indian or Alaska Native	1.4	More likely
	Hispanic/Latino	0.7	Less likely
	Asian	0.8	Less likely
	Multiple Races	0.8	Less likely
	Black or African American	1.0	As likely
IDEA Part B (6–21 years)	White	0.9	Less likely
	Native Hawaiian/Other Pacific Islander	1.6	More likely
	American Indian or Alaska Native	1.6	More likely
	Hispanic/Latino	0.9	Less likely
	Asian	0.5	Less likely
	Multiple Races	0.7	Less likely
	Black or African American	1.4	More likely

Note. Adapted from "2013 Annual Reports to Congress on the Individuals With Disabilities Education Act (IDEA)," by USDE, 2013. Retrieved from http://www2.ed.gov/about/reports/annual/osep/2013/index.html.

and discipline of children in these groups. If the state does find that a local education agency is disproportionate in these areas, it must require the LEA to reserve the maximum amount of funds (i.e., 15%) to provide comprehensive early intervening services to these students. In addition, the LEA must publicly report how they have revised their policies, practices, and procedures in this area (34 C.F.R. § 303.646).

Speech–language pathologists may be involved in determining eligibility, providing early intervening services, or helping develop policies and improved practice to address the needs of students from ethnic minority groups. Although system change will be necessary to improve practices and change how a system can assist students without making special education identification, the important influence that any individual member of the team can make in these situations cannot be overstated. Most likely, the assessment of students from ethnic minority groups who may be referred for eligibility determination will require performance or dynamic measures in order to ensure that the students receive an objective evaluation. The early intervening services provided to these students, including RTI programs, will need to be documented. Cultural competence will be required to create successful solutions for students.

The National Education Association (2007, pp. 19–20) document suggested the following as practices that will lead to positive change:

- Increasing academic language proficiency
- Ensuring quality early childhood opportunities
- Providing early intervening services (EIS)
- Employing an response to intervention (RTI) process
- Implementing school-wide positive behavioral supports (PBS) programs
- Increasing access to culturally responsive, school-based mental health services
- Enhancing classroom management skills
- Using authentic, culturally responsive assessment techniques
- Developing culturally responsive teaching skills
- Using culturally appropriate curriculum
- Strengthening parent and family involvement and community partnerships

Students Who Are English Learners or Dual-Language Learners

In addition to the concerns about the overrepresentation of students from ethnic minority groups, speech–language pathologists and multidisciplinary team members will face special concern about the appropriateness of identification and services for students who are English Learners (ELs) or Dual-Language Learners (DLLs). For this population, the concern is both the possible overidentification and the possible underidentification. In terms of eligibility determination, limited English proficiency is one of the exclusionary factors for specific learning disability. In other words, a student may not be identified as having a specific learning disability if the reason for the determination is limited English proficiency. The term *Dual-Language Learners* is introduced here. It was reported, "This term has been adopted by the Office of Head Start and the United States Department of Education to highlight and promote the linguistic assets of young children and families who speak languages other than English" (Espinosa, 2013).

The ASHA Web site has a page specifically dedicated to English-language learners in schools (www.asha.org/practice/multicultural/ELL/), which can assist speech–language pathologists and audiologists in approaching these cases appropriately. Issues of under- and overidentification have social justice implications. The subjects of diversity, ethnicity, race, poverty, language variation, achievement, and opportunity gaps are difficult and emotionally driven (Cochran-Smith, 2004; Howard, 2010; Hudley & Mallinson, 2011; Milner, 2012).

One of the major factors in eligibility determination is considering whether a child has a language disorder or a language difference. Although ASHA calls on speech–language pathologists to be culturally competent, determining special education eligibility may be challenging because of the many factors related to whether an individual student has received an appropriate educational experience in addition to his or her own cultural and linguistic background.

The first consideration facing educators is to examine the student's educational history and the educational programming required to address his or her specific types of needs. Distinguishment considerations include the following:

- Students with formal academic learning
- Students with limited formal schooling
- Long-term English Learners (Freeman, Freeman, & Mercum, 2003)

Long-term English Learners are of the greatest concern to educators. This term refers to students who have attended schools in the United States for 7 years yet have not been academically successful. Characteristics of long-term English Learners include the following (Menken & Kleyn, 2009):

- They are typically found in Grades 6–12.
- They speak different languages and come from all over the world.
- They are often orally bilingual and sound like native English speakers. However, they typically have limited literacy skills in their native language, and their academic literacy skills in English are not as well developed as their oral skills are.
- They fall into two main groups: (a) transnational students who have moved back and forth between the United States and their family's country of origin and have attended school in both countries, and (b) students who have received inconsistent schooling in the United States, moving in and out of bilingual education, English as a second language, and mainstream programs in which they received no language support services.
- They have often not resided in the United States continuously, despite the fact that they may have been born in this country. So the "U.S.-born" label can be misleading.
- They have experienced inconsistent schooling because of frequent moves or incoherent language programming within and across the schools they have attended. Thus, many have significant gaps in their schooling.
- They perform below grade level in reading and writing and, as a result, struggle in all content areas that require literacy. The overall school performance of long-term English-language learners is low, with poor grades and grade retention commonplace, making this population at high risk for dropping out.
- They have needs that are different from those of newly arrived English-language learners, yet language programming at the secondary level is typically intended for new arrivals. In addition, most educators are unfamiliar with the specialized needs of this population, a problem compounded by poor data about these students in their school records.

A California document titled "Reparable Harm: Fulfilling the Unkept Promise of Educational Opportunity for California's Long Term English Learners?" (Olsen, 2010) chronicled issues that face all states, not just California, which is home to the largest number of English learners in the nation. The report (2010, p. 2) analyzed the disturbing reality that several factors seem to contribute to becoming a long-term English Learner, including the following:

- receiving no language development program at all
- being given elementary school curricula and materials that weren't designed to meet English Learner needs
- enrollment in weak language development program models and poorly implemented English Learner programs
- histories of inconsistent programs
- provision of narrow curricula and only partial access to full curriculum
- social segregation and linguistic isolation
- cycles of transnational moves
- inappropriate placement in mainstream (no program)
- being placed and kept in classes with newcomer English Learners
- being taught by largely unprepared teachers
- overassigned and inadequately served in intervention and support classes
- being precluded from participation in electives
- limited access to the full curricula

These educational challenges mean that students may not have had the educational opportunities to develop language and/or academic proficiency. The educational experience of these students is complicated. They may present as if they have a disability because of their experiences within the educational system.

The other consideration is the development of the student's bilingualism, either simultaneous or sequential.

- *Simultaneous bilingualism* occurs when a young child has had significant and meaningful exposure to two languages from birth. Ideally, the child will have equal, quality experiences with both languages.
- *Sequential bilingualism* occurs when an individual has had significant and meaningful exposure to a second language, usually after the age of 3 years and after the first language is well established. These second-language learners are referred to as "English-language learners" in U.S. schools (www.asha.org/practice/multicultural/issues/bll.htm).

Marian and other researchers (2009, p. 13) reported on the consequences of bilingualism in cognition, language, and brain development:

Cognitive Development
- Bilingualism in children is associated with increased meta-cognitive skills and superior divergent thinking ability, better performance on some perceptual tasks and classification tasks.

- Although some studies report bilingualism has a negative impact on language development and lexical acquisition, bilingual children score on par with their monolingual counterparts on tests of verbal ability by middle school. There is no evidence that bilingual children have lower intellectual abilities than their monolingual counterparts.
- Bilingual children learn earlier than their monolingual counterparts that objects and their names are not the same.
- In vocabulary testing, we count conceptual representations, not lexical labels ("milk" and "grandma" for the monolingual child vs. "milk," "leche," and "grandma" for the bilingual child).
- RECOMMEND: "best performance" technique for bilingual assessment – examine highest level of development regardless of the language.
- Bilinguals may be able to inhibit irrelevant verbal and nonverbal information with greater ease than monolinguals.
- Inhibitory control ability is slower to decline with age in bilinguals than in monolinguals.
- Bilingual children have been found to exhibit superior performance in divergent thinking, figure–ground discrimination, and other related meta-cognitive skills.

Lexical Organization
- Bilingual children are found to respond taxonomically more often than monolingual children (e.g., *chair–table*; *chair–sit*; *chair–legs*); it is interesting considering bilingual children are often found to have smaller English receptive vocabulary. Bilingual children are found to have an advantage in taxonomic responses.
- Bilingual children develop an earlier understanding of taxonomic relationships than their monolingual peers (e.g., *car* and *bus* are vehicles). This understanding is not dependent on vocabulary size, but could be influenced by structural features of the speaker's language.
- Bilingual adults are better than monolingual adults at learning new words. Bilinguals use a variety of word-learning strategies with similar efficiency and are less susceptible to interference from conflicting orthographic information during word learning.
- Linguistic input coactivates both languages in bilinguals; when bilinguals hear or read words in one language, partially overlapping structures in the other language are also activated.

Neural Differences
- Bilateral processing of language (and other nonverbal tasks) is most likely to occur only in early bilinguals.
- Monolinguals and bilinguals use similar neural regions for language processing. However, late bilinguals are likely to activate the LIFG [left inferior frontal

gyrus] differentially for processes in which the LIFG plays a crucial roles, such as phonologic and syntactic processing.

- Bilinguals have greater gray matter density than monolinguals in certain left hemisphere regions.

Peña (2012) reported that Latino children are underidentified in preschool compared to their mainstream peers (3.21% vs. 2.03%), yet the situation changes when they become school aged. Latino children are enrolled in special education at higher rates than mainstream students (1.75% vs. 1.52% in the category of learning disabilities, and 4.69% vs. 3.98% in the category of speech–language impairment).

Professional associations may provide helpful documents and other resources to ensure appropriate practices in this area. The Texas Speech–Language–Hearing Association's document "Linguistically Diverse Populations: Considerations and Resources for Assessment and Intervention," for example, addresses appropriate practices that may be helpful to professionals working with linguistically diverse students. In an issue dedicated to the topic of English-language learners in *Educational Leadership* (Scherer, 2009), the Association of Supervision and Curriculum Development called for consideration of who these children are, including the diversity among them, as well as the need for collaboration among "researchers, practitioners and policymakers" (Garcia, Jensen, & Scribner, 2009, p. 12) to close the implementation gap, meaning that known effective evidence-based strategies either are not being implemented or are being poorly implemented.

Whether effective evidence-based programs are available for English Learners is a critical consideration for IEP teams who are asked to identify some of these students as having disabilities. Biases, lack of information, or old beliefs often affect how these children are viewed, as well as what types of services they might receive (Howard, 2010; Pransky, 2009; Riquelme, 2013; Torres, 2013). The Foundation for Child Development (Espinosa, 2013) identified myths that often plague educators and policy makers in providing appropriate services and making appropriate educational decisions for these children:

- *Myth 1:* Learning two languages during the early childhood years will overwhelm, confuse, and/or delay acquisition of English.
- *Myth 2:* The language development of Dual-Language Learners looks the same as monolingual language development.
- *Myth 3:* Total English immersion from prekindergarten through third grade is the best way for a young Dual-Language Learner to acquire English.
- *Myth 4:* Because schools do not have the capacity to provide instruction in all the languages represented by children who are Dual-Language Learners, programs should provide instruction in one common language: English.
- *Myth 5:* Spanish-speaking Latinos show social and academic delays when entering kindergarten.
- *Myth 6:* Native English speakers may experience academic and language delays in dual-language programs.

- *Myth 7:* If the instruction in a program is delivered primarily in English, educators do not need to worry about the progress of children who are Dual-Language Learners in their home language.

In reminding educators to "look at who English language learners are," Scherer (2009, p. 7) said,

> They are, in fact, a very diverse population, made up of different subgroups requiring different instructional strategies. The variety of languages spoken by the nearly 5.1 million English language learners in U.S. schools is not the only difference among then. Their parents' English language proficiency and literacy levels in their first language matter, and so does family financial and social status. How long students have been in the country matters, as does the kind of education they have received in the past. Although students from immigrant families are the fastest growing segment of the ELL population, they don't account for all of the children who are labeled English language learners. . . . One statistic that reverberates, however, is that 42 percent of them drop out of high school. (Scherer, 2009, p. 7)

When a student fails to make academic progress, the school team will likely consider referring the student for a special education assessment to determine whether he or she has a disability. Speech–language pathologists receive training as part of their educational program in the field and often also as part of professional development in their jobs in schools. Regardless, one study examined speech–language pathologists' comfort level in providing assessment and intervention to English Learners and concluded, "Despite a new emphasis on culturally responsive pedagogy, educators and communication disorders professionals often feel they are ill-equipped to provide serviced to ethnically and linguistically diverse students" (Kimble, 2013). At the same time, new research from WestEd (U.S. Department of Education Regional Education Laboratory West) found that long-term English Learners had a higher percentage of students eligible for special education (WestEd, 2014).

Once a student is identified, providing appropriate services is vital. IEP teams must be aware of ensuring that students who are English Learners or Dual-Language Learners continue to have access to the general education curriculum and have robust opportunities for language development. These students must have many, many opportunities to receive instruction and practice with academic vocabulary and high expectations related to their achievement. The Office of Special Education Programs (2000) suggested the following culturally relevant instructional principles that remain important today:

- Link assessments of student progress directly to the instructional curricula rather than to abstract norms for standardized tests.
- Examine not only the individual child but also his or her instructional environment, using direct observational data.

- Create classroom environments that reflect different cultural heritages and accommodate different styles of communication and learning.
- Develop and implement family-friendly practices to establish collaborative partnerships with parents and other caregivers, including those who do not speak English.

Development of Goals and Short-Term Objectives or Benchmarks

The second step in the IEP meeting process is to develop goals and short-term objectives or benchmarks. At least one goal should be established for each identified area of need. Goals are written in only the identified areas of need and not for curricular or developmental areas that will be addressed in the scope of the classroom instruction at the student's grade level or above. In addition, because the IEP process requires first to identify the areas of need, next to develop goals to address those areas of need, and finally to determine program, placement, and services to address these goals, there should never be services that are not attached to goals. (See the section "Determination of Program, Placement, and Services" later in this chapter.)

IDEA 2004 regulations require each IEP to include the following:

(i) A statement of measurable annual goals, including academic and functional goals designed to—

  (A) Meet the child's needs that result from the child's disability to enable the child to be involved in and progress in the general curriculum; and

  (B) Meet each of the child's other educational needs that result from the child's disability.

(ii) For children with disabilities who take alternate assessments aligned to alternate achievement standards, a description of benchmarks or short-term objectives. (34 C.F.R. § 300.320 [a][2])

IDEA 2004 requires annual goals for students with disabilities and only requires short-term objectives or benchmarks for students who are taking alternate assessments. The rationale for dropping benchmarks for most students in special education is that the goals need to be aligned to standards, so benchmarking is not necessary. Because students who take alternate assessments are working on more functional goals, short-term objectives or benchmarks are needed. It should be noted that in some school systems, local practice is to include benchmarks for all students in special education.

The emphasis on standards, curriculum, and educational results directs the course of what IEP teams need to consider in their goal setting for students. With the advent of the Common Core State Standards (CCSS), there should be no doubt about what students are expected to learn. Many electronic IEP programs have pull-down menus to help IEP teams in developing standards-based goals. The IEP team, however, still must be sure that the goals are individually determined. The academic orientation of the standards might be limiting for students whose goals must include functional or social–emotional skills. However, for the majority of students on the speech–language pathologist's caseload, using standards as a guide for IEP goal development should be an everyday practice. (See the discussion on the CCSS in Chapter 2.)

Speech–language pathologists in public schools have expertise in speech and language acquisition, development, and disorders. Curricula and standards are constructed based on the developmental levels (e.g., cognitive, linguistic, social–emotional) that children are expected to have reached at any given grade level. When writing a goal or developing short-term objectives/benchmarks for a student working on either academic or alternate curriculum, the speech–language pathologist will need to examine the learning expectations and classroom instructional environment to determine how the student's identified disability or delay will affect his or her achieving such expectations. From this information, goals and short-term objectives or benchmarks can be developed. The speech–language pathologist must consider what underlying skills students need in order to accomplish the academic expectations. This will drive the goals that will be written.

Local guidelines or forms will give the speech–language pathologist direction in how each LEA requires measurement to be reflected for the goals or objectives or benchmarks. IEP goals should always describe in measurable terms what the team determines the student is expected to achieve 1 year from the date of the IEP meeting. Goals and short-term objectives should never identify what adults (i.e., teachers, instructional assistants, or parents) do; they should always have the "who" identified as the student. In addition, they should always be written in positive language, not in a way that reflects a decrease in negative behavior. If the desired behavior is identified, then the competing negative behavior will correspondingly decrease or disappear. A good format for writing IEP performance goals and objectives is to answer these six questions: who, does what, when, given what, how much (criteria, mastery), and how will it be measured (Association of California School Administrators, 2006, p. 42).

Who: The student

Does what: Observable behavior

When: By reporting date

Given what: Conditions

How much: Mastery or criteria

How will it be measured: Performance data

Writing curriculum-relevant, standards-based goals for students receiving speech–language services is sometimes confusing. Understanding the interface of curriculum demands and student needs will help guide the speech–language pathologist and IEP team members in their development of appropriate goals. This is increasingly important with the CCSS.

The history of special education (discussed in Chapters 1 and 2) demonstrates Congress's intention to provide opportunity to learn for students with disabilities. In both the 1997 and 2004 reauthorizations, Congress expressed concerns that low expectations for students with disabilities have impeded achievement. This sentiment is sometimes reflected in conversations about CCSS. In the initial implementation phases of CCSS, educators may express the concern that the standards are too difficult for children with disabilities.

A report from the International Center for Leadership in Education (McNulty & Gloeckler, 2011) examined the implications of common core and special education. These authors noted that the CCSS will require all students "to use higher order thinking skills and apply what they have learned to unique situations, and bring together knowledge from a variety of content areas to solve problems. Students will be expected to engage in performance-based events, some of which will take place over long periods of time" (p. 4). Knowing what will be expected of students in the classroom will allow speech–language pathologists to create similar experiences for students during intervention and assessment.

> The goal of the Common Core State Standards is to focus on the knowledge and skills needed by all students so they can be successful in college and careers. This goal applies for all students. Students who are receiving special education services are no exception. They too are expected to be challenged to excel within the general education curriculum based on the Common Core State Standards. (McNulty & Gloeckler, 2011, p. 4)

The majority of students with disabilities receiving special education and related services are students with average intellectual abilities. Students with specific learning disabilities represent the largest category, and students with speech impairments represent the second-largest category; the third-largest category is "other health impairment," according to national data (McNulty & Gloeckler, 2011; USDE, 2014). These students represent nearly half of the students who receive special education supports and who are being educated in the general education program in the general education curriculum. To ensure that these students have an opportunity to develop the knowledge and skills expected in the general curriculum, supports and related services, such as speech–language services, are provided when needed to implement goals aligned to grade-level standards. These services are intended to provide access to the curriculum based on individual student needs. The International Center for Leadership in Education (McNulty & Gloeckler, 2011) stated, "Too many educators believe that students receiving special education cannot perform at higher levels, and the programs offered reflect that attitude, from elementary school all the way to high school" (p. 7). To counter low expectations, the center identified five key elements that schools must address to support achievement for students receiving special education services:

1. Ownership
2. High expectations
3. Intervention systems
4. Inclusion and collaborative teaching
5. Organization and professional development

These elements will create an environment where IEP teams can successfully develop meaningful goals and intervention that will create access to curricula, resulting in improved student achievement.

The IEP process, as it has been explained, provides the opportunity to identify student needs and then develop goals that will create access to the curriculum that students need to master. The IEP is meant not to restate the content standards but to specify skills for students to acquire so that they will meet the standards. In addition, the goals will provide direction to teachers and specialists that will promote meaningful academic instruction, which will eventually tie to state assessment (Courtade & Browder, 2011).

Speech–language pathologists will see many connections with language demands and the common core (Dodd, 2014a; Moore, 2014a; Rudebusch, 2012). Rudebusch (2012, p. 18) recommended, "Prior to developing IEPs, all IEP team members need to be familiar with general education curriculum, including common core state standards. [Speech–language pathologists] need working knowledge of the speech and language complexities expected at each grade level as outlined in the common core state standards, especially in the English language arts and literacy standards in the areas of language, listening and speaking, and writing" (see Table 4.6).

To develop standards-driven IEP goals, then, IEP teams and speech–language pathologists must have a clear understanding of how the standards are constructed and what the requirements are of each grade level. (See the boxed section "Cultivating the Landscape of the Common Core State Standards" [Moore & Nishida, 2014].) Many authors have suggested similar processes to answer the question "How do I know what goals to write?" Consider the similarities between the recommendations of Rudebusch (2012), Power-deFur and Flynn (2012), and Dodd (2014a), as seen in Table 4.7.

Cultivating the Landscape of the Common Core State Standards

1. The landscape of the Common Core State Standards (CCSS) lays a foundation of high expectations for all students.
2. The landscape of the CCSS supports the learner through its design.
3. The landscape of the CCSS is built to nurture 21st-century learners through the four "Cs" of *communication, collaboration, critical thinking,* and *creativity.*
4. The landscape of the CCSS includes listening and speaking standards.
5. The landscape of the CCSS builds the foundation for the development of alternate assessment and alternate achievement standards on communicative competence.
6. The landscape of the CCSS is supported by universal design for learning.
7. The landscape of the CCSS extends access through text complexity and academic vocabulary (Moore & Nishida, 2014).

(text continues on p. 156)

TABLE 4.6. Common Core State Standards for English Language Arts and Literacy in History and Social Studies and Science and Technical Subjects (Grades K–5)

	Kindergarten	First grade	Second grade	Third grade	Fourth grade	Fifth grade
Conventions of standard English	Use frequently occurring nouns and verbs, regular plural nouns, question words, prepositions (to, from, in, out, on, off, for, of, by, with), and complete sentences in shared language activities.	Use common, proper, and possessive nouns; singular and plural nouns with matching verbs; personal, possessive, and indefinite pronouns; past, present, and future verb tenses; adjectives; conjunctions (and, so, but, or, because); articles; and prepositions (during, beyond, toward). Complete simple and compound declarative, imperative, and exclamatory sentences.	Use collective nouns, irregular plural nouns, reflexive pronouns, irregular past tense, adjectives, and adverbs. Produce, expand, and rearrange complete simple and compound sentences.	Explain the function of nouns, pronouns, verbs, adjectives, adverbs, regular and irregular plural nouns, regular and irregular verbs, verb tenses, subject-verb and pronoun–antecedent agreement, comparative and superlative adjectives and adverbs, and coordinating and subordinating conjunctions. Use simple, compound, and complex sentences.	Use relative pronouns (who, whose, whom, which, that), relative adverbs (where, when, why), progressive verb tenses, modal auxiliaries (can, may, must), prepositional phrases, and complete sentences. Correct fragments and run-ons. Correctly use frequently confused words (to, too, two, there, their). Order adjectives within sentences.	Explain the function of conjunctions, prepositions, and interjections. Form and use perfect tenses. Use verb tense to convey various times, sequences, states, and conditions. Recognize and correct inappropriate shifts in verb tense. Use correlative conjunctions (either-or, neither-nor).
Knowledge of language			Compare formal and informal uses of English.	Choose words and phrases for effect.	Choose words and phrases to convey ideas precisely. Differentiate contexts for formal English and informal discourse.	Expand, combine, and reduce sentences for meaning, reader and listener interest, and style. Compare and contrast the varieties of English used in stories, dramas, and poems.

TABLE 4.6. (continued)

	Kindergarten	First grade	Second grade	Third grade	Fourth grade	Fifth grade
Vocabulary acquisition and use	Determine or clarify the meaning of words. Identify new meanings for familiar words (*duck* as a noun or a verb). Use inflections and affixes as clues to meaning (-*ed*, -*s*, *re*-, *un*-, *pre*-, *full*). Explore word relationships and nuances by understanding frequently occurring verbs and adjectives by relating them to antonyms and identifying real-life connections between words and their use and distinguishing shades of meaning among verbs by acting out meaning.	Use sentence-level context as a clue to the meaning of the word or phrase. Demonstrate understanding of word relationships and nuances by defining words by category and one or more key attributes, identifying real-life connections between words and their use, and distinguishing shades of meaning among verbs differing in manner and adjectives differing in intensity by defining them or acting out the meanings.	Use sentence-level context as a clue to the meaning of the word or phrase. Demonstrate understanding of word relationships and nuances by identifying real-life connections between words and their use (describe foods that are spicy or juicy) and distinguishing shades of meaning among closely related adjectives (*thin, slender, skinny, scrawny*).	Use sentence-level context as a clue to the meaning of the word of phrase. Demonstrate understanding of word relationships and nuances by distinguishing literal and nonliteral meanings of words and phrases in context, identifying real-life connections between words and their use, and distinguishing shades of meaning among related words that describe states of mind or degrees of certainty (*knew, believed, suspected, heard, wondered*).	Use context as a clue to the meaning of the word of phrase. Demonstrate understanding of figurative language, word relationships, and nuances by explaining the meaning of simple similes and metaphors; recognizing and explaining the meaning of common idioms, adages, and proverbs; and relating words to their antonyms and synonyms.	Use context as a clue to the meaning of the word or phrase. Demonstrate understanding of figurative language, word relationships, and nuances by interpreting figurative language, including similes and metaphors in context; explaining the meaning of idioms, adages, and proverbs; and using the relationship between particular words to understand the words (synonyms, antonyms, homographs).

Note. From "Common Core State Standards to Standards-Based IEPs: A Brief Tutorial," by J. Rudebusch, 2012, *SIG 16 Perspectives on School-Based Issues, 13,* pp. 17–24. Copyright 2012 by the American Speech–Language–Hearing Association. Reprinted with permission.

TABLE 4.7. Using the Common Core State Standards in the Development of Goals and Intervention

Seven-step process for utilizing the Common Core State Standards in the development of an IEP (Rudebusch, 2012)	To design and unpack the standards (Power deFur & Flynn, 2012)	Write IEP goals that core-inform (Dodd, 2014a)
Consider the content standards for the grade in which the student is enrolled or would be enrolled based on age. Ask what the intent of the content standard is and what the student must know and be able to do to meet the standard.	Read the content standard for the student's grade.	Consider current grade-level language requirements.
Examine classroom and student data to determine where this student is functioning in relation to grade-level standards. Include current assessment data, student work samples, prior year's IEP, and other pertinent information.	Determine where the student is functioning in relation to the standards.	Identify the student's present level of academic performance in communication and language areas.
Determine the student's present level of academic achievement and functional performance. Describe the student's strengths and needs in relation to accessing and mastering the general curriculum. Consider progress monitoring data and response to intervention data. What patterns are presented?	Review the student's IEP.	Conduct a "gap assessment" and develop goals to support the student in achieving grade-level standards.
Develop measurable goals. Four critical components include the following: • Time frame • Conditions • Behavior • Criterion	Review classroom materials.	Choose from several approaches to writing standard-specific goals.
Assess progress.	Collaborate with teachers.	
Identify special instructions.	Design and implement intervention.	
Determine the most appropriate assessment options.		

Note. Adapted from "Common Core State Standards to Standards-Based IEPs: A Brief Tutorial," by J. Rudebusch, 2012, *SIG 16 Perspectives on School-Based Issues, 13*, pp. 17–24; "Unpacking the Standards for Intervention," by L. Power-deFur and P. Flynn, 2012, *Perspectives on School-Based Issues, 13*, pp. 11–16; "Taking Measure," by J. Dodd, 2014a, *The ASHA Leader, 19*, 56–59. IEP = Individualized Education Program.

Rudebusch (2012) specifically provided helpful information about writing measurable goals and identified time frame, conditions, behavior, and criterion as necessary components (see example in Table 4.8).

To write goals that are truly useful and meaningful for students, Dodd (2014b, pp. 6–7) suggested using a SMART-goal format:

TABLE 4.8. Application

Time frame	Condition	Behavior	Criteria
In 18 instructional weeks	When provided with an action series depicted in four picture cards and prompted to tell a complete story	Kelly, a third-grade student, will produce a story.	That the story is a true narrative with all story grammar components and at least two episodes, and that it includes complete simple, compound, and complex sentences with fewer than five errors
By May 15, 2016	Given a fourth-grade story prompt and 30 minutes to write	Kevin, a fourth-grade student, will write a story.	A three-paragraph essay using both compound and complex sentences and transition words in sentences between paragraphs with five or fewer errors

Note. Adapted from "Common Core State Standards to Standards-Based IEPs: A Brief Tutorial," by J. Rudebusch, 2012, *SIG 16 Perspectives on School-Based Issues, 13*, p. 22. Adapted with permission.

- SMART goals are *specific*. Specific goals include clear descriptions of the desired outcome or behavior the student is to achieve following a designated period of time (e.g., a year).
- SMART goals are *measurable*. Measurable goals include a clear statement of how attainment of the goal will be determined and are generally written in terms of accuracy of target behavior (e.g., with 80% accuracy) or frequency of occurrence (e.g., four out of five times, decrease in undesirable behavior).
- SMART goals are *attainable*. Attainable goals consider the present levels of the student without underestimating or overestimating his or her learning potential.
- SMART goals are *relevant*. Relevant goals, in light of the common core, target applicable skills pertinent to grade-level standards.
- SMART goals are *timely*. Timely goals are written with the expectations of what the students will learn within a specified time frame.
- SMART goals state *who* (referring to the student by name), *given what* (how target behavior will be elicited), *does what* (observable behavior described in action terms), *how much* (level of proficiency), and *when* (specified date of accomplishment).

Students with moderate or severe disabilities, as well as those with complex communication needs (CCN), also must have IEPs that are standards based. Many of these students will be taking alternate assessment based on alternate achievement standards (AA-AAS). For these students, like all other students, aligning IEPs with standards is important, for the following reasons (Courtade & Browder, 2011, pp. 12–13):

1. IEPs aligned with state standards can prepare students for state assessments.
2. For students to show progress in academic content, they need academic instruction.
3. Well-aligned IEPs can promote meaningful academic instruction.

Students with severe intellectual disabilities and complex communication needs have not historically received direct instruction in academic content areas but instead receive functional curriculum only. The National Center and State Collaborative (NCSC) is responsible for the development of alternate assessment and alternate achievement standards. It bases the foundational principles of alternate assessment on communication competence, noting the number of students who require augmentative and alternative communication (AAC) to communicate. (See the following box, "National Center and State Collaborative (NCSC) Communication Beliefs.") Speech–language pathologists and special educators must lead the way in ensuring the IEP goals set high standards and academic expectations for students who are accessing alternate achievement standards. Knowing these standards is as important as knowing the general common core.

National Center and State Collaborative (NCSC) Communication Beliefs

- All individuals communicate regardless of age or disability.
- All output (gestures, cries, noises) can be communicative.
- Communication at some level is possible and identifiable for all students regardless of functional "level."
- Every step toward improved communication, attention, and interaction leads to enriched quality of life and independence.
- Students with significant cognitive disabilities can improve their skills with appropriate communication interventions and instruction linked to grade-level standards.
- Communication programming goals should improve students' opportunities for increased integration and interactions with peers and the community in general.
- Students with the most significant disabilities benefit from interactions with typical peers.
- Typical peers benefit from interactions with students with the most significant disabilities!
- No more fundamental outcome of education exists than the right and the ability to communicate. (NCSC, n.d.).

IDEA 2004 has a reporting requirement that aligns reporting on IEP goal progress with the reporting periods of general education. This requirement mandates that IEPs include a statement that includes the following:

(i)   How the child's progress toward the annual goals will be measured; and
(ii)   When periodic reports on the progress the child is making toward meeting the annual goals (such as through the use of quarterly or other periodic reports, concurrent with the issuance of report cards) will be provided. (34 C.F.R. § 300.320 [a][3])

How school districts demonstrate and document progress is central to documenting the provision of FAPE. The legal standard for progress is "educational benefit," or the *Rowley* standard. In the *Rowley* case (see Chapter 2), the Supreme Court provided a two-pronged test to show educational benefit: (a) procedural compliance and (b) designing the IEP so that it is reasonably calculated to ensure educational benefit. *Endrew F.* (2017) added "in light of the child's circumstance."

Advancing from grade to grade may be considered evidence of educational benefit but not necessarily exclusively so. The law requires IEP teams to meet at least annually to review the IEP, but it is important to note that the law also requires the IEP team to address a lack of expected progress, which means if a student is not making progress, the team should reconvene and address the issue. Goals must be based on past data showing need. Have objective data available (e.g., test results, classroom portfolio work, teacher observations) to support expectations. In addition, the IEP must specify how progress toward goals will be measured.

Goals Reflective of the Common Core (Dodd, 2014b)

It is not the intention for content standards to be written as goals but rather goals to be written so standards are accessible to a student with exceptional needs. This can be accomplished in many ways and the following are just a few examples of how IEP goals can be written to reflect content of grade-level standards.

Write a goal that addresses more than a single standard:

"By 3/15/2015, given grade-level text, Charlie will use regular and irregular past tense verbs (CCSS.ELA-Literacy.L.3.1D, CCSS.ELA-Literacy. L. 3.1E) to describe characters in a story (e.g., their traits, motivations, or feelings) and explain how their actions contribute to the sequence of events (CCSS.ELA.Literacy.RL.3.3) with 80% accuracy."

Write a goal to reflect the entire content of a single standard:

"Given grade-level text, Darren will demonstrate understanding of the words and phrases including figurative forms of language based on how they are used in the text (CCSS.ELA-Literacy.R.5.4) by either providing a definition of the word or using the word correctly in a sentence on 4 out 5 opportunities."

Write goals with scaffold supports embedded that teach students how to use strategies (e.g., graphic organizer):

"Given two texts on the same topic presented orally with illustrations and guidance in completing a compare and contrast graphic organizer, Samantha will identify two similarities and two differences between the two texts (CCSS.ELA-Literacy. RL.1.9) with 80% accuracy."

Write a goal to target a single aspect of a standard. Consider the grade-level standard for reading information text for second grade: *Ask and answer such questions* as who, what, where, when, why, and how to demonstrate understanding of key details in a text (CCSS.ELA-Literacy.RI.2.1).

> "Given grade-level text presented orally, Ava will demonstrate understanding of key details in the text by answering who, what, and where questions with 80% accuracy."

Write a goal to target prerequisite foundational skills. Consider a student who is working towards the kindergarten ELA standards for language: Use the most frequently occurring prepositions (e.g., to, from, in, out, on, off, for, of, by, with) (CCSS.ELA-Literacy.L.K1.E).

> "Given objects Mario will follow one-step directions containing prepositions (i.e., in, on, under, off, next to, above) with 80% accuracy."

The common theme is that goals must be customized to meet the individual needs of the student.

Language skills such as comparing and contrasting as well as those skills related to determining and describing word meanings from context are among some of the linguistic skills necessary for execution of the *Literature* and *Informational* substrands of the Reading standards. Writing standards require students to use precise language and domain-specific vocabulary in their composition of various narrative genres. While Language standards facilitate a student's execution of syntax and morphology to levels consistent with the complexity and sophistication of academics, Speaking and Listening standards require students to possess language skills that allow them to effectively respond to and ask questions to contribute meaningfully to group discussions following an agreed-upon set of rules. Mathematics, once viewed as a strength for many of our language-impaired students, has itself evolved into a language task with the introduction of the common core. Students can no longer simply recall math facts; they now must explain their problem-solving and reasoning skills. A task which is even difficult for typically developing students taps into the core challenge of students with language impairments. The common core are here and affords our students with language impairments multiple opportunities to practice the targets we have long seen as necessary for not only academic success but success in life as well. (p. 7)

Determination of Program, Placement, and Services

Once a student has been identified as being eligible for special education by meeting eligibility criteria, that student is entitled to receive any service that the IEP team determines is needed to help the student meet the established goals. The IEP team must follow the requirements and philosophy of the least restrictive environment (LRE) when determining placement and services and ensure the following:

(i)   To the maximum extent appropriate, children with disabilities ... are educated with children who are nondisabled; and

(ii) Special classes, separate schooling or other removal of children with disabilities from the regular educational environment occurs only if the nature or severity of the disability is such that the education in regular classes with the use of supplementary aids and services cannot be achieved satisfactorily. (34 C.F.R. § 300.114 [2])

One of the most important considerations for IEP teams in making determinations of placement is to keep children in the neighborhood school, or as close to home as possible, and attending the school that they would attend if they did not have a disability, unless their IEP requires some other arrangement. IDEA 2004 regulations specifically direct the following about placement:

(a) The placement decision—

   (1) Is made by a group of persons, including the parents, and other persons knowledgeable about the child, the meaning of the evaluation data and the placement options; and

   (2) Is made in conformity with the LRE provisions.

(b) The child's placement—

   (1) Is determined at least annually;

   (2) Is based on the child's IEP; and

   (3) Is as close as possible to the child's home.

(c) Unless the IEP of a child with a disability requires some other arrangement, the child is educated in the school that he or she would attend if nondisabled;

(d) In selecting the LRE, consideration is given to any potential harmful effect on the child or on the quality of services that he or she needs; and

(e) A child with a disability is not removed from education in age-appropriate regular classrooms solely because of needed modifications in the general curriculum. (34 C.F.R. § 300.116)

For children with "speech only" disorders (e.g., articulation, fluency, or voice disorder), speech and language services may be the only special education provided to the student. If this is the case, then the speech–language services are considered the student's special education. This may also occur periodically for students with language disorders for whom speech and language services are the only service provided through the IEP. For children with language impairments that have an academic impact, support may be provided with the addition of specialized academic instruction (SAI). As the nature of the student's disability becomes more complex, it is more likely that the student will receive additional services. Sometimes the speech–language pathologist will be the only provider of special education services. At other times, the speech–language pathologist will be a member of a larger service team. The service provider who is with the student the most usually assumes case management responsibility. Service delivery and how to make these decisions are discussed in Chapter 5.

Speech–language services are identified as a related service (i.e., a service necessary for the student to benefit from special education) under federal law. Speech–language services can also be identified as special education if they are considered so under state guidelines.

Speech–language services are defined as follows:

(i) Identification of children with speech or language impairments;

(ii) Diagnosis and appraisal of specific speech or language impairments;

(iii) Referral for medical or other professional attention necessary for the habilitation of speech or language impairments;

(iv) Provision of speech and language services for the habilitation or prevention of communicative impairments; and

(v) Counseling and guidance of parents, children, and teachers regarding speech and language impairments. (34 C.F.R. § 300.34 [c][15])

Audiology services are defined as follows:

(i) Identification of children with hearing loss;

(ii) Determination of the range, nature, and degree of hearing loss, including referral for medical or other professional attention for the habilitation of hearing;

(iii) Provision of habilitative activities, such as language habilitation, auditory training, speech reading (lip reading), hearing evaluation, and speech conservation;

(iv) Creation and administration of programs for prevention of hearing loss;

(v) Counseling and guidance of children, parents, and teachers regarding hearing loss; and

(vi) Determination of children's needs for group and individuals' amplification, selecting and fitting an appropriate aid, and evaluation of the effectiveness of amplification. (34 C.F.R. § 300.34 [c][1])

The determination of the services a student requires to meet his or her identified goals and receive educational benefit is a most important responsibility of IEP teams. Issues such as caseload management and service delivery options are also tied to placement determination but should be discussed at the IEP meeting only if the issues pertain to the student. In other words, caseload size is an issue for the speech–language pathologist but is not an IEP issue. Figure 4.2 recaps the IEP meeting process.

Recordkeeping and Documentation

Documentation is an essential component of a speech–language pathologist's responsibilities in any setting (Moore, 2013). In the school setting, documentation demonstrates compliance with legal requirements and clearly explains the course of intervention to parents, teachers, the student, and others. To verify which activities were completed with the student and how these activities were designed to meet IEP goals, speech–language pathologists must maintain records for each student. The standard for documentation

IEP Meeting Process

Determination of Present Levels of Educational Achievement
- Review evaluation data
- Review classroom performance
- Review other related information
- Consider input from parents, teachers, and specialists

↓

Determination of Goals and Short-Term Objectives or Benchmarks
- Based on identified areas of need
- Designed to enable the child to progress in the general education curriculum
- Must be measurable

↓

Determination of Program, Placement, and Services
- Includes services needed in order for goals to be achieved
- Designed to confer meaningful educational benefit

FIGURE 4.2. The IEP meeting process.

in public schools is no different than it is in any other sector of our field (Moore, 2013). The following list provides examples of what might be recorded in this documentation:

1. Therapy notes that identify the schedule of when students were seen for service and for how long (be sure to initial the notes)
2. Log of intervention activities and outcomes
3. Portfolio of student performance/student work
4. Records of communication with parents, teachers, and others regarding the student
5. Student file with all IEP and assessment information, as well as IEP procedure documentation and progress report cards

Participating as a member of the IEP team, writing and developing an IEP, and conducting intervention based on the plan outlined in the IEP document is a complex process. Speech–language pathologists who are new to the field or new to a school system should seek a mentor to learn the specifics of the IEP process for the system in which he or she works. If the speech–language pathologist is a clinical fellow (CF), then his or her CF supervisor may be able to serve in this capacity. Other special education professionals in the school district may also be able to assist a new staff member learning the way.

Confidentiality

All educators must be aware of the confidentiality requirements under the Family Educational Rights and Privacy Act (FERPA, 1974, § 513 of P.L. 93-380 [The Education Amendments of 1974]), which applies to IDEA 2004 and all school records. Under FERPA, students' and parents' rights to privacy are protected with regard to personally identifiable information in education records. An IEP is an educational record; therefore, to disclose improperly the contents of an IEP would be a violation of FERPA.

Speech–language pathologists and other special educators need to be aware of the interface between IDEA 2004, FERPA, and the Health Insurance Portability and Accountability Act (HIPAA) of 1996 and 2003. HIPAA covers protected health information, which is individually identifiable health information, both oral and recorded. Under HIPAA, records, such as educational records, that are protected under FERPA are excluded. Professionals need to be clear as to which records are considered educational records and which ones are not.

Educational records covered by FERPA and IDEA 2004 include the following: (a) records directly related to the student and (b) records maintained by an educational agency or institution or party acting for the agency or institution. Educational records covered by FERPA and IDEA 2004 exclude the following: (a) personal notes, (b) employee records, (c) law enforcement records, (d) certain adult/student treatment records, and (e) records not maintained by the registrar.

In practical terms, all educators must be extremely careful when they discuss cases. Revealing the names of children and parents would be considered a violation of their rights, if the receiver of the information is not involved in the case by virtue of his or her position with the LEA. Speech–language pathologists should make it a personal rule not to reveal the names of children or families to anyone who does not have direct involvement in the case, and never to use the names of children on their caseloads in public, even when discussing a case with a team member. If speech–language pathologists make this their personal habit, they will not have to worry about being overheard by a child's relative or family friend. Professionals need to be vigilant about not engaging in conversations in the lunchroom or around the teacher's break room regarding children or their families when the other faculty members do not have a legitimate interest in the case. School-based personnel must also be careful not to unintentionally leave documentation with children's names on it lying in common areas of the school. All documents need to be kept in a secured, locked location.

Parental Access to School Records

Parents also have the right to access and examine school records as part of their procedural safeguards ensuring participation (34 C.F.R. § 300.501 [a]). If parents request to review their child's records, the LEA must respond without reasonable delay, which is typically defined in state law and is often 5 school or business days. In addition, if parents need someone to interpret the records for them, the district must provide someone to do so. Districts must also allow a parent's representative to review the records if so requested (34 C.F.R. § 300.613). School districts must provide parents with copies of school records if requested but can charge a fee. Parents are typically provided copies of IEPs and reports at IEP meetings, and, of course, there is no charge for that. However, when a parent requests a full copy of the student's educational records, then the special education office has procedures to complete the request. School districts generally have a school board policy outlining the procedures for record requests and charges. It would be unlikely that the service provider, such as the speech–language pathologist or teacher, would be required to gather the fees.

Three points are important with regard to student records. One is that if a parent does request records from the speech–language pathologist or classroom teacher, an immediate response is required because of the timeline. In addition, it is important to remember that all records are considered part of a student's record, so confidential, cumulative student discipline records, health records, and teacher files will all need to be copied or available for inspection. One additional point is that sometimes parents request that the service provider generate letters or documentation for some purpose. A general rule is that no record that is not a student record should be generated without consulting with a district administrator. This would prevent the record from being used inappropriately, such as in a child custody situation or other court action that was not the intended purpose for the document. School district personnel should be very cautious about generating any records that are not part of the typical documentation. Last, the use of e-mail is increasingly common as a method to communicate with parents and other teachers regarding students. All educators need to be cautious about the use of e-mail, as has been previously mentioned. E-mail may be printed and placed in the file, at which point it becomes part of the pupil record. E-mail can also be subpoenaed.

Sometimes parents request to have documentation changed or removed from a school district file. The procedures for responding to this type of request are outlined in the district's school board policy. Again, this type of request requires administrative attention and should be referred to the appropriate personnel.

When creating documents for the student's records, such as evaluation reports or IEPs, school district staff can and should be open to input from the family, especially in terms of developmental history and the child's level of functioning from the family's perspective. However, if there is a disagreement in terms of professional opinion, the speech–language pathologist and other school district personnel should always report their findings and interpretations according to their professional judgment. If there is a disagreement about interpretation, conclusion, and recommendations, then the parent can dissent, submit a document to be attached to the IEP, or use procedural methods to challenge the interpretation. If there is a disagreement of this nature and it is discussed in the IEP, of course this should be documented in the notes of the IEP meeting.

Speech–language pathologists and other special education personnel often complain about paperwork demands. Paperwork can be overwhelming; however, all requirements are procedurally driven. To comply with the law, personnel must complete documentation. In addition to completing forms correctly and following appropriate procedures, personnel must keep timelines. Teams that work closely together find that the process moves along smoothly, ensuring compliance and quality.

Many questions can arise in terms of documentation. Always seek guidance in terms of documentation, as there are legal consequences resulting from poor documentation or missed timelines. See the ASHA Web site on documentation in schools  for more information (www.asha.org/Practice-Portal/Professional-Issues/ Documentation-In-Schools/). Also see the article "Five Common Documentation Questions—Answered" (Moore, 2012).

Annual and Triennial Assessments

IDEA 2004 requires that students who are eligible for special education have their progress reviewed at least annually by the IEP team. This requirement is called the *annual review* and must take place within one calendar year of the last IEP. Every 3 years, the IEP team needs to conduct a triennial assessment to determine whether the student continues to be eligible and require special education. Evaluation is the foundation for developing a standards-based, educationally relevant IEP.

An annual review of the student's IEP is conducted each year to measure and record the amount of change that occurred for each of a student's written annual goals. In addition, goals and objectives are reviewed to determine progress and continued area(s) of need that may require goals. Goals must be relevant to the general education curriculum. Annual assessments of students using standardized tests are not required and are not recommended. The results of standardized tests are useful for qualifying students for services, because these tests compare a student's abilities with the expected abilities of other students his or her age, usually nationwide. However, these tests do not offer results in functional terms. When used to measure change, test scores offer a numerical value of how a student responded to a testing probe but not of his or her actual performance in the classroom, with peers, or in other true-life situations. Speech–language pathologists use nonstandardized tests, observations, checklists, portfolios, and other formal and informal measures to determine progress toward goals in a year. IDEA 2004 requires that IEPs report on the results of statewide assessments. The results of any district-wide-administered assessments should also be reported on an IEP. Because IDEA 2004 focuses on the general education curriculum, report-card-type grades, progress toward standards, or periodic narratives should be part of both annual and triennial reports. Therefore, all student annual reviews, as well as evaluations, should be conducted and interpreted using multiple means of assessment.

Every 3 years, an IEP team must determine if a student continues to meet criteria and require special education. In some cases, standardized testing may be used. The same evaluation measures used for annual assessments may be used at the triennial assessment, with the same cautions. IDEA 2004 allows the IEP team to determine if additional data are actually necessary to make the determination of the student's continued disability. If the IEP team determines that special education is not necessary, the district must notify the parents, and the parents have the right to request an assessment. Presumably, this determination would be conducted at an IEP meeting, with the parent present. However, if there is a determination that is not agreed to by the parent, then the district may need to send prior written notice (PWN) to the parent (see the discussion on PWN in "Parental Consent" in Chapter 3).

The district is required to assess all students whose parents request these services. Because parents are a part of all decision making for their child's program, they are involved in the discussion of which, if any, triennial assessments are needed. At times, student needs are clear without formal testing. For example, a child making year-to-year progress on speech–language goals for communication disabilities related to cognitive impairment would not need to have a triennial assessment to determine whether he or she still has a cognitive impairment. The disability would not have to be reaffirmed unless parents specifically request that to be done. However, the student's communication needs are continuing to change, so appropriate data to examine these changes would be necessary in order to make appropriate determinations about the student's needs.

The school district must administer the tests and other evaluation materials needed to produce the data identified by the IEP team. Parents are asked to help define the data needed for their child. The IEP is the vehicle that links this vital evaluation information to the desired outcomes for each child. These outcomes become the basis for determining the particular services that the student needs, which professionals can best provide them, and in what setting they should be offered. Annual reviews and triennial reevaluations, whenever needed, serve this purpose for students and families. Local policy directs procedures for assessments. (See also the discussion on assessments in Chapter 3.)

Some school districts require a report for the annual review; however, others just have the documentation information on the IEP. Sometimes, the dates for the annual review and the triennial assessment become misaligned. IDEA 2004 encourages IEP teams to consolidate these meetings when a reevaluation occurs (34 C.F.R. § 300.324 [a][5]). In fact, it makes sense to revise the IEP when new evaluation information is available.

Exit or Dismissal Criteria

Although this chapter emphasizes how to develop IEPs for students who are eligible and in need of special education services, of equal importance is to consider the criteria for successfully completing that intervention. It is good practice to think about exit criteria at the beginning of the intervention cycle, because the criteria should serve as the "beacon" that guides the intervention process.

Evaluation updates of a student are required by IDEA to make a dismissal decision (34 C.F.R. § 300.305 [e][2]). The student should be dismissed when his or her communication no longer has an adverse effect on educational progress. This can be difficult to ascertain unless functional outcomes have been collected throughout the intervention. Focusing on reducing the effect of the impairment (i.e., the disability) will provide the information needed to decide on dismissal. The data that were gathered while the student was receiving speech–language services can be used for the dismissal decision.

Intervention should not continue until a student is "perfect" or "100%." This is often not realistic. Goals generally should be written to 75% or 80%. If an individual is able to complete tasks at that level, he or she no longer needs intervention to master the skill; he or she simply needs practice.

Dismissal may occur before a student demonstrates complete mastery of all targeted skills. Reassessment for dismissal requires the speech–language pathologist to revisit the options of standardized, performance-based, and dynamic assessment (as discussed in Chapter 3) to determine which will provide the most useful information. Dismissal criteria should be functionally based, not test based.

Some states have criteria for dismissal, but many do not. Some school districts have developed their own dismissal criteria to help support their statements to parents and teachers that a student has made sufficient progress or may benefit more from a different service. In a few instances, a decision to terminate speech–language services may be based on mutually agreed-on circumstances, such as the student's interest, motivation, or available time.

The ASHA (2004a) document "Admission/Discharge Criteria in Speech–Language Pathology" provides guidance to the field in this area. Speech–language pathologists should also check with their local agencies to see whether state or local guidelines exist. In all cases, an evaluation report must be completed, as that is federal law, as described earlier.

CHAPTER 5

Service Delivery Options in Schools

● *In This Chapter*

When viewing service delivery in speech–language and special education in the broadest sense, every activity on behalf of, or in contact with, a student—screening, consultation, assessment, identification, goal setting with functional outcomes and links to the curriculum, intervention, collaboration, reevaluation, parent contacts, and dismissal—is service delivery. This chapter scans the larger picture of special education, of which speech–language services are a critical part. The role of school-based speech–language pathologists in inclusive education, models of speech–language intervention, good practice issues, working with a school team, functional outcomes, linking services to consumer satisfaction, and the importance of Common Core State Standards are discussed. Response to intervention (RTI) is described as a service model rather than a framework.

● *Chapter Questions*

1. What are the components of service delivery in speech–language programs in schools? What are the primary driving considerations in designing service delivery for students receiving speech and language services?
2. If you worked in an elementary school, describe a role you could play to support inclusion of a 6-year-old student on the autism spectrum.
3. What resources can you use to respond the four basic questions that center on functional outcomes?
4. Discuss with a colleague how emerging evidence-based systematic reviews (EBSR) assist speech–language pathologists when selecting service delivery models. How can this be helpful at an Individualized Education Program (IEP) meeting with teachers, parents, and attorneys?
5. How can a speech–language pathologist learn more about counseling and guidance as a component of service delivery? What resources might be available at a school site?
6. What program characteristics may be used to show consumers that a student will receive appropriate benefit from an IEP? Give examples of measures that would demonstrate educational benefit.

7. Review the concept of clinically significant change. Design a graphic that shows the three basic elements and their relationship to each other and to the process of evaluating students who are receiving speech and language interventions.

8. Describe three situations in which telepractice would enable speech-language therapy to occur or enhance limited therapy services.

The Concept of Service Delivery

Deciding what to do in therapy and how to deliver effective services is at the core of intervention. Both the Individuals With Disabilities Education Improvement Act of 2004 (IDEA 2004) and effective practice documents dictate that these choices must be made based on the student's identified needs, determined through assessment and data collection, and correlated with the evidence from the field. The following questions are intended to guide such choices (adapted from Kamhi [1999] and Ehren [2006] in Wallach, 2008):

- Is the intervention method based on a theoretical principle?
- Is the intervention based on current research? Are there data to support the approach? Is it evidence based? Are there studies that provide evidence?
- Was it chosen with student's strengths and skills in mind?
- Are the intervention choices curriculum relevant?
- Is the intervention strategically focused?
- Do the tasks integrate oral and written language systems?
- Are you as the therapist knowledgeable about how to conduct the intervention?

Wallach (2008) recommended asking two basic questions—"Why am I doing this?" and "Where does this technique or approach 'come from'?"—along with the previous questions to guide intervention choices. The answers to these two basic questions should relate directly to the student, academic expectations, and sound therapeutic principles.

Service Delivery for Prevention Services

The American Speech–Language–Hearing Association (ASHA, 2010a) "Roles and Responsibilities" document, Practice Portals in each disorder area and the IDEA 2004 call for speech–language pathologists to be engaged in prevention activities. Response to intervention (RTI) and prereferral are discussed in Chapter 3 as part of the referral and assessment process. This section considers prevention and RTI as a service delivery model.

Roles and responsibilities change in a system that seeks to prevent children from struggling and also to prevent them from needing special education. Engaging in prevention is a concept that speech–language pathologists have supported for many years;

yet, until the IDEA Amendments of 1997, and specifically until IDEA 2004, speech–language pathologists and other special educators did not work with students who were not identified as being eligible for special education. Because of this restriction, and the application of cognitive referencing (ASHA, n.d.-b) (see section on "Normative Reference Points" in Chapter 4), special education was known as a "wait to fail" system.

To change this system, IDEA 2004 instituted provisions to allow for RTI as an alternative method of identifying students as being learning disabled but also created a provision for *early intervening services*, or the utilization of special education resources, including assessment and services, by students who were struggling, to potentially prevent them from needing special education and related services (ASHA, n.d.-m).

In examining the roles they can play in RTI or prevention activities, speech–language pathologists will find that there will be "fundamental changes in the way speech–language pathologists engage in assessment and intervention activities" (Ehren, Montgomery, Rudebusch, & Whitmire, 2006, p. 1). These authors suggested that RTI will bring both challenge and opportunity and that the new and expanding roles for speech–language pathologists will specifically be in the areas of program design, collaboration, and work with individual students. Rudebusch (2008) stated that the speech–language pathologist "can play a number of important roles in an RTI framework: team members, technical assistance provider, curriculum and instruction advisor, problem solver, [and] direct service provider for assessment and intervention activities" (p. 5). These roles, then, also support system change.

RTI is typically considered within a three-tiered model of services, outlined in Chapter 3 (Rudebusch, 2008, p. 77):

- *Tier 1:* Mostly indirect services to support quality instruction in the classroom and participation in prevention activities
- *Tier 2:* A combination of direct intervention and indirect service
- *Tier 3:* Mostly direct intervention and identification services

The expectation that speech–language pathologists will be involved in RTI is well established and previously discussed in the section on assessment and prereferral (see the section "Multi-Tiered System of Supports: Response to Intervention and Early Intervening Services" in Chapter 3). Because RTI is building based—not district based—and locally organized, states have created unique projects to encourage and oversee local plan areas as they develop systems that work, often displaying local or regional project titles. The ASHA Workload Approach is strongly recommended for use as part of RTI (Ehren, 2007; Rudebusch, 2008; Rudebusch & Wiechmann, 2011).

In 2010, Bourque Meaux and Powell conducted a study of the speech–language pathologist caseloads in schools in two states and reported the following:

- Twenty-one percent used a workload approach, whereas 79% use a caseload approach.
- The median caseload size was 46 students.

- Of 309 respondents,
  - 73% reported participating in alternative service delivery models, whereas 27% reported that they do not participate in alternative service delivery models;
  - 93% reported spending more time in pull-out therapy, whereas 7% reported spending more time in push-in therapy;
  - 95% reported participating in RTI in their school, whereas 5% reported not participating in RTI at their school; and
  - 92% reported advocating and supporting their role in RTI in their schools.
- Of 308 respondents,
  - 72% reported using a caseload approach (82% nationally) to caseload management, whereas 28% reported using a workload approach (18% nationally).

The researchers noted that speech–language pathologists were serving fewer articulation and language students than the national mean but that they were also participating in RTI at a much higher level than figures at the national level. It was suggested that this higher participation of speech–language pathologists in RTI could be a result of state initiatives that promote speech–language pathologists serving all students through RTI and not solely through special education. While these data served as a positive indicator, speech–language pathologists in the study still predominantly used traditional service delivery model and caseload approaches to caseload management (Bourque Meaux & Powell, 2010).

Recommended practices for speech–language pathologists in the RTI model are identified in Table 5.1.

Service Delivery in Special Education

The majority of the work that speech–language pathologists in schools do will be under IDEA 2004. In some cases, the services that are provided in an RTI model to students not eligible under IDEA may appear similar to those used for identified students under IDEA. Services provided to a student identified for special education and related services must be documented on an Individualized Education Program (IEP) and through appropriate documentation procedures. Service delivery models that are used in the delivery of speech–language services are reviewed later. Although IDEA requires linking services to the curriculum, and the literature in the field also guides speech–language pathologists to use collaborative and consultative service delivery (Ehren, 2007; Wallach, 2008), ASHA's surveys of school-based members shows that pull-out remains the predominant service delivery model used by speech–language pathologists in schools.

As the law requires, assessment drives intervention. In the area of language, a comprehensive assessment will determine which underlying factors contribute to the student's language delay or disorder. Regardless of the causation, intervention that will lead to increased functional outcomes is recommended (Kaderavek, 2011). In addition, regardless of the causation, intervention should be meaningful and linked to literacy and the curriculum.

TABLE 5.1. Response to Intervention Activities for Speech–Language Pathologists

Tier	Speech–language pathologist role	Activity or intervention	Reference
Tier 1	Direct service provider	• Provide expanded speech and language screening • Organize materials • Organize groups • Provide tutoring • Suggest modifications for the classroom • Offer classroom time with a small group of struggling students • Provide classroom lessons	Rudebusch (2008) Roth, Dougherty, Paul, and Adamczyk (2010)
	Indirect service provider	• Make classroom observations • Assemble school improvement team • Assist with parent education • Offer a homework program • Provide curriculum and instruction consultation • Provide professional development	Rudebusch (2008) Troia (2005) Wallach (2008)
Tier 2	Direct service provider	• Provide directed instruction for diagnostic and therapeutic instructional purposes • Offer an articulation intervention program • Offer a language and literacy intervention program • Administer and interpret language assessments (spoken and written) to plan and provide small-group instruction	Troia (2005) Rudebusch (2008) Roth et al. (2010) San Diego City Schools (2004–2005) Montgomery and Moore-Brown (2005) Wallach (2008)
	Indirect service provider	• Be a consultant for teams delivering targeted instruction and interventions • Make observations • Assist with progress monitoring • Participate in problem-solving teams	Troia (2005) Rudebusch (2008) Roth et al. (2010)
Tier 3	Direct service provider	• Provide intensive, individualized intervention for articulation and language • Provide specialized treatments for poor readers with language deficits who have not responded to universal instruction and targeted interventions	Rudebusch (2008) Wallach (2008) Troia (2005)
	Indirect service provider	• Select research-based literacy interventions • Observe Tier 3 students • Assist with progress monitoring • Participate in problem-solving team to make decisions about referral to special education • Consult with special educators to help them make their services maximally beneficial	Rudebusch (2008) Troia (2005)

An expanded list of service delivery models used to deliver speech–language services is presented in Table 5.2. It is noted that some of these models may overlap in their description, but these are the actual terms used in the field.

Telepractice

A rising new area of service delivery is telepractice. The ease of using technology in literally every aspect of our lives has made it possible to extend services to remote or underserved areas. ASHA defined *telepractice* as "the application of telecommunications technology to the delivery of speech language pathology and audiology professional services at a distance by linking clinician to client/patient or clinician to clinician for assessment, intervention, and/or consultation" (2016b). The speech–language pathologist is at one site directing the therapy, and the client is at another school, building, home, or hospital responding to the therapy in real time. The interaction is two-way, with clear audio and video, often including an aide, progress monitoring, and assigned homework.

Telepractice is a new service delivery model that has addressed the difficulties of providing services when the speech–language pathologist and student are not in the same room. Telepractice has become a viable option for the provision of services in a variety of situations, including shortages, maternity leaves, need for specialty services, and/or difficulty with providing face-to-face services because of various logistic challenges including transportation, geography, or weather. At one time students simply did not get the speech and language services they were entitled to under the law. Now they do.

Speech–language pathologists need to have training in how to conduct therapy online, and students need to focus their attention on the moving screen and the voice of the clinician, but early reports have indicated that this is easily accomplished (Jakubowitz, 2013). Research has shown that telepractice—a form of telehealth—may resolve many of the remote service delivery problems we have had as a profession. Although adult clients do well without a support person, children need frequent redirection in telepractice, just as they do in conventional face-to-face therapy. An entire inventory of therapy tasks, worksheets, reinforcement games, and homework for telepractice is now available. Schools have responded to this new technology enthusiastically in most states, and state licensing agencies have produced clarifying statements about this form of billing for services and consumer protections. For example, a speech–language pathologist needs to hold a license in any state in which he or she provides services. If the speech–language pathologist lives in one state and provides services to a child in another state, he or she must hold a license in both states.

Components of Service Delivery

Service delivery models, or how a speech–language pathologist delivers service to students, is dynamic and ever evolving. In the era of accountability, service delivery

(text continues on p. 179)

TABLE 5.2. Service Delivery Models for Speech–Language Services

Service delivery model	Description	Recommended population or area of intervention
Coteaching: Lead and support (Friend & Bursuck, 2002)	One teacher leads and another offers assistance and support to individuals or small groups. In this role, planning must occur by both teachers, but typically one teacher plans for the lesson content, while the other does specific planning for students' individual learning or behavioral needs.	Students with learning and language disabilities Services in a self-contained or general education classroom Support for academic interventions (reading, math, social studies, science) Fully included students
Coteaching: Station teaching (Friend & Bursuck, 2002)	Students are divided into heterogeneous groups and work at classroom stations with each teacher. Then, in the middle of the period or the next day, the students switch to the other station. In this model, both teachers individually develop the content of their stations.	All grades and ages Articulation or speech–sound intervention at the speech–language station Vocabulary or syntax intervention at the speech–language station Allows for creativity and also smaller groupings
Coteaching: Parallel teaching (Friend & Bursuck, 2002)	Teachers jointly plan instruction, but each may deliver it to half the class or small groups. This type of model typically requires joint planning time to ensure that as teachers work in their separate groups, they are delivering content in the same way.	This method is effective with middle and high school students with learning and language disabilities and/or fully included students. Students do not feel isolated or singled out. Other students benefit from the intervention.
Coteaching: Alternative teaching (Friend & Bursuck, 2002)	One teacher works with a small group of students to preteach, reteach, supplement, or enrich instruction, while the other teacher instructs the large group. In this type of coteaching, more planning time is needed to ensure that the logistics of preteaching or reteaching can be completed; also, the teachers must have similar content knowledge for one teacher to take a group and reteach or preteach.	This method is effective for delivering curriculum-based interventions so that students can receive support specific to their needs (i.e., vocabulary instruction, text-based instruction, written language support) but not be removed from the classroom for core instruction.
Coteaching: Team teaching (Friend & Bursuck, 2002)	Both teachers share the planning and instruction of students in a coordinated fashion. In this type of joint planning time, equal knowledge of the content, a shared philosophy, and commitment to all students in the class are critical. Many times teams may not start with this type of format, but over time they can effectively move to this type of coteaching, if they have continuity in working together across 2–3 years.	This method is effective for classrooms where there is a variety of learner needs in the classroom. It is appropriate for any academic core area.
Consultation	The speech–language pathologist consults with the general or special education teacher, and/or other related service providers (OT, PT, psychologist, adapted PE, behavior specialist, social worker, counselor, etc.), to exchange information about student's functioning and also to make recommendations for enhancement of instructional practices.	This method is appropriate for all ages and grades, but it is especially important when students have many service providers and/or at the secondary level, when students have many teachers.

(continues)

TABLE 5.2. (*continued*)

Service delivery model	Description	Recommended population or area of intervention
Collaboration	This may be the same as or similar to the other coteaching models. The speech–language pathologist works with other professionals, both general education teachers and special education teachers and specialists, to collaborate on the coordination and design of a student's program, as well as the interventions provided.	This method is appropriate and necessary for all students but especially those who have complex or specialized needs to ensure continuity of care. It may also help to have regularly scheduled team meetings. It may also include parents. Key research study: Throneburg, Calvert, Sturm, Paramboukas, and Paul (2000) demonstrated that the collaborative model was more effective for teaching curricular vocabulary than the classroom-based parallel teaching model or pull-out.
Cotreatment	The speech–language pathologist and another related service provider provide service together. This allows for integration of interventions so the student is receiving simultaneous input. This is particularly beneficial for students who have complex disorders, so the specialists are not missing an unidentified component that is interfering with progress when it is outside of the specialist's area of expertise.	This is a good model when there are multiple needs being met. For example, for students with pragmatic or social skills disorders, the speech–language pathologist and psychologist may cotreat; or a music therapist or behavior analyst and speech–language pathologist may work together for students with autism or selective mutism; or a speech–language pathologist and OT may work together for students with multiple disabilities or intellectual disabilities.
Small group	Groups of two or more deliver speech–language intervention. Groupings can be variable: done by age, disability, and goals; homogeneous or heterogeneous. Groupings may be for the convenience of the therapist or specifically to use the group for modeling or to meet the goals of the individual student. This provides opportunity to provide directed intervention on a specific speech–language skill.	Small group may be used within a classroom setting or in a pull-out setting (i.e., the speech room). This method may be used for any type of speech–language intervention. It is often used for directed instruction on common goals and for articulation, fluency, language, and pragmatics. It also may be used for age or class groupings with students who have different goals but come from the same classroom or who are the same age. Small group may be used to have children serve as models for other children and to increase their social skills.
Pull-out	Speech–language intervention is delivered in an isolated setting, other than the classroom, typically in the speech room. It may be individual or small group.	Pull-out is still the service delivery model of choice for speech–language pathologist intervention, especially when addressing fluency, intelligibility, voices, speech-sound production, emergent literacy, pragmatics, spoken language production, and spoken language comprehension (ASHA National Outcomes Measurement System, 2005–2009).

TABLE 5.2. (*continued*)

Service delivery model	Description	Recommended population or area of intervention
Individual treatment	One-to-one intervention is done in a pull-out model. It is often perceived to be the "best" type of service delivery, but it is not necessarily, depending on the student's needs and goals.	This is appropriate when teaching specific intervention targets that are highly specialized and/or when the student has attentional or other needs that require reduced distraction in the therapy room, which is accomplished through 1:1 interventions.
In-class	Speech–language intervention is provided in the general or special education classroom. It can be provided in a coteaching model, collaboration, or consultation. (See descriptions in this table.)	This self-contained classroom model is used more predominantly when addressing areas such as composition, reading comprehension, word recognition, and writing accuracy (ASHA National Outcomes Measurement System, 2005–2009). Key research study: Systematic review investigating classroom-based interventions found that there was little research on these models but that classroom intervention models were at least as effective as pull-out. It notes the preference for least restrictive environment and curriculum interventions (Cirrin et al., 2010).
Telepractice	ASHA defined telepractice as "the application of telecommunications technology to delivery of professional services at a distance by linking clinician to client, or clinician to clinician, for assessment, intervention, and/or consultation" (http://www.asha.org/Practice-Portal/Professional-Issues/Telepractice/).	Telepractice is an appropriate model of service delivery for audiologists and speech–language pathologists. ASHA requires that individuals who provide telepractice abide by the ASHA Code of Ethics, including Principle of Ethics II, Rule B, which states, "Individuals shall engage in only those aspects of the profession that are within their competence, considering their level of education, training, and experience" (ASHA, 2010c). Telepractice is constantly evolving. Ongoing education and training is required to maintain expertise and familiarity with changes in technology and potential clinical applications.
Speech–language pathology assistant	Speech–language pathology assistants are support personnel who, following academic and/or on-the-job training, perform tasks prescribed, directed, and supervised by ASHA-certified speech–language pathologists. There are typically two levels of support personnel: aides and assistants. On the basis of the level of training, these support personnel may have a different scope of responsibilities in the work setting. Aides, for example, have a *(text continues)*	Speech–language pathology assistants can be used to provide direct intervention. They will require supervision by a speech–language pathologist. There are specific duties and responsibilities outlined regarding what they can and cannot do. They cannot conduct assessments or develop intervention plans. They can *(text continues)*

TABLE 5.2. (*continued*)

Service delivery model	Description	Recommended population or area of intervention
Speech–language pathology assistant (*continued*)	different, usually narrower, training base and a more limited scope of responsibilities than speech–language pathology assistants. States may use different terminology to refer to support personnel in speech–language pathology (e.g., communication aides, paraprofessionals, service extenders) (ASHA, 2016b).	provide direct intervention, which allows for direct services to be provided to a broader number of students. All intervention must be approved by the supervising speech–language pathologist.
3 in 1	The speech–language pathologist provides direct service for 3 weeks and then indirect services for 1 week. This is designed to allow for consultation, meetings, assessments, and so on during the fourth week.	This model uses the other service delivery models during the 3 weeks of interventions.
Self-contained classroom	Self-contained classrooms are taught by a speech–language pathologist.	This may be used at any grade level but is most commonly at preschool. It is intended for intense speech–language intervention and strategies throughout the day and may require specialized credentialing.
Language lab	This is a lab setting for language and/or literacy interventions. It may have small group stations to assist students with homework, class assignments, or strategies instruction. Students may be assigned specific times or may come on an as-needed basis.	The speech–language pathologist, speech–language pathology assistant, and/or other interventionists (Title I teacher, other specialists) may staff this setting. Labs are most typically used at the secondary level.
Writing lab	This lab setting or classroom provides instruction for students to receive assistance on writing assignments. Written language instruction is an important part of literacy intervention. This includes spelling. Spelling should be considered through a phonological approach.	
Articulation lab	This lab setting provides for students to receive articulation intervention. It may be for response to intervention or Individualized Education Program services.	See the Articulation Differences and Disorders Manual (San Diego City Schools, 2004–2005).
Social skills class	This is a special class to teach social skills to students who need this intervention. It is done within the schedule of a middle or high school but can also be done at the elementary level within a self-contained setting. The speech–language pathologist provides instruction in these skills. This class may be cotaught or cotreated with another professional. If within a classroom, teacher and aides should be present to learn the interventions, so that they can be reinforced.	This is appropriate for groups of students with autism, learning disabilities, and emotional disturbance.
Study skills class	This is a special class to teach students strategies for specific language-based study skills.	This is for students on a diploma track at the secondary level.

should be "effective, efficient, economical and evidence-based" (Moore-Brown, 2007a). A framework for designing service delivery models takes into account all the conventional criteria and allows speech–language pathologists to embrace new models as they became necessary. A speech–language pathologist's role is continually evolving with an increased understanding of individuals with communication disorders and the effects on learning and daily living tasks. Throughout the field, consumers of speech–language services have become more involved in their own treatment. In schools, partnerships are formed with parents and community agencies, technology has made the improbable likely, and documentation of student outcomes drives education and rehabilitation. Speech–language pathologists need a framework that encompasses all service delivery models, not a proliferation of more and more models.

Every service model should address four ideas: overall effectiveness, coordination with other programs and services, commitment of all parties, and resources available. A student should receive services that are matched to his or her needs at that point in time and are flexible to changing conditions. This requires flexing the provider, the activities, and the context. In the following descriptions, the provider arrangement changes, the range of activities is broad but primarily curriculum centered, and the contexts are school related. Flexibility among the provider, activities, and context is important in the following models, as in the curriculum models in Chapter 6 and the expanded and specialized service delivery models presented in Chapter 7. Whitmire (2002) encapsulated the "contemporary vision of school-based practice" (p. 71) as converging on three fundamental elements of school-based speech and language therapy: contextually based assessment, educationally relevant intervention plans, and increased collaboration and consultation.

Intensity and Dosage

IEPs require that services be described in terms of the frequency and duration of the service, as well as the location of service. Speech–language pathologists in schools may describe frequency and duration according to a workload model, describing minutes per year or per semester, and should check with their local district to determine what the preferred format is for the local education agency (LEA). Within the field, there is increasing discussion regarding the required intensity and dosage that should be necessary to remediate certain communication disorders. Although treatment outcomes are based on evidence-based practice (see the section "Evidence-Based Practice and PICO Statements" later in this chapter), *intensity* and *dosage* are defined currently not by evidence-based practice but rather by convention, resources, and clinical craft (Ukrainetz et al., 2008). Intensity and dosage can be considered as follows (Warren, Fey, & Yoder, cited in Ukrainetz et al., 2008):

Quantifying Intensity
- *Dose:* Number of properly administered teaching episodes during a single intervention session (e.g., 20 response opportunities in 30 minutes)

- *Dose form:* The physical manner in which the active ingredient is dispensed (e.g., in play format)
- *Dose frequency:* Number of times a dose is provided per day or week (e.g., two times per week)

Intervention Dosage
- *Total intervention duration:* Time period over which the intervention is presented (e.g., 10 weeks)
- *Cumulative intervention intensity:* Product of dose $\times$ dose frequency $\times$ total intervention duration (e.g., $20 \times 3 \times 10 = 600$ teaching episodes)

As with other advances in the field, the question of intensity and dosage is receiving greater attention in the field. These discussions will assist speech–language pathologists in supporting their IEP recommendations.

Counseling and Guidance

Although many speech–language pathologists feel uncomfortable with counseling and guidance as an aspect of their practice, it is very important because of the many overlays that come from communication disorders and the sense of loss or life complications that may come as a result of the disability. Flahive (2006) reminded us that speech–language pathologists are not just specialists in communicative disorders but also members of a helping profession. As such, speech–language pathologists are helping their students manage their problems and helping them learn better ways to live their lives. In the therapeutic relationship, trust is built. Through counseling, which is a dynamic process, speech–language pathologists are acknowledging the person and not the disorder (Roth & Worthington, 2013). Roth and Worthington (2013) instructed the following:

> In speech–language pathology intervention, counseling is an essential aspect of the therapeutic process and fulfills several important functions:
> - It allows the clinician to impart basic information to clients and their families.
> - It provides opportunities for clients to verbalize feelings, fears, and uncertainties.
> - It serves as an emotionally supportive milieu in which clients are comfortable making attitudinal and behavioral changes. (p. 296)

> The nature of counseling includes three main phases:
> - Establishing the Therapeutic Relationship
>   ~ Clinician directed initially; establish parameters of relationship
> - Implementing Counseling Intervention
>   ~ "work" stage that addresses the primary deficits
>   ~ More non-directive
>   ~ Client encouraged to take more responsibility in setting the agenda of the therapeutic relationship

- Terminating the Therapeutic Relationship
  - ~ Clinician lays groundwork
  - ~ Client responsible for maintaining new behaviors learned

Understanding the reactions that students may have to their communication disability is valuable in the treatment of young people and interventions in the school settings. Students with disabilities often are labeled "uncooperative" or such, indicating that the problem lies in the student. However, consideration of the impact the student's disability may have on his or her social–emotional development allows for more of a therapeutic and supportive approach that will engender greater understanding and, in the long run, have a positive impact.

Flahive (2006) recommended a simple counseling mode that includes two stages: (a) informational, for gathering and giving information; and (b) personal adjustment. Methodologies in this model are included in Table 5.3.

Some of the possible emotional reactions to communicative disorders are presented in the following box. These reactions may be on the part of the student or the family. As the individual or family makes personal adjustments, emotions (anger, anxiety, fear, guilt) and defensiveness (denial, altruism, intellectualization, displacement) emerge (Flahive, 2006).

Client and Family Emotional Reactions to Communicative Disorders

- Grief
- Anger
- Depression
- Guilt
- Shame
- Anxiety
- Inadequacy
- Isolation

Source. Adapted from Roth and Worthington (2013).

Because of the emotional aspect of the situation, as well as the disorder itself, being intentional about how to present information is pivotal. Margolis (2004) recommended the following strategies for maximizing retention. These were modified to be useful for children aged 8 to 18 years.

- In giving advice, use concrete and positive instructions. "Tell the teacher if another child takes your paper" is more effective than "Don't hit other children in your class!"
- Use easy-to-understand language with short words and sentences.

TABLE 5.3. A Simple Counseling Model

Stage 1: Informational

Getting information: Use various question types.

- Use closed questions to discover facts.
- Use open-ended questions to discover understanding, concerns, values, expectations, goals, dissonance, perceived frustrations, and impediments.
  - Direct questions
    - ~ *How are things going?*
    - ~ *How did that feel?*
    - ~ *How well did that work?*
    - ~ *How do (or did) you . . . ?*
    - ~ *What happened next?*
    - ~ *Tell me why . . . ?*
    - ~ *Was there . . . ?*
    - ~ *What do you mean?*
    - ~ *Where are we now?*
    - ~ *Where do we go from here?*

  - Indirect questions
    - ~ *Are you okay?*
    - ~ *Tell me more.*
    - ~ *Tell me about . . .*
    - ~ *Tell me what you mean by . . .*
    - ~ *I hear you saying . . .*
    - ~ *Please describe . . .*
    - ~ *Show me how.*

Giving information: The client will not remember most of what is given.

- Recall depends on the client.
- Recall depends on the presentation.
- Recall depends on the clinician.
- Look for the balance between emotion and intellect.
- Effective strategies for presenting information:
  - Give advice as specific, concrete instructions.
  - Use short statements.
  - Present the most important information first.
  - Stress the importance of what you want remembered.

Stage 2: Personal adjustment

Things to remember:

- Loss is the intentional or unintentional parting with something of value.
- Deprivation or harm results from such a loss.
- Loss is individual; we react in our own ways.
- Clinician skills
  - Facilitating skills (listening, reflecting, affirming)
  - Referring skills (resources available to student and families)

Note. Adapted from "Counseling? But I Work in Schools!" by M. Flahive, 2006. Invited presentation, Annual Schools Conference, American Speech–Language–Hearing Association.

- Present the most important information first (the primacy effect). Often the most important information is a recommendation such as "Go to the school nurse or the office when this happens."
- Stress the importance of recommendations or other information that you want the student to remember: "Ask the teacher to repeat the directions one more time before you begin."
- Use the method of explicit categorization. Tell the student, "We are going to go over recommendations, then we will talk about your learning problem [diagnosis], then we will go over test results, then we will talk about how your learning problem may change in the future [prognosis]." Ask for questions before moving on to the next category.
- Repeat the most important information.
- Do not present too much information. Present only what the student needs to remember.
- Be sure you understand what students want from the evaluation and what their beliefs are concerning the problem. Specifically address the person's desires and beliefs.
- Supplement verbal information with written, graphical, and pictorial materials that the student can take home and share with parents or families.

When students are presenting these issues, consultation with the school psychologist and/or other mental health professionals is in order. Although counseling is a part of the therapeutic process for speech–language intervention, it may be that cotreatments are also indicated, particularly for students with emotional disturbance or other concomitant disabilities. The following counseling techniques were offered by Roth and Worthington (2013) as appropriate for communication disorders:

- Desensitization
- Relational
- Counterquestion
- Reframing
- Open-ended and indirect questions
- Role playing
- Empathetic listening
- Silence

The Concept of Good Practice

The term *good practice* is used in school-based programs (and other settings) to denote the use of research-based, effective, and measurable techniques to provide intervention or instruction for students who experience communication disorders and disabilities. In contrast to *best practice*, which establishes one intervention as better than all others, good practice can be defended successfully in legal proceedings and mediations. What is best for one student's circumstances may not be best for another. Professionals in speech and language and other educational pursuits are ethically bound to apply good practice principles to all their responsibilities, maintaining vigilance for new evidence and research. "To use only one [approach] . . . is not malpractice. To use more than one is merely enriched practice" (Rosenbek, 1984, p. 361).

Some speech–language pathologists teach classrooms of students with communication disorders, some may coteach with education specialists or general education teachers, and others use multiple approaches of pull-out therapy (i.e., removing children from a classroom for speech–language services), coteaching, and classroom support. There are many models based on students' needs, the culture of school districts, and the innovative ideas and skills of speech–language pathologists everywhere.

Good practice in schools requires speech–language pathologists to recognize the commonalties and differences among three macrodelivery systems—classroom instruction, conventional therapy, and collaborative intervention—and to choose the system or combination of systems most likely to result in progress for a student. Progress in speech–language skills was initially the goal of school-based speech–language pathologists, but with the reauthorization of IDEA 2004, this progress must be linked to academic achievement at a student's appropriate level (Brannen et al., 2000).

Speech–language pathologists may choose one or more of the macrodelivery systems or may alternate from one to another over the period of time a student receives speech–language services. "Service delivery is a dynamic concept and should change as the needs of the students change. No one service delivery model should be used exclusively during treatment" (ASHA, 1999, p. 58). State education agencies (SEAs), through their consultant staff and committees of speech–language pathologists from the field who volunteer their time, publish guidelines for assessment, eligibility, and service delivery for speech–language and hearing services in their states (see "Whom to Ask When You Have a Question on the Job" in Chapter 9).

Classroom instruction is typically delivered by a classroom teacher, a supervised instructional aide, or a subject area specialist (e.g., music, art, biology).

- In self-contained classrooms for students with special needs, this person can be a special education teacher or a speech–language pathologist.
- The intent in this setting is to teach students the grade- or age-level curriculum.
- Speech–language skills are directly or indirectly taught by a teacher as part of the subject area (e.g., auditory attention skills, opposites, descriptive labels, public speaking, oral book reports, noun–verb agreement in written discourse, vocabulary, narrative scripts).
- The instruction is directed to the ability level of the middle of the class, and although students earn individual grades on report cards, whole class improvement is sought. Individual instruction is planned; however, an entire class is taught subject matter together. This is challenging when students present a wide range of skills and abilities.

Conventional therapy is typically delivered in individual or small-group pull-out sessions in a small room or area designated for intervention.

- A speech–language pathologist or a supervised speech–language pathology assistant (SLPA) presents a task, introduces the directions, and often interacts directly with a student during the session.
- The intent in this setting is to modify a student's specific deficient communication skills. Some groups are composed of students who all have the same type of deficiency, whereas others may have different areas of need.
- The skills are selected from developmental hierarchies, standardized testing levels, and expectancies for children at various ages. Speech–language skills are directly modeled, encouraged, and reinforced using a wide range of materials and interest areas (e.g., toys, games, books, cards, practice workbooks).
- The therapy is designed for a particular student, and only that individual's improvement is measured and recorded.

Collaborative intervention is typically delivered in a classroom in a coteaching arrangement with a teacher or in a less distracting environment or pull-out session using materials from the classroom.

- A speech–language pathologist or speech–language pathology assistant (using tasks from the classroom) modifies the presentation or scaffolds a student's responses, or both to ensure success.
- The intent is to increase the amount of interaction a student has with the curriculum and thereby address deficient speech–language skills in a way that will rapidly affect grade-level work. New skills are taught using the student's areas of strength.
- Speech–language skills are directly modeled by a speech–language pathologist and peers and then encouraged, facilitated, and reinforced by a student's successful completion of the assigned curriculum. Examples include the following:
  - Class plays
  - Cooperative learning group assignments
  - Question-and-answer sessions
  - Journal writing
  - Recalling facts from a textbook
- The intervention is directed at the juncture of a student's deficient communication skills and the requirements of the curriculum. The intention is to create access to the curriculum through the development of skills and strategies that will assist the student in learning the grade-level curriculum and/or standards.
- Although advancement of the whole class is the focus, an individual student's progress on predetermined communication goals is also monitored and recorded. Service delivery options should focus on functional intervention based on students' needs.

All social, political, and professional influences shaping the practice of speech–language pathology in schools have emphasized consideration of the array of service delivery options when designing an intervention plan that will best meet a child's individual needs. These options may be combined and should be seen as flexible, depending on changing student needs. Regardless of the service delivery models deemed appropriate for any given student, the focus of the interventions should be functional and content based, integrating intervention with the meaningful activities of the child's educational experience (Whitmire, 2002).

Consistent with this concept of service, Vicker's (2009) article titled "The 21st Century Speech Language Pathologist and Integrated Services in Classrooms" suggested the term integrated services, as opposed to "push-in," and claimed that this service delivery model will yield more functional outcomes for students on the autism spectrum. (See more at www.iidc.indiana.edu/?pageId=495#sthash.EQh2abLk .dpuf.)

The Role of a Case Manager in Service Delivery

Decisions regarding the nature (direct or indirect), type (individual, group, or class), and location (resource room, classroom, home, or community) of service delivery are based on the need to provide a free appropriate public education (FAPE) for each student in the least restrictive environment that is consistent with a student's individual needs as documented on an IEP. The speech–language pathologist's role is to help an educational team in selecting, planning, and coordinating appropriate service delivery using various scheduling options throughout the duration of services. This begins with the initial placement decisions, extends through all reevaluations and special circumstances, and culminates when the student is dismissed from the speech–language program.

Speech–language pathologists serve as case managers for students whose primary need is communication or whose program is constructed around speech–language goals. They may also serve as case managers for students who are included in a general education program and monitored by one or more special educators, or if, for some reason, it makes sense for the speech–language pathologist to manage the case. As a case manager, a speech–language pathologist may

- serve as the point of contact for a student's special education services;
- schedule and coordinate both school-based and community-based assessments;
- assume a leadership role in developing an IEP or Individualized Family Service Plan (IFSP);
- help families in identifying available service providers and advocacy organizations within a community;
- coordinate, monitor, and ensure timely delivery of special education services, related services, or both;
- schedule and coordinate any requested reevaluation processes;

- facilitate the development of IDEA-required transition plans at any level; and
- coordinate services or provide consultation for students in charter schools, private schools, or other educational agencies off a school campus (ASHA, 1999).

If a speech–language pathologist is not a case manager, he or she remains an active team member, providing appropriate services to identified students and following through on all joint responsibilities coordinated by the case manager. The speech–language pathologist is the most knowledgeable person to select the service delivery model for speech–language services; however, input from parents and other team members is always considered. When selecting the service delivery model, the speech–language pathologist acting as case manager must give consideration to a student's goals and what the most efficient and effective way is to meet these goals, specifically considering the curriculum need, educational environment, and functional outcomes desired. Many times, it may seem that one type of service delivery model would be indicated, but a different approach will garner greater benefit. Speech–language pathologists must be prepared to discuss the rationale for recommending specific service delivery models. It should also be remembered that the recommendation should be based on student need and not convenience for the adults. Factors such as communication opportunities in authentic settings, students' needs and functioning level, proximity and benefit of peer modeling, access to and demands of the curriculum, student preference, and evidence base for the intervention provided should be considered.

Evidence-Based Decision Making in Service Delivery

The need for a full continuum of services for students with disabilities underlies the mandate to provide for a least restrictive environment (LRE) to all students with disabilities. For some students, the LRE required to ensure their free appropriate public education will be more restricted than that of others. Because there is no single special education setting that benefits all students, a number of options should be available with different levels of support and opportunities for independence. The review of special education models in this text, the mandate for providing access to the general education curriculum for students with disabilities (Karger, n.d.), and ASHA's (1996) position statement on inclusive practices enable speech–language pathologists to conclude that "an array of speech, language, and hearing services should be available in educational settings to support children and youths with communication disorders" (ASHA, 1996, p. 35).

How to Include Children With Disabilities

The Lieberman and Houston-Wilson (2002) model demonstrated options that allow students to move from a *totally inclusive environment* to a *segregated environment* for including students with disabilities. This gives teachers options to have their students move from one environment to another based on their unique needs. The following outlines the Lieberman and Houston-Wilson model of continuum of supports and placements (Lieberman & Houston-Wilson, 2002):

- Inclusion options
  - Full inclusion with no adaptations or support
  - Full inclusion with curriculum adaptations
  - Full inclusion with trained peer tutors
  - Full inclusion with teacher assistants
  - Full inclusion with interpreter
- Part-time segregated placement options
  - Split placement without support
  - Split placement with support
- Community-based options
  - Part-time (community- and school-based activities)
  - Full-time
- Full-time segregated placement options within a regular school district
  - Small group
  - One to one
- Segregated placement options
  - Day school for specific disabilities
  - Residential school for specific disabilities
  - Home schooling
  - Hospital setting

The IEP team's offer of FAPE in the LRE will identify the programs and services needed to meet the student's needs and implement the agreed-on goals. The speech–language pathologist will consider all aspects of the student's needs and services so as to provide services in a manner that will be effective and efficient (Gierut, 2001; Justice, Gillam, & Dolleghan, 2010; Moore, 2010).

> *Effectiveness:* Doing the right things.
> *Efficiency:* Doing things right.

During the course of his or her intervention, a student might participate in many different service delivery models. Research on effectiveness of various service delivery models is an emerging area in the field. Throneburg, Calvert, Sturm, Paramboukas, and Paul (2000) conducted a comparison study of three service delivery models, examining the results to determine the effect on vocabulary growth. In this study, the collaborative model was more effective for teaching curricular vocabulary than were the other two models. In addition, both collaborative and classroom-based models increased vocabulary skills to a significantly greater degree for students in the classroom who were not IDEA eligible than did receiving only regular instruction from the classroom teacher.

A 2010 systematic review addressed the following clinical question: What is the most effective system of speech–language intervention service delivery in a school-based setting? The conclusions reported were as follows:

(a) Collaborative-classroom models of service delivery sometimes may hold some advantages compared to pull-out programs, but the success of collaborative-classroom models may be determined by the target of treatment as well as the student's unique attributes. Further there is no evidence that one model holds a resource reduction advantage over another model. Though the collaborative-classroom model of service delivery is an option, it may not be appropriate for every child or every disorder.

(b) No one service delivery model is likely to work best for every child. Instead, different models may fit different children's needs, or a combination of service delivery models should be used; minimal evidence supports parent training for delivering language programs to children with autism. In as much as the evidence is weak, the use of parent training in such cases should be monitored regularly to assess its efficacy.

(c) Given the state of available research, [speech–language pathologists] should gather their own data and develop local solutions that work best for the school or district to meet the needs of their students. (Meline & Kauffman, 2010, p. 6)

Cirrin et al. (2010) also conducted a systematic review to examine the effects of service delivery on vocabulary development. In addition to the conclusions suggested in the Meline and Kaufman review, these authors commented,

[Speech–language pathologists] must provide services that are consistent with the requirements of federal policy. Service delivery models for students with disabilities are not directly addressed in IDEA (2004). Instead, IDEA states that children must be provided a free, appropriate public education in the least restrictive environment (LRE). LRE stipulates "to the maximum extent appropriate, children with disabilities are educated with nondisabled children" (34 C.F.R. § 300.550). This implies the need for an array of environments and services that meet the evolving learning requirements of children with disabilities. In addition, federal regulations state that "placement decisions must be based on the individual needs of each child with a disability. Public agencies, therefore, must not make placement decisions based on a public agency's needs or available resources, including budgetary considerations and the ability of the public agency to hire and recruit qualified staff." (Federal Register, 1999, p. 12471)

Schmitt and Justice (2011) observed, "School-based [speech–language pathologists] do not operate in a vacuum, nor do the students with whom they are concerned" (p. 11). They conceptualized schools as "complex host environments" in which services are provided:

The students with whom speech–language pathologists work are nested in classrooms; these classrooms, in turn, are nested in school buildings and districts. At each level of nesting, students have experiences that deeply influence their development. As professionals who are invested in changing students' developmental trajectories, we must be aware of features of the school environment that exert influence on students' development and thus may serve to reinforce or, alternatively, circumvent our efforts to serve students' needs. (p. 8)

By considering the following features that can significantly affect a student's development, speech–language pathologists can develop strategies to create environments supportive of student success (Schmitt & Justice, 2011).

Strategies to Maximize Quality Classrooms for Children With Language Impairment

Classroom quality and composition
- Assess the quality of the environment to ensure optimal conditions for students with language disorders in classroom management, emotional support, and instructional support.
- Recommend peer groupings for children with language disorders to ensure exposure to appropriate, language-rich models.
- Advocate for children with language disorders to be placed in high-quality classrooms.

Teacher self-efficacy
- Empower teachers by providing strategies to support language learning in the classroom.
- Be aware how the speech–language pathologist's own self-efficacy may affect speech–language intervention.

School climate
- Support teachers' efforts within the classroom.
- Partner with teachers and school-based personnel for challenging students.
- Develop a personal rapport with school personnel.

Functional Outcomes and the School-Based Speech–Language Pathologist

Functional outcomes are defined as "the results of care" in health-care circles and the "results of intervention" in educational settings. They are considered evidence of progress. The bottom line for all service delivery programs is contained in this question: When you provide services for a student with communication disorders, *how do you determine that the intervention has made a meaningful difference in that student's life*? This may seem like a straightforward question, but in identifying the tools and procedures speech–language pathologists need to find the answer, several other questions are raised:

- Should speech–language pathologists rely on standardized test scores to capture the improvement?
- Is it more authentic if persons other than speech–language pathologists report the changes they observe?
- Do others besides the student know whether the intervention was helpful?
- Do speech–language pathologists know whether most students with similar diagnoses make similar improvements? How can this be determined? If students do not make improvements, why not?
- Does the student's rate of improvement change with different speech–language pathologists?
- Does one service provider see results more quickly or more slowly than another? How can speech–language pathologists alter that rate?

Speech–language pathologists have responded to questions about individual effectiveness. Researchers and speech–language pathologists have investigated the efficacy of one clinical approach over another (Cirrin & Gillam, 2008; Fey et al., 2011; Loeb & Gillam, 2010; Schooling, Venediktov, & Leech, 2010). Speech–language pathologists have asked whether clients receiving a certain type of intervention scored higher on the same battery of tests at the end of a cycle of treatment. The profession has queried itself about whether clients actually had less communication difficulty at the conclusion of therapy, whether clients regressed or maintained their skills, or whether clients received direct assistance from a speech–language pathologist a second time. In schools, questions relate to the benefit of speech–language services on advancements in the curriculum and on functional skills, especially listening and speaking skills, as well as social skills. Parents and teachers are also frequently concerned with the potential loss of skills should a student be dismissed from services, and speech–language pathologists may question whether speech–language services are necessary if a student is receiving intense interventions through other service providers working on the same or similar goal area. These closely related and interesting questions do not adequately address an underlying concern in health care and education posed in the 21st century: Is there a research base to show that speech–language pathology services are valuable and necessary for persons with communication disorders?

According to ASHA, the answer is a strong yes. (See Evidence-Based Practice at www.asha.org/Research/EBP/ and Evidence Maps at www.asha.org/Evidence-Maps/.) Measuring and reporting that value and then linking it directly to a speech–language pathologist's intervention process is the purpose of functional outcomes. (See also "Evidence-Based Practice and PICO Statements" later in this chapter.) The Early Childhood Technical Assistance Center (2016) provided a clear definition of *child and family outcomes* and *functional outcomes* that can be applied to all ages:

What are child and family outcomes?

An outcome is a benefit experienced as a result of services and supports provided for a child or family. The fact that a service has been provided does not mean that a positive outcome has been achieved. Likewise, an outcome is not the same as satisfaction with the services received. The impact that services and supports have on the functioning of children and families constitutes the outcome. Consider the example of a child with autism who receives therapy services to increase communication skills. Receiving the services is not an outcome, but, if the child learns words he can use to convey his needs to others, then he has achieved an outcome. Similarly, a family may receive information about their child's disability. Although this information is a service provided to the family, it is not an outcome. However, if the information enables them to assist in their child's learning and development more effectively, then the family has achieved an outcome.

What is a functional outcome?

Functional outcomes describe children's mastery and appropriate application of behaviors, knowledge, and skills in a meaningful way in their everyday lives. The three child outcomes refer to actions that children need to be able to carry out and knowledge that children need to use in order to function successfully across a variety of settings. To be successful in these settings, it is important for children to be able to, for example, get along with others, follow the rules in a group, continue to learn new things, and take care of their basic needs in an appropriate way. Ultimately, achieving these outcomes will help children thrive at home, in school, and in many settings throughout their communities.

What's an outcome? (Rooney, 2009)

- Outcomes are the benefits that children and families experience as a result of early intervention/early childhood special education services.
- The three child outcomes, as measured for accountability purposes, are different from IFSP or IEP outcomes in that
  - the three child outcomes reflect global functioning in three broad areas of development (social–emotional, knowledge and skills, getting needs met), and
  - IFSP or IEP outcomes are specific to an individual child, based on his or her individual needs.
- Each outcome is a snapshot of
  - the whole child,
  - the status of the child's current functioning, and
  - functioning across settings and situations.

But what makes it *functional*?

- Functional outcomes
  - refer to things that are meaningful to the child in the context of everyday living, and
  - refer to an integrated series of behaviors or skills that allows the child to achieve the important everyday goals.

The entire IEP team must think about the functional outcomes that will be targeted for the student during the development of the IEP. The speech–language pathologist can contribute to this discussion by considering the broader picture of the functional parameters of the student's experience in schools. School-based speech–language pathologists must ensure that IEP goals are well written and truly reflect the outcomes desired for the student in order to demonstrate attainment of the skills needed to progress in the academic environment.

Well-written goals that list academic skills and the degree of improvement expected are required in schools. Speech–language pathologists in schools use these "smart goals," as they are often called, to clearly measure the positive impact of speech–language service delivery for children attaining the Common Core State Standards (Dodd, 2014b; Moore & Nishida, 2014). (See Chapter 4, "Development of Goals and Short-Term Objectives or Benchmarks.")

Functional Outcomes Defined as Results of Intervention

The employers, agencies, insurance companies, school boards, legislators, and clients who pay for speech–language services want to know when meaningful change can be attributed to the speech–language pathologist's services. These payers want to know consumers' functional outcomes. Because speech–language pathologists are primarily employees of a school district or a regional system, the idea of these agencies as service payers may seem out of place at first glance. Speech–language pathologists and all professionals who work in school systems must remember that taxpayers support all educational services. Documentation of accountability in schools helps in developing reasonable cost–benefit ratios for program planning purposes. Use of this documentation can be persuasive when seeking the value added by speech–language pathologists. Cost–benefit ratios and similar methods of accountability determine whether school-based speech–language pathologists are hired and receive the respect of fellow professionals, and how workloads are assigned.

Functional outcomes are not scores on standardized tests, nor are they lists of the objectives an individual has mastered. Instead, they are an accounting of the cost, time, and resulting restoration (or newly acquired performance) of the student. They are treatment tools that show the close relationship of service delivery to reimbursement in all work settings. The use of functional outcomes has been noted in the professional literature for several decades.

Functional outcomes for adults are measured in terms that reflect a life context beyond therapy. An adult may return to work or previous social activities, interact with family and friends, and be independent at selected tasks again after treatment for a communication disorder. These changes are called *restorative*. For children and youth, functional outcomes are framed in broader educational standards: progress in academics or a life-skills curriculum, friendship development, and age-appropriate interdependence and interaction with family members and care providers. Functional outcomes for children are habilitative, or newly acquired performances. An exception to this might be an acquired brain injury in which the focus of speech–language therapy would be to both reach previous functioning levels and learn new academic information at the student's grade level.

Functional Outcomes: Relationship to Health Care

School administrators watched the evolution of functional outcome measures in health care during the early 1990s. Speech–language pathologists providing services through health care were jarred by the sudden restrictions on reimbursement imposed by health maintenance organizations (HMOs) and fee capitation. In an even tighter managed care system introduced in 1998, speech–language pathologists were expected to share the risk rehabilitation of a client with the parties paying for the intervention services. Significant change in patient-functioning level was required in a prescribed amount of time to receive a maximum payment. If it took longer to reach the expected level of function, in most cases, there were no additional payments.

The restrictions required health-care administrators to accurately estimate the time it would take for speech–language pathologists to meet patients' goals; otherwise, speech–language pathologists or health-care facilities found it was not cost-effective to offer services. Insurance companies did not deny services, but they did deny payment. Speech–language pathologists were expected to know how many sessions would be needed for a client to reach a certain performance level. Conversely, they had to decide how much patient progress was reasonable in the amount of intervention time that was covered by insurance. Speech–language pathologists also needed to recognize clients who were not expected to make meaningful change in a short time and to judiciously not schedule them for therapy reimbursed by a particular payer. Although many speech–language pathologists decried this health-care environment as fiscally driven, it was apparent that this fiscal pressure fueled the need for accurate outcome data in speech–language pathology and audiology. Functional outcomes were measured therapeutically, fiscally, and emotionally in adult health care before the term reached the schools. Health-care reimbursement had a direct effect on school speech–language pathologist service models.

As a result of the Patient Protection and Affordable Health Care Act of 2010 (ACA), the health-care system continues to evolve and change how rehabilitative services, including speech–language pathology and audiology services, will be provided. As health-care reform rolls out, the goals of improving the patient experience of care (including quality and satisfaction), improving the health of populations, and reducing the per capita cost of health care, known as the Triple Aim, set the course. From the experience of colleagues in health care, school-based personnel can see the focus on "value," which realizes quality and safety based on the intersection of the use of evidence-based practice, functional outcomes and outcome data, and patients' needs and goals. This conceptualization of patient-centered care in health care may provide school-based personnel a view of how government agencies are beginning to examine outcomes and costs to realize outcomes or benefits for those covered under funded programs (Cornett, 2012). As speech–language pathologists in schools, we are members of a broader community of colleagues who provide services in other settings. Attending to the trends in these settings is wise, as it may preview impending future changes in schools.

Functional Outcomes as Reflected in IDEA 2004

According to IDEA 2004, all special educators are mandated to link intervention with a general education curriculum and proficiency in core subject areas. Furthermore, special educators must report student progress to parents on a schedule that is similar to that of general educators and address progress in the curriculum on an IEP. IDEA 2004 requires that educators write comprehensive goals for students; they do not have to write short-term objectives or benchmarks. Some states continue to write both goals and objectives or benchmarks.

Speech–language pathologists may write short-term objectives for improving a child's auditory processing skills to build a foundation for curriculum skills, or they may write goals to show the level of spelling and literacy skills that are found in the grade-level Common Core State Standards. Goals that relate to academic or school behaviors identify functional outcomes, whereas those that relate to underlying processing deficits usually do not. Benchmarks and short-term objectives serve as points along a path to a goal. If the early parts of intervention are focused on changing underlying skills only, a speech–language IEP may not appear to be connected with the student's use of these new skills. Speech–language pathologists need to link skills with daily functional activities from the beginning. If speech–language pathologists use a method of sampling improvements called progress monitoring, it is not necessary to write lengthy statements of objectives the student will "touch" along the path toward his or her goal. Examples of functional outcomes written as measurable annual goals can be found in Chapter 4.

Four Basic Questions for Functional Outcomes

The systematic search for practical intervention benchmarks has inspired speech–language pathologists in all settings to use functional outcomes. The four basic questions illustrated in Figure 5.1 characterize these functional outcomes:

- Question 1 asks, "How much time does it take to show meaningful change?"
- Question 2 queries, "How will each assessment streamline the costs of serving this student?"
- Question 3 poses, "Have I selected the most cost-effective way to provide this service?"
- Question 4 asks, "Can I prove that the services I provided made a difference for this student?"

By answering one or more of these questions with confidence, the speech–language pathologist has ventured that much closer to restructuring services around a student's

after-reading

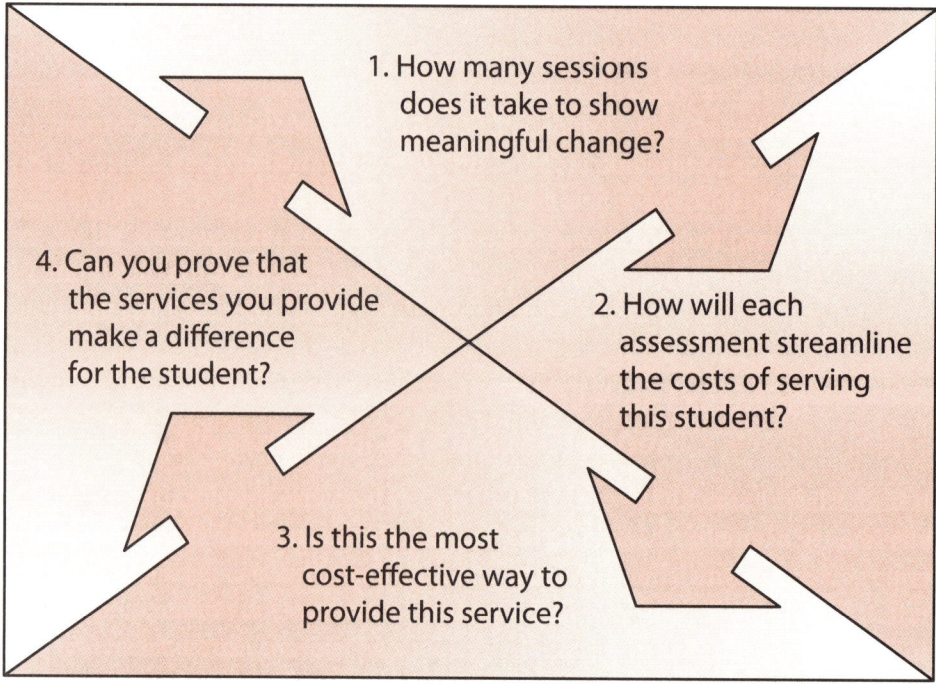

FIGURE 5.1. Four essential questions for functional outcomes in school-based service.

and payer's expectancies, which leads to greater customer satisfaction and more consistent remuneration for speech–language pathologists. Although tying speech–language services so closely to the payment system has been considered lacking in professionalism, it is precisely this results-based approach that demonstrates the speech–language pathologist's value in health care and schools. Keeping track of the individual's functional outcomes (academic learning), instead of reporting more trivial changes in discrete communication skills or comparing scaled scores on pre- and posttests, has demonstrated that the speech–language pathologist was applying resources wisely.

Speech–language pathologists in schools must align their intervention with students' academic or developmental progress. Results must document increased functional performance levels for students who receive speech–language services. Increasingly, the functional outcome that is needed is academic achievement. For students with more significant disabilities, other types of functional outcomes will be sought and measured, which is equally functional for them. This means that the assessments to determine areas of need should also be functional (see Figure 5.2). The measure of value-added service is currently realized in terms of grades, promotion, participation in the academic curriculum, a high school exit exam, and a high school diploma, as well as social skills and transition skills.

Functional Communication Assessment Summary

Functional communication skills are forms of behavior that express needs, wants, feelings, and preferences that others can understand when individuals learn functional communication skills, and they are able to express themselves without resorting to problem behavior or experiencing communication breakdown. Functional communication includes spoken and written communication, gestures and pointing, and other forms of communication.

This Functional Communication Assessment Summary may be used to document the functional communication skills of any student in the education setting and may be helpful when examining the educational impact of a suspected communication impairment.

Functional Communication Categories include:

Communicative Interaction

Evidenced by: initiation, topic maintenance turn-taking, opening/closing conversations

Communicative Intention

Evidenced by: requesting objects/actions, commenting on objects/actions, etc.

Communicative Methods

Evidenced by: use of one or more modes of communication (e.g., verbal, manual sign, AT or AAC system, gestures, pointing)

Comprehension of Language

Evidenced by: appropriate actions or communicative responses indicating comprehension of what others say, sign, or show

Effect on Educational Performance

Student demonstrates communication skills adequate for participation in current educational setting

Data collected from known and novel communication partners in a variety of settings should be used when examining functional communication. Data should reflect interactions with persons other than the speech–language pathologist.

(continues)

FIGURE 5.2. Functional Communication Assessment Summary.

Functional Communication Assessment Summary

Name _____ Date _____

This form may be used to document functional communication skills in the education setting and may be helpful when evaluating students when a valid comparison to a normative sample cannot be made or a student has significant impairments. Data collected from a variety of communication partners in a variety of settings should be used to complete this form.

Communicative Interaction Evidenced by: initiation, topic maintenance turn-taking, opening/closing conversations	☐ Successful	☐ Usually Successful	☐ Frequently Unsuccessful	☐ Not Successful
	Data Sources: Describe Performance:			
Communicative Intention Evidenced by: requesting objects/actions, commenting on objects/actions, etc.	☐ Successful	☐ Usually Successful	☐ Frequently Unsuccessful	☐ Not Successful
	Data Sources: Describe Performance:			
Communicative Methods Evidenced by: use of one or more modes of communication (e.g., verbal, manual sign, AT or AAC system, gestures, pointing)	☐ Successful	☐ Usually Successful	☐ Frequently Unsuccessful	☐ Not Successful
	Data Sources: Describe Performance:			
Comprehension of Language Evidenced by appropriate actions or communicative responses indicating comprehension of what others say, sign, or show	☐ Successful	☐ Usually Successful	☐ Frequently Unsuccessful	☐ Not Successful
	Data Sources: Describe Performance:			
Effect on Educational Performance Student demonstrates communication skills adequate for participation in current educational setting.	☐ Successful	☐ Usually Successful	☐ Frequently Unsuccessful	☐ Not Successful
	Data Sources: Describe Performance:			

Virginia Department of Education, Office of Special Education and Student Service.

FIGURE 5.2. *(continued)*

Clinically Significant Change

Functional outcomes must be the paramount product of speech–language pathologists' planned intervention for students. Speech–language pathologists must design measurable goals and select meaningful benchmarks for students, families, and the systems educating students. Speech–language pathologists want to be sure that their work results in clinically significant change for individuals with communication disorders. The classic criteria for clinically significant change from Bain and Dollaghan (1991) are widely cited in the field. They proposed that clinically significant change must be

- due to intervention, not maturation;
- real, not random; and
- important, not trivial.

Bain and Dollaghan's (1991) guidelines continue to help speech–language pathologists in selecting consumer-driven goals. The documentation of clinical significance is used in prospective, online, and retrospective decision making for service delivery in schools. IEPs must be designed to confer educational benefit. What better way to do this than to use functional outcomes?

Unlike the fiscally based decisions of cost and length of speech–language services, functional outcomes (also called *performance outcomes*) evolve directly from a speech–language pathologist's assessment of a student's functioning level. Functional or performance outcomes are the best estimate of the student's anticipated communicative status. Functional outcomes for students actually vary little by practice setting because all the statements focus on how individuals will have more effective and satisfying lives. In education, curricular goals are the focus; in health care, life, or the workplace, expectancies are emphasized. Schools use both. Eventually functional outcomes may actually draw together education and health care and also draw together private and public sector speech–language pathologists in common benchmarks and common agreement of termination points for therapy. Functional outcomes have a universal appeal to interdisciplinary teams, families, and payers (i.e., insurance agencies and state taxpayers). When students' IEPs are designed to confer educational benefit, functional outcomes are easy to document and ensure clinically significant change. Requirements to develop Individualized Transition Plans (ITPs) for students once they turn 16 years of age reflect IDEA's commitment to ensuring functional outcomes for students in postsecondary years. Increasing state and federal focus on indicators such as drop-out rate, graduation rate, and postsecondary indicators for education and employment demonstrates the importance of functional considerations leading to positive outcomes for students well beyond their school experience.

Evidence-Based Practice and PICO Statements

Evidence-based practice (EBP) has been defined as "the conscientious, explicit, and judicious use of current best evidence in making decisions about the care of individual patients . . . [by] integrating clinical expertise with the best available external clinical evidence from systematic research" (Dollaghan, 2004). EBP derives from evidence-based medicine and has been the standard in the medical field. The use of EBP in the delivery of services was deemed necessary and ethical by ASHA (2005b).

Speech–language pathologists need to select appropriate intervention strategies for the students who receive speech and language services at their schools. Appropriate speech and language interventions will weigh the student's age, interests, and skill level; the clinician's expertise; and the current research in the field on the specific communication disorder that was assessed. This process leads the school-based speech–language pathologist toward evidence-based practice and more defensible goals, objectives, and IEPs.

The process is now taught in graduate programs to enable first-year clinicians to be fully prepared for their responsibilities in schools. One widely used approach, called PICO, has helped clinicians frame four important questions: What is the population? What is the proposed intervention? How does it compare to one or several alternatives? What are the expected functional communication abilities? The initials refer to *population*, *intervention*, *comparison*, and *outcome*. The four categories are written in this order as a four-part question. Here is an example:

> Are 8-year-old students with resistant [w/r] substitutions more or less likely to remediate in individual or pull-out treatment in one 30-minute session per week? (See Table 5.4.)

The first challenge is determining the specificity of each cell. Should we consider the number of years of previous therapy? Should we specify the size of the group? Should we use a vocalic /r/? Should we accept any improvement in [w/r] substitution? In any position? In reading but not conversational speech? Sixty percent of the time?

The second challenge requires the clinician to spend considerable time searching and reading a large amount of data or, perhaps more likely, to discover there is only a small number of articles available, and it may be necessary to expand the criteria to all age groups or specify an alternative strategy to decide on the most promising evidence-based practice. The data may not be available yet. The PICO statement must be adjusted to fit the student, speech–language pathologist's skills, and desired functional outcome.

TABLE 5.4. PICO Categories

Population	Intervention	Comparison	Outcome
Characteristics, conditions	Types, approaches, amount of time	Alternatives for this population	Degree of functionality
Eight-year-old students with resistant [w/r] substitutions in all three positions in words	One 30-minute pull-out session per week for 18 weeks	Individual sessions versus group sessions	/r/ used in initial position in words in conversational speech 80% of the time

Today's speech–language pathologists are committed to using evidence-based practice for the following reasons:

1. *Accountability*. Evidence-based practice (EBP) means conducting therapy that can assist students in meeting standards and functional goals.
2. *Due process*. Using EBP makes the work legally defensible.
3. *Student–clinician time*. Being efficient in treatment means that everyone's time is maximized, that students are not in therapy longer than they need to be, and that the clinician is available for the next student or project that needs his or her attention.
4. *Challenges from the outside*. EBP builds a response to questions and challenges.
5. *Parent, teacher, and student satisfaction*. EBP will mean increased satisfaction with speech–language pathology services and increased consumer satisfaction.
6. *Enhanced professionalism*. Because EBP is the standard for the field, the evidence will be there that the speech–language pathologist is conducting himself or herself according to the highest professional standards.

Linking Services to Consumer Satisfaction

Consumer satisfaction is a fitting conclusion to a discussion of functional outcomes. Speech–language pathologists may be unaware of how their services appear to consumers. In infant and preschool services provided by schools, children and families are primary consumers. School-aged consumers also include teachers, administrators, peers, and state legislatures. They are all seeking satisfaction, often from diverse outcomes.

When a speech–language assessment indicates the need for an intervention program, a parent wants to know the best program available for his or her child. Finding what is best for each client means focusing on consumer satisfaction. "Best" is a thoughtful combination of what functional outcomes are desired, when and where services are provided, and the amount of time and resources needed. IDEA 2004 requires schools to provide intervention that is of educational benefit for a student. It does not require that the "best" or maximum intervention be sought. School-based personnel know that "best" is a highly subjective standard. IDEA 2004 and state education agencies (SEAs) require highly qualified personnel to use research-based practices and adequate resources to ensure that all students have access to the curriculum and can benefit from their education. Speech–language pathologists recognize that this may translate into good practice instead of best practice.

Selecting more effective interventions, with some individual variance, is easier if we use the academic outcome data gathered on elementary- and secondary-level students. All students in special education should receive appropriate services resulting in clinically significant change and educationally functional outcomes. A parent's or guardian's observation of student change subsequent to services showed 97% satisfaction with speech–language services in schools, and 92% believed there was improvement (Whitmire, Karr, & Mullen, 2000; Whitmire, Rivers, Mele-McCarthy, & Staskowski, 2014).

Though more data are needed to reach broader conclusions, speech–language pathologists who respond to the four basic questions in Figure 5.1 for students on their caseload will be able to address consumer satisfaction. Outcome data for school-age children continue to be collected nationwide from school-based speech–language pathologists serving individuals with communication disorders (www.asha.org/NOMS/).

Additional Resources

The following are excellent Web sites for speech–language pathologists and RTI:

- RTI Action Network: "Speech–Language Pathologists and RTI" by Barbara Ehren and Maureen Staskowski (www.rtinetwork.org/professional/rti-talks/transcript/talk/31)
- Georgia Organization of School Based Speech–Language Pathologists: "Speech–Language Pathologist's Role in RTI" (www.tcse.us/wp-content/uploads//2011/01/SLPsRoleRTITiers2011.pdf)

Also see the ASHA Web site and put "response to intervention" in the search engine. Convention presentations and other resources are available there.

The following are some excellent references for service delivery models:

- *Story Grammar Marker* by Rooney Moreau and Fidrych-Puzzo (1994) (https//:mindwingconcepts.com/)
- *The Writing Lab Approach to Instruction and Intervention*, by Nickola Nelson, Christine M. Bahr, and A. M. Van Meter (2004)
- *Ten Steps to Writing Better Essays*, by J. Montgomery and N. Kahn (2007)
- *What's Your Story?*, by J. Montgomery and N. Kahn (2005)
- "EmPOWER: A Strategy for Helping Students With Language Disorders Learn to Write Expository Text," by B. D. Singer and A. S. Bashir (2004), in Language and Literacy Learning (pp. 239–272), edited by E. Silliman and L. C. Wilkinson, New York, NY: Guilford.
- http://es-learningsupport.ism-online.org/2011/03/04/empower-a-method-for-teaching-expository-writing-by-bonnie-singer-and-anthony-bashir/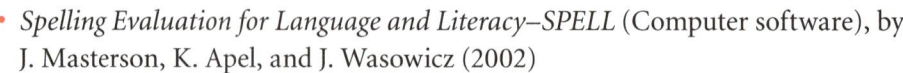
- *Spelling Evaluation for Language and Literacy–SPELL* (Computer software), by J. Masterson, K. Apel, and J. Wasowicz (2002)
- *Conversation Framework*, by B. Hoskins and K. Noel (2011)
- Michelle Garcia Winner's social thinking models (www.socialthinking.com/home)
- *Spelling Evaluation for Language and Literacy–2* (SPELL-2) (Computer software), by J. Masterson, K. Apel, and J. Wasowicz (2006)

- *How Much Is Enough? The Intensity Evidence in Language Intervention* (ASHA convention presentation), by T. Ukrainetz et al. (2008)
- *How Much Is Enough? Dosage in Child Language Intervention* (ASHA convention presentation), by R. Gillam, E. Baker, and L. Williams (2012)

Within the specialization of each disorder practice area, there are also counseling resources available. For example, Wolter, DiLollo, and Apel (2006) presented "A Narrative Therapy Approach to Counseling: A Model for Working With Adolescents and Adults With Language-Literacy Deficits" and Bill Murphy's DVD on *Dealing With Guilt and Shame* produced by the Stuttering Foundation of America (www.stutteringhelp.org/).

The following are excellent resources on counseling skills:

- *Counseling Skills for Speech–Language Pathologists and Audiologists*, by Lydia V. Flasher and Paul T. Fogel (2004)
- *Counseling Persons With Communication Disorders and Their Families*, by David Luterman (2017)

Professional journals and other resources focus on evidence-based topics and evidence-based systematic reviews, including ASHA's Practice Portal, which contains evidence-based maps on a variety of clinical topics (see www.asha.org/Evidence-Maps/). Evidence-based reviews are also provided through Pearson at SpeechandLanguage.com (www.speechandlanguage.com/ebp-briefs).

CHAPTER 6

Providing Successful Intervention and Access to Curricula

● *In This Chapter*

This chapter introduces issues that surround and affect service delivery. One section focuses on managing caseloads and workloads. Service delivery is discussed in the form of specific intervention models that are based on American Speech-Language-Hearing Association guidelines, incorporate both direct and indirect forms of contact with students, and link to the curriculum. Helpful grouping strategies and specific models for consultation and collaboration are described. Examples of literacy support from the speech-language pathologist in schools and preschool programs, plus a focus on secondary students, are included.

● *Chapter Questions*

1. Why is there a feeling of urgency in professionals when working with pre-schoolers? How does that urgency affect the delivery of services? Plan a series of questions to ask a parent to help you understand how the child communicates at home.
2. Should high school students receive speech-language services if they previously have had more than 3 years of service in the elementary grades? Defend your answer.
3. From your viewpoint, discuss the effect of year-round education (YRE) on all students, students with disabilities, and the professionals who work with them, especially speech-language pathologists. Would YRE affect functional outcomes? In what way?
4. What factors would you consider when deciding how to group students for intervention? Select one grouping arrangement described in the text and plan a lesson using it.
5. Collaborative consultation assumes cooperativeness among professionals. Cooperation does not always occur in schools. Why is it important to have a plan to handle resistance? What are some of the causes of resistance to

new service delivery models? Suggest what might be done when resistance to the process exists.

6. Practice writing a speech and language goal that is linked to a child's general education curriculum. If you do not know how, what resources might you tap to locate the curriculum?

7. Find the documents that give guidance on the increase of inclusive programs for preschoolers. Why would the federal government encourage such placements if a school district does not have inclusive preschool programs?

8. Interview a high school student about how speech and language services help support his or her academic needs. Ask the student what his or her opinion is of the services and the service delivery model.

Caseload, Workload, and Service Delivery

Caseload refers to the number of individual students for whom the speech–language pathologist is providing services at any point in time. There are many service delivery models operating within a single caseload. Speech–language pathologists are responsible for providing appropriate services to all students on their caseloads. Speech–language pathologists in schools have the same responsibilities as all employees in a school district. They must enforce the academic standards of state education agencies (SEAs) and local education agencies (LEAs) to enable students with communication disabilities to be successful in school. The American Speech–Language–Hearing Association (ASHA), researchers, and speech–language pathologists in schools have developed many effective service delivery methods that speech–language pathologists may use with confidence.

Service delivery takes on many forms in the school environment (discussed in detail in Chapter 5). Speech–language pathologists should not only use a variety of methods and delivery models but also be able to categorize or describe them to fellow professionals to build administrative support at the school or district level. Using and advocating for a range of service delivery models promotes new ideas and gains support for speech–language pathologists as school team members. These models also guide speech–language pathologists to become an integral part of their school team, enabling them to apply their expertise to the goals of the school and the curriculum. Teachers do not have caseloads; they have one or more classes they are responsible for teaching. Speech–language pathologists (and some other related services providers) select and manage caseloads. Typically, the term *caseload* is exclusively used in schools. Speech–language pathologists base most of their clinical decisions on information they glean from three places: their graduate programs, their clinical experience, and the opinions of their colleagues (Zipoli & Kennedy, 2005). This may be viewed as contrary to the principles of evidence-based practice (EBP), in which professionals should use research evidence, sound theory, and client needs (Gillam & Gillam, 2006). Therefore, the effective school-based speech–language pathologist must give careful thought to the service delivery environment. This chapter will offer other ways for professionals to make clinical decisions in the educational workplace.

ASHA Workload Approach

In 2002, ASHA promoted a new concept in caseload and service delivery management: *workload.* Central to this approach is the understanding that although providing services to students is the main function of a speech–language pathologist, there are many other duties and responsibilities that are demanding, necessary, and time-consuming. These activities are accounted for in Figure 6.1.

The ASHA position statement on workload (www.asha.org/policy/ PS2002-00122/) does not include a recommended maximum caseload number. Any arbitrary caseload maximum is inconsistent with a workload analysis approach to setting caseload standards. Instead, it is necessary for education agencies to consider how the amount of time available in each school day, week, or month can be

Workload

Administer new assessments

Analyze response to intervention

Supervise assistants, interns, or clinical fellows

Attend school or district meetings

Travel to other sites or student homes

Perform interprofessional practice on-site

Provide parent education and aide training

Screen for speech, language, or hearing
   issues on-site

Attend mediations and due process
   hearings

Observe classrooms

Attend required legal and clinical
   training

Assist with student projects and
   special events

Analyze speech data

Create materials for intervention

Caseload

Provide direct intervention for students

Work with teachers and core curriculum

Reassess students on caseload
(3-year reevaluation)

FIGURE 6.1. Workload vis-à-vis caseload of speech–language pathologists.

divided across services to children. It is also important to consider that the expanding responsibilities imposed on school speech–language pathologists reduce the time available for face-to-face services to students. Furthermore, setting a caseload maximum number may be misused as a caseload minimum. Speech–language pathologists who work with students with high needs may be functioning at capacity yet serve significantly fewer students than an arbitrary maximum number because of the array of intensive direct and indirect services their students need.

Traditionally, the workload of school speech–language pathologists has been conceptualized as being almost exclusively synonymous with *caseload*. Caseload is more accurately conceptualized as only one part of speech–language pathologists' total workload. The job is much more than the number of students with Individualized Education Programs (IEPs) or Individualized Family Service Plans (IFSPs). In some school districts, the speech–language pathologist's caseload may also include students who do not have identified disabilities and who receive prereferral intervention and other services designed to help prevent future difficulties with language learning and literacy. Speech–language pathologists may also serve as case managers for all or some students on their caseload, which adds significant responsibilities and time for writing and managing IEPs, as well as ensuring compliance with special education regulations. *Workload* refers to all activities required and performed by school-based speech–language pathologists. Workloads include considerable time for direct services to students. Workloads also include many other activities necessary to support students' education programs, implement evidence-based practices for school speech–language services, and ensure compliance with the Individuals With Disabilities Education Improvement Act (IDEA 2004) and other mandates.

ASHA members have reported that large caseloads constrain the speech–language pathologist's ability and capacity to engage in the expanded roles that are necessary for meeting the individual needs of today's diverse and complex student population. Research has indicated that large speech–language caseloads are related to poorer student outcomes and to the availability of fewer service options for students with disabilities (American Occupational Therapy Association, American Physical Therapy Association, & American Speech–Language–Hearing Association, 2014; Mullen, 2000). This suggests that large caseloads impede the intent of IDEA from being fully implemented, given that federal legislation mandates the use of a continuum of services tailored to students' individual needs and collaboration between special education and general education teachers.

Workload and caseload size issues for school speech–language pathologists are difficult to resolve because of the complex interaction of the many factors that influence the number of children and adolescents speech–language pathologists serve. School personnel, including administrators, human resource departments, collective bargaining units, site personnel, and special education staff, should work in partnership to ensure that caseload size does not negatively affect speech–language pathologists' ability to meet the needs of their students. Setting caseload standards on the basis of an analysis of speech–language pathologists' total workload activities can help ensure that students with disabilities receive the services they need to support their education programs.

Caseload size remains the biggest influence on the work of a speech–language pathologist, but through the workload approach, the other activities are also recognized as being part of the duties and responsibilities that need to occur during the workday.

Speech–language pathologists around the country have adopted this model and adjusted it to what works for them. Their success stories are also available on the ASHA Web site, as are worksheets, frequently asked questions, and other resources.

Caseload Size

Examining school-based speech–language pathologists' typical caseloads by day and by week has long been considered a factor in choosing models of service delivery. The authors believe that this factor should not be the focus. ASHA's "2014 Schools Survey" (ASHA, 2014a) reported a median average caseload size ranging from 35 to 60 in this survey. The authors and others recognize that individual speech–language pathologists across the country may have caseload sizes that range in further extremes than is reported here. States, not federal law, determine their caseload minimums and maximums, thus the extremely wide variations. Caseload size and management have been the number-one issue of concern for speech–language pathologists in schools for many years. Advocating for a reduction in the size of caseloads for public school speech–language programs is a politically and economically volatile issue because of competing needs and limited resources.

Good practice and good service delivery, however, are not based on political and economic issues. Regardless of caseload size, consumers expect speech–language pathologists to make professional decisions that must include choosing interventions wisely, matching students' performance levels with available services, and measuring progress with functional outcomes. (See "Functional Outcomes and the School-Based Speech–Language Pathologist" in Chapter 5.) Nevertheless, speech–language pathologists do need to advocate for reasonable caseloads so that they can perform their duties. As will be discussed in "Professional Organizations" in Chapter 9, maintaining a political voice through membership in professional organizations and being on alert for proposed legislation are speech–language pathologists' responsibilities. Vigilance and tenacity in reshaping state caseload maximums do reap benefits for students and their families.

Although maintaining a lower caseload may allow speech–language pathologists to schedule more frequent or intensive services for some children (ASHA, 2006a), data on improved outcomes in these circumstances are not collected in a standardized manner from state to state. Data collection is a state task; it is not federally managed or funded. Therefore, such data have not yet been used to persuade lawmakers to reduce caseload size nationwide. Speech–language pathologists also need to be vigilant in the management of their caseloads by ensuring that they are using current practices and service delivery models and exiting students who no longer need services (Moore-Brown, Nishida, & Laverty-Reeves, 2003).

Scheduling and Organizing Services

Caseload size can significantly influence the service delivery choices that speech–language pathologists make; however, individual student needs must be the overriding factor. This can be anxiety producing and requires flexibility from everyone involved. No single method of delivering services is appropriate for the entire intervention period, as student needs, demands, and expectations will change as the years progress. Service delivery model changes are inherent in the scheduling process and should be based on students' needs, not on the time of year, space, or other external factors. Practically, of course, all these factors must be worked into a schedule. For example, a student may need one-to-one service for a phonological disorder for 6 weeks, then an in-class model to begin the generalization process with meaningful classroom-based cues for 8 weeks, and finally a once-a-month "drop-in group" (i.e., checkup) for reinforcement for the remainder of the school year.

Speech–language pathologists need to be able to make adjustments whenever necessary. As long as a student is making steady progress toward IEP goals, the existing service model may be maintained. Lack of progress mandates a need for change in one or more aspects of service delivery. A considerable advantage of a school-based service model is the many options available that are not found in hospital programs, day clinics, or private practice settings. In these other settings, the pool of typical peers is simply not there, and the learning environment provides limited opportunities for naturalistic practice.

Organizing service models by communication disability is a frequently seen practice in schools. The authors believe that this approach restricts creativity in service delivery for speech–language pathologists and students. ASHA Practice Portal provides more information (www.asha.org/practice-portal/). Variations in service delivery are recommended throughout this text. Children participate in school programs with a variety of peers and partners. Grouping students exclusively according to their disability will not provide them with good communication models, so speech–language pathologists are encouraged to consider age, disability, grade, and peer variations when setting up groupings.

Figures 6.2 and 6.3 provide practice advice on this aspect of the speech–language pathologist's responsibilities. Table 6.1 offers ideas for how to schedule programs in elementary and secondary schools and programs for speech–language pathologists who serve multiple school sites. Schedules must allow for some assessment and meeting time and use every available minute of the school day to serve students. Direct interventions to students generally will occupy the largest portion of a speech–language pathologist's day, although other activities, such as assessment, meetings, report-writing, IEP preparation, professional development, and teacher consultation, will also consume time during the week. There are several different types of schedules that must be created by speech–language pathologists each year. They serve as the evidence of delivery of services as specified in student IEPs. Each schedule has a distinct purpose, a different audience, and a corresponding format. Some features will be found in every schedule, whereas others are unique to a specific format. Schedules with student names on them are considered a part of confidential records and are not shown to unauthorized persons. Types of schedules used in school programs are outlined in Table 6.1.

Despite the pressure to use every available minute for intervention, speech–language pathologists must wisely allocate time for assigned duties that are expected of all school personnel.

What to Do First!

Get a list of speech–language students.
Remember to check with teachers if you are missing anyone.
Make your own assessment of student needs.

Read the Files!

Determine the types of needs and how you need to serve the students to meet those needs.

Building the Schedule

Ascertain what history you need.
Outline the day.
Put first things first: What time blocks do you need?

- Assessment
- Meeting
- Individual sessions
- Response to intervention
- Collaboration
- District and/or other meetings

FIGURE 6.2. Creating your schedule.

Tips for Creating Your Schedule

The referral process is critically important for management of your workload, caseload, schedule, and life!

- Don't think that your schedule is going to be the same every week. Make a monthly and/or quarterly schedule.
- Be able to describe why you are managing your schedule this way. Have individual meetings if necessary.
- Remember that you are the one who makes this decision, but what you do affects others.
- Talk to your principal ahead of time!
- Don't tie yourself into 2 × 30 for every student!
- Examine groupings.
- Be flexible!

FIGURE 6.3. Scheduling tips to consider.

TABLE 6.1. Creating Schedules for Service Delivery

Type of schedule	Purpose	Audience	Format
Daily	Used to record daily activities at a specific location	Education team, site administrator	By time and names
Daily with assistant	Used to record daily activities of the speech–language pathologist and assistants at a specific location	Education team, site administrator, assistants, supervisors	By time and names
Weekly	Used to track weekly locations for services if more than one location; week at a glance if one location Important for block scheduling and monitoring students	Speech–language pathologist, education team, district administrators, parents	By time and names
Weekly with assistant	Same as above with assistants added when appropriate	Same as above, classified staff administrators, assistants	By time and names
Monthly	Kept for documenting monthly responsibilities, such as school staff meetings, out-of-district or agency meetings, district meetings, professional growth conferences, continuing education units, and so on Important if using block scheduling, curriculum-based instruction (off campus), or monthly monitoring and checking	Same as above	By month and activity; usually includes contact information, such as names and phone numbers
Yearlong	Primarily used for documenting long-range planning, evidence of contacts with agencies, out-of-district commitments, and so on May have screening dates, Individualized Education Programs, triennial reevaluations, school-based teams for prereferral, and special education interventions	Administrators, hearing officers, court orders, subpoenaed records	By activity and contact time expended; may include names of others at meetings

Alternate School Schedules and Year-Round Education

Traditional school calendars were established to meet the needs of an agrarian society in which entire families needed to devote uninterrupted time to harvesting crops each year. Although we are no longer driven by crop harvests, the traditional school calendar is still in wide use today. As part of school reform and greater consideration of time in schools, alternate schedules have been implemented in a variety of ways. These include varying time schedules within a traditional calendar and varying school schedules. Year-round education (YRE) may provide an alternative to the traditional 180-day, September-through-June schedule. Some school districts have adjusted their start and end times to start school in August and end in May because of state testing in the spring. Others have examined their schedules to vary timing during the day, moving to block schedules to enable students to have longer periods of time for classes so that teachers can go deep into subject areas and not be affected by time limitations. Block schedules and other time variations are seen more at secondary levels than at elementary ones. Speech–language pathologists find that these alternate schedules can allow for greater flexibility in service delivery.

YRE sites reorganize the school year to provide more continuous learning by dividing summer vacation into shorter, more frequent vacations throughout the year. It does not eliminate the summer vacation, but reduces it and redistributes it as vacation, or intersession, time during the school year. Students attending a year-round school attend the same classes and receive the same instruction as students on a traditional calendar. The year-round calendar is organized into instructional periods and vacation weeks that are more evenly balanced across 12 months than they are in the traditional school calendar. The balanced calendar minimizes the learning loss that may occur during a typical 3-month summer vacation (Alexander, Entwisle, & Steffel Olson, 2007; Huebner, 2010; National Association of Year-Round Education, www.nayre.org/index.html).

YRE schools use several calendar variations that typically schedule three quarters of the students to attend "on track," while one quarter of the students are "off track." Although YRE was begun, in part, to maximize facility usage in crowded buildings, academic benefits may be realized for students, especially those in need of special education, because of shorter nonschool breaks.

Educators generally follow the same track or schedule as their students, but scheduling becomes more difficult for support services providers. Speech–language pathologists need a work calendar that provides service to students throughout the school year. Some solutions include the following:

- Speech–language pathologists' contracts and salaries are extended, covering between 200 and 230 days of the school year.
- Certain days of the year are identified as "no speech" days and are nonwork days for speech–language pathologists, such as the first week of school, the 3 days before the Thanksgiving holiday, the week before the winter holiday break, or the last 2 weeks of the school year.
- Speech–language pathologists coordinate schedules to provide coverage for each other during these off-track times.
- Speech–language pathologists work a 4-day workweek.

Other creative solutions have been used to ensure that students receive speech and language services and speech–language pathologists receive either pay or vacation within the YRE schedule.

Once a work calendar is established for speech–language pathologists, the challenge of how to serve students must be addressed. The most significant difference for speech–language pathologists in a YRE school is the fact that the groupings of students can change every month (if on a multitrack YRE schedule). Although this may sound like a daunting task (and it is at first), thoughtful scheduling may allow speech–language pathologists to realize greater variation and effectiveness in service delivery. The changing mix of students on the caseload will allow for greater intensity at times with certain groups and will also allow children greater opportunities to work with different peers.

Speech–language pathologists working in YRE schools must learn how to calculate special education procedural timelines according to the various tracking systems in the schools. Mandated timelines are on hold when students are off track but not when speech–language pathologists are. Most YRE school districts publish a timeline calendar to make this calculation easier for staff.

Other members of a team may not have the same vacation schedule as a speech–language pathologist, so planning forward and backward is a good idea when working in a YRE school. Scheduling meeting dates when everyone will be available should be done at the beginning of the year. Some assessments may need to have plans signed early to accommodate vacation schedules. Moving a timeline up is always acceptable practice, but being late on completing an assessment or IEP, especially because of vacation schedules, is never acceptable and would be considered noncompliant with IDEA 2004. Team coordination takes exceptional planning in a YRE school.

Tables 6.2 and 6.3 show schedules for a speech–language pathologist who serves a multitrack YRE school. There are four tracks: A, B, C, and D. One track is always "off," and three are always "on." Table 6.2 shows A, B, and D on, and Table 6.3 shows B, C, and D on. When A-track students are on vacation, C-track students replace them on the schedule. For example, in Table 6.2, in the 11:00 a.m. to 11:30 a.m. slot on Monday, four children in kindergarten are seen for intervention. In Table 6.3, two of the children, Matt and Chris, continue in the second schedule, while Jason and Gabriel, who go on vacation, are replaced by Tabitha and Adam.

There is great potential in YRE for positive effects for students and greater flexibility in service delivery models. Remember that although the YRE schedule may seem like a greater amount of time, it is really the same amount, spread over a 12-month period.

There are two keys to ensuring successful implementation of alternative scheduling. The first is to remain open and creative. School-based speech–language pathologists have met numerous challenges with patience, understanding, and creativity. The second key is to stay involved and be proactive. YRE may provide time for intensive interventions that are more efficient for some students, reducing their overall time receiving services. One of the authors worked in YRE schools for many years and found it highly beneficial for students and staff.

Another issue that has been raised about schedules and calendars is the way the school day is scheduled. Typically, the same learning block is presented for all subjects. But with the need to go deeper into core content area, some schools have also adopted alternate time schedules and/or block schedules. The National Education Association (n.d.-b) described this type of a schedule:

> In contrast with the traditional daily six-, seven-, or eight-period schedule, a
> block schedule consists of three or four longer periods of daily instruction.

TABLE 6.2. Year-Round Education Schedule for Speech–Language Services, Calle Lakeview School: Part 1, Tracks A, B, D

	Monday	Tuesday	Wednesday	Thursday	Friday
9:00–9:40 Response to intervention	Austin Casey Chase Andrew Nadia	Austin Casey Chase Andrew Nadia	Austin Casey Chase Andrew Nadia	Austin Casey Chase Andrew Nadia	Austin Casey Chase Andrew Nadia
9:45–10:15 Primary-level class	Artesia Andrea Denise Rebecca	Steven Mattie	Chrissy Missy	Andrew	Assessments
10:30–11:00 Pull-out	Denise	Daniel Andrew	Chrissy Nikki Ennis	Daniel Nikki Alex	
11:00–11:30 Kindergarten	Matt Chris Jason Gabriel	Travis	Matt Chris Jason Gabriel	Travis	
11:30–12:00 Pull-out/class	Darren Brian	Special education class	Darren Chris	Natalie Juan	Will Emily
1:00–1:30 Primary-level class	Andrew Kevin Bura	Bernice Joanna Nick Kristine	Andrew Kevin Brian	Lonnie Joanna Kevin Nick Kristine	Instructional support team meeting
1:30–2:00 Coteach upper-level class	Sofia Bryan Dereck Robert Jimmie	Justin Tearah Christine	Sofia Bryan Dereck Robert Jimmie	Justin Tearah Christine	
2:00–2:30 In-class	Courtney Heather Darryl	Gabriel	Courtney Heather Darryl	Jill Toya	Consultation
2:30–3:00 Pull-out	Kristin Matt Ashlee	Kevin Andrea Marlie Cody	Kristen Matt Ashlee	Andrea Marlie Cody Kevin	

The three most common forms of block scheduling are as follows (National Education Association, n.d.-b):

1. The *alternate day schedule,* where students and teachers meet every other day for extended time periods, rather than meeting every day for shorter periods
2. The *"4 × 4" semester plan,* where students meet for four 90-minute blocks every day over four quarters
3. The *trimester plan,* where students take two or three courses every 60 days to earn six to nine credits per year

TABLE 6.3. Year-Round Education Schedule for Speech–Language Services, Calle Lakeview School: Part 2, Tracks B, C, D

	Monday	Tuesday	Wednesday	Thursday	Friday
9:00–9:40 Response to intervention	Jose Griffin Travis Hunter Nadia	Jose Griffin Travis Hunter Nadia	Jose Griffin Travis Hunter Nadia	Jose Griffin Travis Hunter Nadia	Jose Griffin Travis Hunter Nadia
9:45–10:15 Primary-level class	Artesia Andrea Denise Rebecca	Steven Mattie Kennisha	Andrew	Chrissy Missy	Assessments
10:30–11:00 Pull-out		Daniel Mikla Ennis Kelly	Kelly	Daniel Mikla Ennis	
11:00–11:30 Kindergarten	Matt Chris Tabitha Adam	Travis	Off-campus Head Start collaborative program	Home visits, curriculum team meetings	
11:30–12:00 Pull-out/class	Brian Chris	Special education class			
1:00–1:30 Primary-level class	Andrew Kevin Bura	Bonnie Kyle Zachary			Instructional support team meeting
1:30–2:00 Coteach upper-level class	Sofia Bryan Dereck	Justin Eric Taylor			
2:00–2:30 In-class	Courtney Tony Nate Barstow	Adolfo Sarah Darryl			Consultation
2:30–3:00 Pull-out	Kristin Matt Ken	Kristin Matt Ken			

There are many reasons why schools consider alternate schedules, including addressing facilities challenges and creating greater learning opportunities for students. Both of these are important variables for school administrators to consider. Speech–language pathologists are increasingly concerned with questions of appropriate dosage and intensity (see Chapter 5), which can be considered as part of the benefit when schools adopt an alternate schedule. Special education laws have provided for "extended school year" (ESY) to be provided to students who have demonstrated issues with recoupment and regression during extended breaks. Alternate schedules may benefit these students, as well as other students, including those in the general population. If a school is on an adopted school calendar that is a nontraditional calendar, this should be noted in the IEP.

Support Personnel Model

Using support personnel in a school speech–language program is gaining support in many states. Although support personnel have been routinely used in other special education settings since the early 1970s, they have had little involvement with speech–language services. Some states established special training and employment categories for speech–language support personnel early, but many states were hesitant to start until the field formally embraced the idea of trained support personnel in 1995 through its national professional organization, ASHA (see "Speech–Language Pathology Assistants and Aides in Schools" in Chapter 9).

The speech–language pathology assistant (SLPA) is typically regulated in a school program by at least two agencies: at the state licensing or certification of training level, and at the local school district employment level. Trained and supervised SLPAs can be very helpful to speech–language pathologists, especially if caseload numbers are high or spread over several sites per week. SLPAs allow greater numbers of children to be seen for more intensive services.

SLPAs may dramatically change the way speech–language pathologists manage the intervention schedule and organize service delivery. ASHA (2016b) outlined the "Speech–Language Pathology Assistant Scope of Practice" of a SLPA in terms of service delivery as follows:

A. Self-identify as SLPAs to families, students, patients, clients, staff, and others. This may be done verbally, in writing, and/or with titles on name badges.

B. Exhibit compliance with the Health Insurance Portability and Accountability Act (HIPAA) and Family Educational Rights and Privacy Act (FERPA) regulations, reimbursement requirements, and SLPAs' responsibilities.

C. Assist the speech–language pathologist with speech, language, and hearing screenings without clinical interpretation.

D. Assist the speech–language pathologist during assessment of students, patients, and clients exclusive of administration and/or interpretation.

E. Assist the speech–language pathologist with bilingual translation during screening and assessment activities exclusive of interpretation; refer to "Knowledge and Skills Needed by Speech–Language Pathologists and Audiologists to Provide Culturally and Linguistically Appropriate Services" (ASHA, 2004d).

F. Follow documented treatment plans or protocols developed by the supervising speech–language pathologist.

G. Provide guidance and treatment via telepractice to students, patients, and clients who are selected by the supervising speech–language pathologist as appropriate for this service delivery model.

H. Document student, patient, and client performance (e.g., tallying data for the speech–language pathologist to use; preparing charts, records, and graphs) and report this information to the supervising speech–language pathologist.

I. Program and provide instruction in the use of augmentative and alternative communication devices.

J. Demonstrate or share information with patients, families, and staff regarding feeding strategies developed and directed by the speech–language pathologist.

K. Serve as an interpreter for patients, clients, students, and families who do not speak English.

L. Provide services under speech–language pathologist supervision in another language for individuals who do not speak English and English-language learners.

The support personnel model enables speech–language pathologists to provide a greater range of services to students on the caseload, but SLPAs cannot maintain their own caseload. They must only serve students who are identified by a speech–language pathologist and an IEP team. They must be directly supervised 10% to 30% of the time they are working with students. Initially, SLPAs will require greater amounts of supervision to ensure that intervention and other activities are conducted accurately and uniformly. However, SLPAs can provide services to students using all available models and may work simultaneously with speech–language pathologists. This allows daily intensive therapy for some students, in-class support for some students, and discrete trial sessions for others. Carryover and generalization sessions can be set up on a routine basis for students about to be dismissed.

The support personnel model is actually a cluster of models that can be managed by a communication team (e.g., the speech–language pathologist and one, two, or three SLPAs). Speech–language pathologists are always responsible for the complete program but may delegate tasks to SLPAs. One speech–language pathologist in a large school district reported that SLPAs are the trained eyes and ears of speech–language pathologists when they are in the classroom, and are equally effective at using the therapy room for small groups when speech–language pathologists are coteaching in the classroom. SLPAs are also able to monitor students who need to be checked each week for hearing aid batteries, motor speech exercises, and written journal entries.

Schedules should remain flexible throughout the year. One method that facilitates flexibility is to use cards with students' names on them in a pocket chart so that assignments can be moved around as conditions change. A master schedule of all students seen for speech–language intervention may be necessary, for sharing with other team members who need to coordinate with an ever-changing schedule that involves several speech–language service providers on the communication team. This model increases the visibility of the speech–language pathologist and connects him or her more closely with the life and mission of the school.

Articulation Resource Centers

Because of the expanded service delivery possible with response to intervention (RTI) (discussed in depth in Chapter 3), speech–language pathologists can now serve some students within general education. If students have impairments, for example, speech-sound errors that do not have an adverse impact on their academic performance, they can be served for brief periods of intense intervention without an IEP. A third grader with a frontal lisp who earns As and Bs in her class does not have a disability. She does have a speech-sound error. She deserves the services of a speech–language pathologist to improve her communication. IDEA 2004 makes it possible to serve these students in a wide range of general education venues, one of which is an articulation resource center. Students who need direction for the specific placement of articulators, intensive supervised practice, and a strong home-to-school generalization program can be served in the resource center. Resource centers serving larger groups of children, aided by SLPAs, have reported significant reductions in the caseload size and overall effectiveness in schools (Taps, 2006). Using a complexity approach to articulation intervention (Morrisette & Geriut, 2002), requiring 150 correct productions of a target sound or word in a session, a large urban district reported that students remediated speech-sound errors in 20 hours or less (Montgomery, Dunaway, & Taps, 2005; San Diego City Schools, 2004–2005; Taps, 2006, 2008, 2009). (See SLPath Web site: http://slpath.com/.)

Sometimes the resource center concept is brought to the students for one-on-one intervention in either general education or special education. Kuhn (2006) reported on a highly intensive program for speech-sound errors in which the clinician saw the student three to four times a day for 5–10 minutes at a table in the hall. Students missed only short portions of the school day and responded rapidly to intensive, explicit intervention, and 69% of students reached their goal in 16 weeks or less.

Variations on the resource center concept hold promise as a new service delivery option since IDEA 2004. Students with IEPs may also be served in these settings; however, the resource center holds the greatest promise for students on Section 504 plans (see Chapter 2) or those with relatively mild articulation impairments who do not meet eligibility criteria for a special education disability label. This model results in a dramatic reduction in paperwork and meetings and an equally dramatic increase in the number of students who can be rapidly dismissed from the caseload as corrected after intensive services.

Service delivery is determined by clinicians' theoretical perspectives on correcting speech-sound errors. Thus, service delivery changes as perspectives change. If speech–language pathologists want to demonstrate that improvements in an individual's communication behaviors are due to interventions, as evidence-based practice would dictate, a range of services is essential. The speech–language pathologist must be mindful of district rules and processes for serving students under 504 or RTI.

Grouping Strategies

Scheduling, professional collaboration, and efficiency can be enhanced by using thoughtful student grouping strategies. An eminent body of research on the effectiveness of grouping strategies exists, linking cooperative learning groups to academic success (Johnson & Johnson, 1989; Kagan, 1994; Slavin, 1990). Children learn in groups throughout their school years. Recognizing that groups are the natural context of the classroom helps speech–language pathologists build collaborative working relationships with teachers and other education professionals. Group learning has several overall benefits. Grouping students for intervention may occur in traditional pull-out models, classrooms, resource or learning centers, and collaborative teams.

On the IEP service section, the IEP team will need to define the service recommendation, including the frequency, location, and format for the services. Families, teachers, and speech–language pathologists may believe that individual treatment is "better" than group sessions for students. The rationale for conducting group treatment should be clear in the mind of the speech–language pathologist so he or she is able to explain why this treatment method (i.e., format) was selected for an individual student. As mentioned, groups are the natural learning setting for children, lending to greater motivation and opportunity for both practicing with peers and having peer models. Studies on individual versus group treatment models have shown limited and mixed results; however, none have concluded that individual treatment is preferred over group sessions to achieve treatment outcomes. These conclusions are reached often because other variables are present in studies, such as what intervention procedures are being implemented, making the results confounded. What is evident, however, is that there is not clinical evidence that individual treatment is a preferred method in terms of treatment outcomes (Law, Garrett, & Nye, 2003; McGinty & Justice, 2006; Schooling, Venediktov, & Leech, 2010; Valdez & Montgomery, 1996). In fact, there are observed benefits in terms of motivation, peer learning, and least restrictive environment that come with group treatment.

This text has advocated for a full continuum of service delivery models, which includes individual treatment sessions along with group sessions. The same would be noted in terms of times per week or the frequency and duration of treatment plans for students, as reflected in their IEPs. As mentioned in other sections (see Chapter 4), an appropriate treatment plan for a student may include a progression of service delivery models that range from individual to group in a pull-out setting to group in a classroom setting to consultation only. What is also important to note is that the rationale for various service delivery, including the decision of setting, which reflects group or individual treatment, must be based on student need and not based on the schedule and/or availability of the speech–language pathologist. Although logistics will come into play when designing the schedule (see "Scheduling and Organizing Services," previously in this chapter), determination of setting and format on the IEP is based on the individual student's needs. Speech–language pathologists must be able to describe the benefits of group work to parents, teachers, and advocates in order to explain the evidence-based rationale for this treatment recommendation. Some parents and advocates have argued that placing a student in a group may mean that the student actually receives reduced service (e.g., if there are four students in a 30-minute group, that means each student is receiving only 7.5 minutes of therapy). The speech–language pathologist must be able to explain that part of the therapeutic process is also listening and practice, in addition to learning while the speech–language pathologist provides instructions to the group as a whole and to other students in the group. Learning occurs then, too. Another key aspect of the rationale for group session is that the ultimate goal of any communication treatment is for the individual to be able to use the skill in a variety of contexts. This is known as generalization. Complexity theory (Gierut, 2001) advocates for intervention to provide complex treatment targets within the treatment design in order to achieve goals more quickly (i.e., treatment efficiency). Learning skills with the communication partners with whom those skills will be used is a preferred method of intervention. Finally, the way to determine whether treatment benefit is being realized is through the data collection and progress monitoring that will occur as part of the session.

Three types of groups are used in schools: skill groups, friendship and classmate groups, and random-purpose groups. Speech–language pathologists can use all three.

Skill Groups

Skill groups are composed of children who cannot independently do an assigned task or lack an underlying skill necessary to complete a task. Educators and speech–language pathologists commonly group children with similar skill levels together. Professionals need to work intensively with skill groups because there are no peer models in these groups who can do the task. Skill groups are often used for reading, with instructors moving from group to group.

Speech–language pathologists frequently use skill groups, assigning children with peers who have the same perceived or tested communication deficits. Perhaps a student does not demonstrate a skill, such as conversational turn-taking or consistent production of a phoneme. All students near that student's age who have the same difficulty would be placed together in a skill group. Skill grouping is labor intensive for speech–language pathologists who do all the modeling, facilitating, and reinforcing. Students must wait, not always patiently, for professionals to provide cues and evaluation. Skill grouping often results in teaching isolated communication skills in an unnatural communication context, which can limit generalization.

However, skill groups are easy to assemble and plan. Progress can be easily measured using only one probe for the group. Once students show improved skills, they are likely moved to another skill group. Students have been known to seek out ways to stay in their skill group. If improvement in the target skill means leaving the comfort and routine of a group of friends, students choose to not demonstrate that they can do the task. Progress dissipates when some students conclude that they like to attend speech sessions just to be with their friends; speech–language pathologists need to observe their skill groups conscientiously to ensure that students are making progress at a steady pace.

Friendship and Classmate Groups

Friendship groups are composed of students who choose to be together or who are assigned together by adults because they are friends. In these groups, students may be highly motivated and often quite social. They enjoy each other's company and will often work much harder just to keep all their friends together. Educators find these group-ings to be full of energy and surprisingly productive. Much work can be accomplished quickly in a friendship group.

Speech–language pathologists rarely group this way, because they are less aware of the social groupings of their students or may not be able to place classmates, let alone friends, together. Grade-level groups are often a preferred method, as they allow the speech–language pathologist to vary service delivery easily, going from pull-out to in-class service delivery depending on the goals of the classroom and therapy. In addition, children spend the most time with their grade-level peers, so this can be supportive to their learning. When speech–language pathologists use social groups, they remark on how exciting the activities are and how supportive the students are of each other, espe-cially considering the variety of target goals a group may have. Friendship and classmate groups often get an extra boost in their effectiveness because students genuinely like each other, enjoy the opportunity to practice together, and are powerful models for each other. The targeted need of one student is a strength of one or more of the other students, providing peer facilitation, social rewards, and motivation. Natural contexts provide many opportunities for practice and generalization of communication skills. These groups may be exuberant and noisy, requiring the speech–language pathologist to monitor the social conversation that occurs. An added benefit, though, is that these groups can also be fun for everyone, including the speech–language pathologist.

Methods for Enhancing the Grouping Process

Educators often assign students who are to be in a random-purpose group (also referred to as "flexible grouping" or "heterogeneous grouping") through some type of matching task. Speech–language pathologists might enhance this grouping process by using lan-guage-oriented sorting methods, such as passing out cards with words, phrases, or pic-tures printed on them. Speech–language pathologists might ask students with picture cards to move around the room and talk to other students to determine what "scene" they belong in, such as a rain forest, desert, grassy plain, or mountain. The picture card belongs to one of the scenes and is part of the grade-level core curriculum. Content from the classroom can be used, such as recent books read, science words, or adjectives that go with nouns. The process of finding one's group should be an authentic language and communication experience. Speech–language pathologists may want to ensure that caseload students receive cards that will place them in the appropriate group. Speech–language pathologists who work in collaborative classrooms use these types of activities often.

Random-Purpose Groups

Random-purpose groups are the most time-consuming to assemble but result in the most facilitative learning environment for children. Even though these groups appear random, speech–language pathologists have a purpose for putting them together. Edu-cators group children by selecting students who can do various aspects of a task so that they must join together to get it done. In the classroom, this usually means a group composed of some students who read easily and some who struggle, some students who write well and some who avoid it, some students who have artistic talent, and some students who can organize others. A group of five to six students can pull together and accomplish something that none of them can do alone. They may or may not be friends, but they recognize that together they can accomplish the task. The term *cooperative learning* is often used for this type of group, in variations known as *jigsaw learning*, *pinwheels*, or *share pairs*.

In speech–language intervention, a group of students with various phonological disabilities can operate like a random-purpose group. Children with multiple articulation errors, sometimes unintelligible, are grouped together and cycled through many phoneme productions. Different phonemes are targets for different children. This enables some students to be models for others in the group rather than depend on an adult model, who is often less motivating than peers. In random-purpose groups, speech–language pathologists structure services to accommodate the strengths and needs of all children. Montgomery and Bonderman (1989) reported that random-purpose groups of four to nine unintelligible children were very successful in phonological remediation programs, with 85% of the students demonstrating significant change in 17 weeks or less of therapy. Groups of this type take considerable time and effort to organize. Changes in the group can upset instructional goals and activities.

Educators have reported to the authors that they often keep effective random-purpose groups together for several subject areas as students become more and more productive and eventually learn to blend and multiply their skills. Speech–language pathologists can use this strategy also, moving previously unsuccessful students into already functioning groups without the limitations of matching a child's specific area of need, as is done in skill groups. One speech–language pathologist found success in grouping students according to grade level. She commented that because the students brought their various needs to and from the classroom, working in a group on various need areas built a support network for the students when they were back in the classroom and the speech–language pathologist was not there.

Effective grouping of students on school caseloads is an important and easily overlooked responsibility of speech–language pathologists. The effectiveness of group therapy lies in the thought behind the grouping, which can result in greater student progress.

Using wise grouping strategies is an important component of collaborative consultation. Flexible grouping of children allows for the provision of services for vastly different communication needs. Random-purpose groupings or friendship and classmate groupings can be a great help to teachers and can bring speech–language pathologists into classes for a wide variety of communication intervention activities.

Consultation and Collaboration

Consultation and collaboration, distinctly different approaches, evolved as models for all aspects of school-based services nationwide focused on the general education curriculum (Flynn, 2010; Montgomery, 1992; Moore-Brown, 2007; Whitmire, 2002). When deciding to work in a consultative and collaborative environment, focus on the student and ask, "What is it about the student's learning or language disability that is preventing the student from performing the skills needed to achieve standards?" The purpose of intervention is to help the student in achieving academic goals.

In response to these concerns about the effectiveness and efficiency of individualized and small pull-out groups, as well as mandates from the Elementary and Secondary Education Act (ESEA) and IDEA 2004, districts attempted to integrate their special education services into the general education program and combine some of the specialized intervention with grade-level academic activities. This integration promoted the idea of professionals working with each other to support students rather than each support staff person working directly with each student. Such speech–language school services have been enthusiastically described in the literature (e.g., Creaghead, 1999; Ehren, 2000; Ferguson, 1991; Flynn, 2010; L. Miller, 1989; Montgomery, 1992; Moore-Brown, 2000, 2007; Prelock, 2000a, 2000b; Roth & Worthington, 2000; Secord, 1999; Secord & Damico, 1998; Whitmire, 2002).

Broadly speaking, speech–language intervention services may be provided in three forms: direct, indirect, or collaborative and consultative.

- A student can be served directly by a speech–language pathologist individually or in a group of students, either separately from the classroom or in the classroom.
- A student can be served indirectly by a speech–language pathologist individually, in a small group, or with the whole class in the student's classroom.
- A student can be served by a trained person, who is directed by a speech–language pathologist, in any relevant setting. This collaborative and consultative arrangement can be with an SLPA, a classroom teacher, another special educator, a peer, a parent, a bus driver, and so on.

IDEA 2004 requires that qualified professionals (e.g., speech–language pathologists) direct service delivery, but it does not have to be administered directly by these professionals. In some cases, intervention is much more effective if it is not directly administered. The support personnel model (i.e., speech–language pathology assistant [SLPA]) reviewed earlier in this chapter, for example, can be an effective consultative model. It is another way to structure meaningful intervention services for students and release speech–language pathologists for assessment, consultation, or work with families. (For another example of indirect services through consultation, see "Infants and Toddlers" in Chapter 7.) Service delivery can happen wherever it is arranged to happen. The essential component is that services are planned, supervised, measured, and evaluated for effectiveness by speech–language pathologists.

Consultation is a *voluntary process* in which one professional assists another to address a third party's problem. It is a process rather than a style. It is voluntary and entails an indirect relationship. It involves shared participation, effective communication, teamwork, sharing, and problem solving.

Collaboration is a *style* in which two coequal parties engage voluntarily in shared decision making as they work toward a common goal. It involves shared participation, resource ownership, accountability, and rewards (Secord, 1999).

Collaborative consultation is an *interactive process* that enables teams of people with diverse expertise to generate creative solutions to mutually defined problems. The outcome is enhanced and altered and produces solutions that are different from those that the individual team members would have produced independently.

Few speech–language pathologists provide their services as sole practitioners. The classroom teacher is the expert on curriculum; the speech–language pathologist is the expert on speech and language acquisition, vocabulary, metalinguistic awareness, and literacy. Putting teachers and speech–language pathologists together has been recognized for many years as facilitating the most efficacious treatment for the student.

IDEA 2004 shifted focus of special education to ensure access to the general education curriculum (Karger, n.d.). When considering the responsibilities and mandates associated with ensuring access and progress in the general curriculum, the speech–language pathologist's service delivery naturally lends to greater opportunities to partner with general education teachers in the environment where instruction is delivered. Vicker (2009) referred to this type of service delivery as *integrated services in classrooms*. Working with teachers in a collaborative relationship requires a different skill set than the skill set required during therapeutic intervention for children based on their disability and identified goals. (See "Stages of Consultation" later in this chapter for tips for building collaborative relationships for consultation with teachers.) Although focusing on discussing the benefits of this model for students with autism spectrum disorders, Vicker's (2009) outline of the various benefits to this model applies regardless of the student's disabling condition:

- Maybe interventions that were provided in the speech room could be offered within the classroom environment (p. 2).
- The speech–language pathologist can provide support to a variety of students at the same time in the classroom.
- Working with students is currently viewed as only part of the equation when providing integrated intervention services. Working with classroom teachers and paraprofessionals is equally important when the end goal is that of automaticity and generalization of language, communication, and literacy skills. Speech–language pathologists can play a variety of roles depending on the learning and support needs of the students, especially those with IEPs; the classroom context; and the needs of the classroom staff (p. 3).
- The first step of providing services in the classroom involves the building of a working collaborative relationship between the two professionals (p. 4).
- Consultation is one way a speech–language pathologist initially works with a teacher on a team within a classroom focus. Consultation services are more typically problem oriented (p. 4).
- The collaborative role opens doors for a more intensive, ongoing involvement with the educational staff than the consultative role. The term *collaboration*

suggests a partnership and willingness to work with one another. The two can focus on improving communication support for many curricular areas for all students for the core level of instruction, targeting skills for a select group of students, or focusing on students with specific challenges that could benefit from the experiences and skills of a speech–language pathologist (p. 4).

Flynn (2010) also provided tips for building collaborative relationships for consultation with teachers.

Stages of Consultation (Flynn, 2010)

In building new collaborative relationships with teachers, consider the stages of consultation (Wesley, Dennis, & Fenson, 2007). Strong, healthy consultative relationships require trust and time. Establishing relationships with these stages in mind may help all parties build the trust required for long-term professional relationships that serve students' best interests. The following are tips for building collaborative relationships for consultation:

- *Initiate and build relationships.* Choose a teacher who you know you can work well with, perhaps someone with whom you already have experienced success, to initiate your effort into collaborative service delivery.
- *Assess by gathering information.* Discuss the strengths and needs of the parties involved. Teachers are experts in curriculum and behavior while speech–language pathologists are experts in differentiated instruction and learning strategies.
- *Prioritize issues and set goals.* Establish what is most important to accomplish through this collaboration and set goals for planning, students, and self-evaluation.
- *Select strategies.* Brainstorm ways to prioritize and implement goals creatively in time-saving and energy-efficient ways.
- *Implement.* Put your good planning to work to improve services to students in the least restrictive environment.
- *Evaluate.* Critique your effort in a risk-free environment, implement the improvements, and continue to refine your collaborative efforts.

ASHA's (2014a) "2014 Schools Survey" revealed that most speech–language pathologists in schools still use the traditional pull-out model as their primary method of providing service. On a weekly basis, the speech–language pathologist spent 18 hours providing services in a traditional pull-out model, 7 hours in recordkeeping and paperwork, and 4 hours a week in classroom-based or curriculum-based direct intervention and other indirect activities. In addition, diagnostic evaluations (3 hours), Multi-Tiered Systems of Supports (MTSS) or response to intervention (RTI) (1 hour), troubleshooting technology, and supervising and providing services to Section 504 students were part of the duties of the speech–language pathologist during the week. In one of a few studies comparing the three service delivery models, the collaborative model was the most effective in teaching curricular vocabulary for students receiving speech–language services (Throneburg, Calvert, Sturm, Paramboukas, & Paul, 2000). The same was found in the evidence-based practice brief comparing classrooms to pull-out intervention models (McGinty & Justice, 2006).

Using any of these consultative constructs with deliberative planning allows speech–language pathologists to work in conjunction with classroom teachers, education specialists, occupational therapists, social workers, and others. The curriculum is incorporated into therapy, and therapy is incorporated into the curriculum. Solutions to taxing service delivery issues present themselves when more than one individual assumes ownership for services and when entire schools assume ownership for all of their students. This ensures more functional interventions, reduces the fragmentation of students' days, and enables speech–language pathologists to take a more active part in schools. Collaboration begets more collaboration as team members begin to rely on each other, meet more often, and reinforce with each other's successes.

Teaming on Goals

IDEA 2004 requires the use of a group of qualified professionals representing different disciplines and parents, often called a *multidisciplinary team* (MDT), to plan and implement a student's IEP. Appropriate service delivery (i.e., planning and implementing the IEP) for the student with communication disabilities is directly linked to how well the various professions work together. This collaborative work is now referred to as *interdisciplinary education*. Interdisciplinary teams extend the effectiveness of school-based services for children and families and enhance generalization to other settings.

An effective way for speech–language pathologists and other educators to begin collaborative and consultative service delivery is to write and implement shared goals for students with disabilities. Teams have used the following methods to write shared goals by using transdisciplinary planning even though their IEP process was still basically multidisciplinary:

- The speech–language pathologist and two special educators meet and plan their actions together, resulting in three joint goals rather than a series of goals from each specialist.
- For some children, only one common goal is most effective. All the team members responsible for the child's program contribute to the writing of this statement and rotate the responsibility for monitoring it throughout the year.
- Educators write goals and objectives in their own areas of expertise (e.g., speech and language, academic areas such as English and language arts, gross- or fine-motor skills); however, many team members are responsible for implementation.
- Parents and educators write goals and objectives together, using a single monitoring system carried back and forth by the child each night in his or her backpack. A separate monitoring system in each setting can be used and routinely compared to measure progress in different settings.

- Teams write embedded skill goals, where all objectives lead to a single goal, such as functional communication, for example, "Theresa will use her communication board to meaningfully respond to an adult greeting once a day." Occupational therapy and physical therapy have embedded motor goals, while the teacher has embedded cause-and-effect cognition goals, and the behavior therapist has embedded goals for appropriate requesting or transition.
- The student's school day is viewed through life domains (e.g., homeroom, hallways, bus stop, scouts, cafeteria, etc.), and service plans and objectives written by the team are taught to the general education or support personnel in each domain, setting, or location. Data are kept on a large chart by all involved adults and one peer.

Creating Access Through Universal Design for Learning: Engagement, Presentation, and Representation

The primary principles of universal design for learning (UDL) are critical for creating classrooms where all students can participate and succeed. Students in general education classes with language and learning problems may have challenges accessing curriculum if the presentation does not consider their learning needs. Within the UDL framework, team members can consider how to ensure that students are engaged through using various engagement strategies and scaffolding the presentation to their learning needs. (See National Center on Universal Design for Learning, UDL Guidelines–Version 2.0; www.udlcenter.org.) Each principle of UDL contains recommendations on how classrooms are able to provide multiple means of engagement, action and expression, and representation, with guidelines for language, expression and symbols (representation), and expression and communication (action and expression). Rather than have the student leave the classroom to receive remedial services, the speech–language pathologist can work with teachers to ensure that classrooms are designed to deliver instruction within a UDL framework. Speech–language pathologists can also coteach the curriculum using the most effective strategies (e.g., listen, repeat, listen, code, and read). In this way, the strategies are taught along with the curriculum, which is less time-consuming for students than learning strategies in one place and content in another. High levels of success have been reported using this approach for struggling readers and writers (Toner & Helmer, 2006). Collaborative approaches through coteaching and differentiation are considered keys to developing inclusive environments where all students have access through instructional supports (California Statewide Special Education Task Force, 2015; Tomlinson, 2006; Villa & Thousand, 2003; Villa, Thousand, & Nevin, 2013).

Recordkeeping Is Critical

Recordkeeping is important with all service delivery models and often serves useful functions for many team members involved with indirect service environments. When speech–language pathologists act as consultants, the use of a recordkeeping form helps to structure the discussion and keep it focused on positive problem solving. The form can also guide a team in setting expectations for each team member's activities, and examining results.

Records of a consultative meeting should include identification information regarding a student, a family, and team participants. A clear description of any difficulties or challenges should be stated in terms that are observable and measurable, along with a statement of the desired behavior or outcome. A review of past attempts to resolve the problem can be helpful. A range of options to address the issue may be listed, and the action that is agreed on should be clearly identified. The consultative meeting adjourns after team members set a date to check on progress or results.

Consultative forms should be used to clearly identify action plans, including persons responsible, what they will do, and the timelines for implementation. These actions should be tied to the functional outcomes desired for a student. (See "Functional Outcomes and the School–Based Speech–Language Pathologist" in Chapter 5 for a discussion of functional outcomes.)

When acting as consultants, speech–language pathologists guide team members to focus on problems, identify successes and concerns, and clearly state the desired functional outcomes for a student. A well-designed form helps draw the discussion away from frustrations and toward a vision of what is desired for the student.

Action plans identify responsibilities, deadlines, and expected outcomes. This format helps reinforce the concept of teamwork and avoids the assumption that consultants have taken on the responsibility of solving problems independently. Consultants may use consultation forms to check back with team members to monitor their progress toward deadlines. When teams meet at their assigned follow-up sessions, they will have the information and make needed adjustments. Increasingly, online programs have integrated these steps for speech–language pathologists to monitor students receiving speech–language services.

Peer Tutors as Part of Intervention

Once planning is focused on a student's environment, peers take on greater significance in the delivery of services. Some students respond much more favorably to peers than adults and can demonstrate faster progress if the work is connected to peer interactions. This is a distinct advantage of school-based intervention that many speech–language pathologists may overlook. Speech–language pathologists can use the collaborative and consultative approach and gradually shift responsibilities for monitoring to peer tutors or cooperative learning groups. This is also effective with adolescents (Flynn, 2013; Larson & McKinley, 2003). Speech–language pathologists need to make the shift gradually, select peer models carefully, orient and train peers, have supports readily available for peers, and monitor and follow up with students and peers conscientiously. The advantages to peer tutoring are numerous and match many overall communication and academic goals designed for target students by speech–language pathologists. Some of these advantages include the following:

- Increased time for support and assistance for target students
- Increased number of contexts in which target students can be supported

- Greater amount of natural intervention, as most students learn with peers not with adults
- More give-and-take interaction between target students and peer tutors
- Collaboration without directly involving other professionals, a first step in a resistive school environment
- Opportunities for incidental learning and social and academic scripts for target students in school and beyond (Friend & Bursuck, 2012; German, 1992; Hardman, Drew, & Egan, 2011; Larson & McKinley, 2003; Thiemann-Bourque, 2010)

Building Relationships With General Educators

General educators will be valuable resources in helping identify and serve children who need services, because children with language disabilities often exhibit concomitant problems with grammar, vocabulary, and conversation skills. Speech–language pathologists may team with teachers to jointly observe a student's interactions in class and other school settings. Teaming facilitates all types of service delivery, especially collaboration. Successful collaboration means all professionals involved with the child's services will attend referral and IEP meetings together. IDEA 2004 requires that each child's IEP team include "not less than one regular education teacher of the child (if the child is, or may be, participating in the regular education environment)" (34 C.F.R. § 300.321 [a][2]). This should be someone who teaches or would have taught the student in a general education class. This person may be a grade-level teacher, a subject-area teacher, or a teacher at the home school of a student placed in a specialized school. The grade-level educator keeps the conversation grounded in general education instruction, curriculum, and Common Core State Standards (CCSS) expectancies. This person's role should add a realistic and thoughtful appraisal of the student in the natural environment.

General Educators at the IEP Meeting

General educators can make great contributions to the development of a student's IEP. Speech–language pathologists will find that "academic language" issues are highly relevant to educators, and therapy is more successful when the whole team is aware of, and working toward, the student's communication goals.

There are specific actions that general educators can take prior to or during meetings to provide the other team members with information as to the academic expectations and instructional methods of his or her classroom. Speech–language pathologists can share therapeutic ideas with general education colleagues appropriate for the student's age and grade. General educators have a unique perspective on education that is often unfamiliar to special education teams. Appropriate decisions for a student's level of inclusion or support can be made at subsequent meetings if facts and opinions are shared early in the process. Again, it is important to have a classroom teacher be aware of the speech–language goals for a student by joint planning.

General education teachers may often be unsure of their role at an IEP meeting. The emphasis on progress in the general education curriculum and the requirement that the student's general education teacher be present at the IEP meeting demonstrate the importance of their contribution. General education teachers should be aware of the requirements for their participation at the IEP meeting. (See the following box, "General Education Teacher Responsibilities at the IEP Meeting.") In addition, the speech–language pathologist can offer the following suggestions of how general education teachers can contribute at the IEP meeting:

- Listen carefully to the discussion of a student's strengths and needs without undue concern about the label or diagnosis the student may carry.
- Bring a copy of the age-appropriate curriculum, such as the CCSS, to the meeting.
- Describe a project or task students accomplish at their grade level.
- Bring or name a few books that are read to students at this grade level.
- Describe how supplies and materials are acquired and stored by students in this classroom.
- Bring a list of what they believe are the five most important concepts students will learn that year.
- Be prepared to answer questions about instructional methods that they use frequently.
- Give examples of the type of instructional support typically provided to students in this class.
- Describe the technology students use in this class.
- Discuss the teaming activities of teachers at this grade level.
- Think about and share experiences they have had with paraprofessionals or other support personnel.

General Education Teacher Responsibilities at the IEP Meeting

It is required to have not less than one regular education teacher of the student if the student is, or may be, participating in the regular education environment.

If more than one regular education teacher is providing instructional services to the individual with exceptional needs, one regular education teacher may be designated.

The regular education teacher, to the extent appropriate, shall participate in the development, review, and revision of the IEP, including assisting in the determination of appropriate positive behavioral interventions and supports and other strategies for the student and the determination of supplementary aids and services, program modifications, and supports for school personnel that will be provided for the student.

Speech–language pathologists can and should take a leadership role in the area of communication with and about students on their caseloads. General educators make important contributions when discussing access, accommodations, modifications, and behavioral support. It is the responsibility of classroom teachers to ensure that all students in their classrooms learn. Special education teams support general educators to meet that expectation based on each student's present level of performance.

The current environment of schools under ESEA, IDEA 2004, and CCSS calls for a coherent system of instruction and supports for students. The mantras "all students will learn" and "special education is not a place" are not just random phrases but truly represent educators' responsibilities. Speech–language pathologists and special educators must know and understand the demands of curricula and how to support students so they can learn. General educators must be able to provide instruction and to create a learning environment for all learners in their classrooms. As a result, teachers and specialists need to work together to ensure practice that will realize these goals and outcomes for students.

Linking Services to the Curriculum

Speech–language intervention services in schools gradually evolved from clinically based therapy to broader-based educationally and developmentally related intervention services. Individual or small-group sessions with speech–language pathologists were once the norm. Larger student groupings with technology-assisted, curriculum-related sessions conducted in classrooms are now used in many districts. Descriptions of these inspiring models are available in the literature, and several will be discussed in this chapter.

Several models have been developed to compare purposes and characteristics of therapy versus instruction. The authors have observed one such model (see Table 6.4) in numerous schools, and it follows the spirit and letter of IDEA 2004. It links all the communication services to a student's educational goals and includes roles for speech–language pathologists to provide conventional therapy and classroom instruction. This approach has been used by many speech–language pathologists who use the student's curriculum as the vehicle for practicing targeted communication skills.

Some states tap the expertise of speech–language pathologists to work as communication teachers in self-contained classrooms. These professionals teach the content of the curriculum, guided by a strong language component, to children who have pervasive communication disabilities. This reduces the fragmentation that occurs with pull-out services. A thorough description of service delivery in schools must include speech–language pathologists who apply all the therapeutic practice directly to the teaching of a content area. This position may require additional course work or another credential in some states. Compatible with IDEA 2004, this model enables educators and parents to be aware of students' evolving communication skills in a classroom setting.

These three macrosystems may use many broad-based instructional strategies. A service delivery model is similar to the outside walls of a house or the fence around

TABLE 6.4. Blended Therapeutic–Educational Role for Collaboration in the Curriculum

Factors to consider	Classroom instruction	Conventional therapy	Collaborative intervention
Learning	Deals with learning new information and skills in the normal course of development	Deals with remediating or compensating for deficient skills that have not developed or that have been lost	Focuses on a combination of learning new information plus research-based intensive strategies using individualized instructional accommodations with a sensitivity for different learning styles and varying levels of student support
Student engagement	Involves a captive audience with varying degrees of active engagement at different times	Depends on a student's ongoing, active participation in a self-help process	Combines the advantages of students working in multiskilled groups of same-age peers with individual empowerment made possible with effective scaffolds
Planning	Uses a teaching sequence based on external criteria, curriculum standards, and progression	Uses a sequence of activities based on individual needs and progress	Uses a sequence based on individual needs and progress within the larger framework of curricular expectations for students at a particular grade level
Needs of learners	Is oriented to group goals and uses a standard approach	Incorporates selection of individual goals and uses a diagnostic approach	Incorporates a selection of individual, measurable annual goals but encourages use of state or local standards as benchmarks under those goals
Pace	Is determined by the majority of the group and average ability	Is determined by a student's mastery and the speech–language pathologist's judgments	Demands more intense efforts and adjusted pace to promote mastery; actions of all members of the team, including the general education teacher, are contingent on the actions of the student
Interaction	Has teachers teach the planned lesson and students provide feedback after specific tasks	Incorporates the speech–language pathologist's actions contingent on a student's reactions; informative and corrective feedback are essential and ongoing	Uses informative and corrective feedback provided in both formal and informal ways from educators, speech–language pathologists, peers, and support personnel

Note. Adapted from *Inclusive Practices in the Middle School*, by J. K. Montgomery, 2000. Presentation at Hewes Middle School, Tustin Unified School District, Tustin, CA. Adapted with permission.

a yard. Each occupant can decorate it to fit his or her tastes, interests, and resources. Once the parameters of service are established, numerous therapeutic strategies will fit. As noted in the many previous examples in this chapter, using evidence-based practices, a wide range of theoretical perspectives will fit comfortably within service delivery models in schools (Flynn, 2010, 2013; Gilliam & Gilliam, 2006; Justice, 2006a; Kader-avek, 2011; Kamhi, 2006; Taps, 2006; Ukrainetz, 2015; Vicker, 2009; Wallach, 2008).

Access to the Curriculum

The single most important feature of access to the curriculum is the ability to read for information and for pleasure. Children who can read have the best access to the broadest range of academic learning. Speech–language pathologists must be active members of the literacy team at their schools. Although speech–language pathologists do not teach reading as a subject, they support its skill acquisition from preschool through adult transition programs. The following section offers many ways that speech–language pathologists are active members of the literacy team in every school setting.

Literacy, Reading, and Writing

ASHA Position Statement

ASHA (2000b) made the following statement concerning the role of speech–language pathologists with respect to reading and writing:

> Speech–language pathologists play a critical and direct role in the development of literacy for children and adolescents with communication disorders, including those with severe or multiple disabilities. Speech–language pathologists also make a contribution to the literacy efforts of a school district or community on behalf of other children and adolescents. (p. 1)

This forthright statement acknowledged the strong connection between spoken and written language, asserting that speech–language pathologists play a major role in supporting students with reading and language difficulties. It was motivated by the national interest in promoting literacy for all individuals, the acknowledgment that speech–language pathologists serve students whose language difficulties involve reading and writing, the role of speech–language pathologists as advocates for these students, the benefits of collaborative partnerships between educators, and the questions that speech–language pathologists had regarding their role in literacy (ASHA, 2000b). There is a body of research from the communication disorders, linguistics, and education fields that confirms the connection between language and reading (Goldsworthy & Peretti, 2013; Kamhi & Catts, 2012). Reading, language arts, and communication skills are linked and interdependent in the educational process.

Reading and Reading Disabilities

Literacy is defined by Section 3 of the National Literacy Act of 1991 as "an individual's ability to read, write, and speak in English and compute and solve problems at levels of proficiency necessary to function on the job and in society, to achieve one's goals and to develop one's knowledge and potential." Literacy encompasses reading, writing, speaking, listening, and thinking in most languages, not just English. Literacy is the purpose of schooling in this country (Goldsworthy & Peretti, 2013). "Of all school learning, nothing compares in importance with reading; it is of unparalleled significance" (Bettelheim & Zelan, 1982, p. 5).

Some descriptions of reading explain the reading event but are not helpful in providing understanding about why some students struggle to learn to read. Definitions typically include the two basic elements of reading: *comprehension* and *decoding*. Kamhi and Catts (2012) called reading "thinking guided by print." Snow, Burns, and Griffin (1998) offered the following description:

> Reading as a cognitive and psycholinguistic activity requires the use of form (the written code) to obtain meaning (the message to be understood), within the context of the reader's purpose (for learning, for enjoyment, for insight). (p. 33)

Goldsworthy (1996), in one of the early texts on intervention for reading disabilities for speech–language pathologists, indicated that some simple definitions were misleading if reading was defined as an event rather than a process:

> During the reading process, information extracted from the printed page, whether at the level of decoding and word recognition or comprehension of text, is analyzed and compared with previously stored information. If it were a simple matter of learning a set of associations between sounds of the spoken language and printed squiggles on a page, learning to read would be relatively easy because it would involve little that is new to the would-be reader with the exception that language will now be presented through the visual modality. The process involved in reading acquisition, however, is far more complex than a simple transfer of meaning from oral to written language. (p. 33)

The National Reading Panel (2000) report contributed the five elements of reading instruction. A meta-analysis of over 10,000 studies led the panel to conclude that a complete reading program needed to include instruction in these areas:

- Phonemic awareness
- Phonics
- Fluency
- Vocabulary
- Text comprehension

Most researchers agree that 80% of children in elementary schools learn to read adequately (Fey, 1999; Kamhi & Catts, 2012; Lyon, 1998). The 20% who struggle do so for many reasons: They may have sensory impairments or developmental or language disabilities or are English Learners, for example (August & Shanahan, 2006; Kaderavek, 2011; C. E. Snow et al., 1998; Ukrainetz, 2015; Wallach, 2008). These students require explicit systematic instruction in the areas outlined by Lyon (as cited in Snow et al., 1998) to be successful.

The past 15 to 20 years have been robust with research in reading and literacy within the disciplines of reading research, learning disabilities, general education, special education, speech–language pathology, and school administration. Numerous approaches to reading and reading instruction have improved practice for developing readers and young children. Kaderavek (2011) asserted the following regarding the role of the speech–language pathologist in reading and writing, agreeing with ASHA (2001) that speech–language pathologists should "indirectly and directly incorporate reading and writing interventions into clinical practice" (p. 306):

- At the younger level, speech–language pathologists may be the first to detect the child's language impairment. Research demonstrates that the presence of a language impairment in preschool and kindergarten is an important indicator of a potential reading disability. Consequently, prior to school entry, the speech–language pathologist is likely to be at the forefront in leading an early literacy and language intervention program (p. 307).
- Primary targets of emergent literacy prevention, assessment, and intervention programs include the following:
  - Phonological awareness
  - Print concepts and alphabetic awareness
  - Oral language skills
  - Emergent writing
- At later ages (first grade and beyond) the speech–language pathologist generally works alongside other education professionals. The speech–language pathologist's role in assessment and intervention is typically domain specific; for example, targeting the student's narrative ability or spelling abilities or focusing on written language skills (p. 307).
- The following are primary targets of literacy assessment and intervention for school-age students with specific language impairment (LI):
  - Narrative assessment and intervention
  - Spelling assessment and intervention
  - Reading comprehension assessment and metaskills intervention
  - Writing assessment and intervention

In the era of Common Core State Standards, all students, including students with significant cognitive disabilities, are expected to be instructed and achieve standards. Students with significant cognitive disabilities may be instructed on alternate achievement standards. The key is that these students will receive explicit direct instruction, just like other students. For many years, individuals with cognitive disabilities were not provided specific instruction in reading or provided literacy experiences beyond functional literacy. The CCSS and current practice require vigilance in providing literacy experiences to all students, including those with significant disabilities and complex communication needs (ASHA, 2005a; Moore, 2014a; Sturm, 2015).

The Literacy Gateway of the ASHA Web site (ASHA, 2016a) stated the following regarding the role of the speech–language pathologist working with students with reading disabilities or literacy issues:

> Speech–Language Pathologists have the specialized knowledge and experience needed to identify communication problems and to provide the help that children need to build critical language and literacy skills. Speech–Language Pathologists are often the first professionals to identify the root cause of reading and writing problems through a child's difficulty with language. Speech–Language Pathologists help children to build the skills they need to succeed in school and in life.

Key elements of a speech–language pathologist's academic training relating to early language and literacy development include skills to

- build and reinforce relationships between early spoken language and early pre-literacy abilities, and consider the influences of parent–child interactions in early shared storybook interactions;
- address difficulties involving phonological awareness, memory, and retrieval;
- teach children to use tactile–kinesthetic and auditory cues in reading and writing;
- analyze how the language demands of textbooks, academic talk, and curriculum may stress a student's capabilities at different age and grade levels; and
- conduct fine-grained analyses of written language, including spelling, to generate intervention that matches the needs of individual students.

The role of speech–language pathologists as compared to other education professionals is often debated in the field. There are clear indications that ASHA, child language researchers, and federal legislation require attention to students' skills in reading and writing. Students with disabilities will be affected in this area. Reading is a language-based skill, so it is vital that speech–language pathologists are vigilant about addressing these needs in intervention and through collaboration with other educators. Reading disabilities have been described as both a cause and a consequence of language impairment (Kamhi & Catts, 2012). Being vigilant about new research and developments in the field related to reading, written language, and literacy should be considered a requirement for those working with children. Speech–language pathologists in schools will find it beneficial to attend in-service trainings on reading and written language with their general education colleagues. As Ehren (2009) suggested, the speech–language pathologist will view all issues through the language lens. This will be very important for issues related to reading.

Areas of Instruction for Successful Readers

In testimony to the U.S. House of Representatives, Committee on Education and the Workforce, July 10, 1997, G. Reid Lyon, Chief, Child Development and Behavior Branch of the National Institute of Child Health and Human Development (NICHD), said: "To learn to read, a child must integrate phonemic skills into learning phonic principles, must practice reading so word recognition is rapid and accurate, and must learn how to actively use comprehension strategies to enhance meaning" (as quoted in Snow et al., 1998, p. 41).

Roles and Responsibilities in Reading

The roles and responsibilities of speech–language pathologists in literacy development are identified in three sources: (a) national literacy recommendations, (b) state guidelines in special education and reading, and (c) ASHA guidelines for roles and responsibilities for speech–language pathologists in facilitating literacy.

The National Council on Preventing Reading Difficulties in Young Children noted in its findings that identification of, and service to, children with language problems by speech–language pathologists was second in a long list of critical recommendations for prevention (as cited in Snow et al., 1998). It reported that identification of preschool children who were at risk for learning to read was based on these research-derived indicators:

- In infancy or during the preschool period, children have significant delays in expressive language, receptive vocabulary, or IQ.
- At school entry, children have delays in a combination of measures of readiness, including the following:
  - Letter identification
  - Understanding the functions of print
  - Verbal memory for stories and sentences
  - Phonological awareness
  - Lexical skills, such as naming vocabulary
  - Receptive language skills in the areas of syntax and morphology
  - Expressive language
  - Overall language development

Most states have robust literacy programs that address the issues of prevention of reading difficulties, philosophies of reading acquisition, the selection of reading books and educational materials, and university teacher education programs. States have documented that 80% of the children referred for special education programs exhibited reading problems (President's Commission on Excellence in Special Education, 2002). The vast majority of goals and objectives on IEPs address needs in reading and writing.

Poor reading skills were preventing these children from accessing meaningful instructional content in their classrooms. For 85% to 90% of poor readers, effective prevention and early intervention can increase their reading skills to within average levels (Justice, 2007; Lyon, 1998). Speech–language pathologists and other special educators have a role to play in service delivery to students with reading and language disabilities.

The ASHA (2000b) guidelines for speech–language pathologists' roles and responsibilities in promoting reading and literacy in school-age children expand the initial technical report and the profession's position paper on reading and writing. These guidelines clarify that speech–language pathologists have the expertise and responsibility to play important roles related to literacy. Collaborative approaches with other school-based professionals are urged throughout the ASHA guidelines, along with close adherence to state and local policies, procedures, and regulations on the subject of reading and literacy. Service delivery for children with a combination of reading difficulties and language disabilities should include prevention, identification, assessment, intervention, coordination with other professionals, and contributions to future research and information. The ASHA document that outlines each of these areas in highly practical detail is almost 60 pages long, which attests to the importance of service delivery in this expanded model (ASHA, 2000b). The guide is available on the ASHA Web site (www.asha.org).

Comprehension and decoding may affect students' reading behaviors in different ways. One skill group without the other is not true reading; however, students with special needs will often acquire skills unevenly. Balancing the teaching of comprehension (e.g., listening, narrative, and retelling skills) with decoding (e.g., sound–symbol matching and pattern-recognition skills) must be a collaborative effort between speech–language pathologists and other educators. Speech–language pathologists provide intervention services in both components of reading (ASHA, 2000b).

Serving Students in Preschool

Assessing and providing therapy for children younger than 5 years of age was a permissive program under the Education for All Handicapped Children Act (EAHCA) of 1975. A *permissive special education program* is one that federal law approves to be funded but does not mandate. Some states immediately began serving very young children, with Michigan offering programs in schools, preschools, and day-care settings for children age 2 years. In other states, parents of children with long-standing conditions, such as hearing loss, cerebral palsy, developmental delays, or syndromes, waited for their children's fifth birthdays to have them assessed by the school district so that they could receive services free and in the vicinity of their neighborhood school. Unfortunately, lack of intervention through the formative preschool years only made the task of appropriate programming that much more difficult in kindergarten.

School districts without preschool intervention discovered a need to know the number of children with disabilities (and with which disabilities) would arrive in their kindergartens each year. Once they knew the children and families, they could prepare suitable programs and have staff hired or trained when necessary. The most compelling reason for early intervention programs was, of course, that successful early intervention ameliorated children's disabilities and enabled them to be a part of a general education class sooner. Because these youngsters would spend the next 12 to 16 years in the school system, schools had a big stake in early and effective intervention.

With the amendments to the EAHCA of 1975 in P.L. 99-457 (1986), preschool and early childhood special education programs became a part of the full special education continuum of services offered by schools. Preschool programs were included in Part B of the act to include services for children with special needs beginning at age 3 years. Districts sought space to set up classes and offer center-based services (i.e., children come to a school facility to receive services), sometimes nudging out privately run preschools that were leasing empty classrooms in schools. In the late 1980s, large preschool programs were created in many states (e.g., Texas, California, Maryland), including transportation systems for very young children and a full staff of specialists to assess children, counsel families, and provide occupational, physical, and speech–language therapy. Communication disorders quickly became the most commonly identified disability, and its intervention became the most frequently provided service in preschools. Most preschool children with identifiable impairments and disabilities demonstrate some type of communication disorder. The U.S. Department of Education (2014) reported to the Congress,

> in 2012, the most prevalent disability category of children ages 3 through 5 served under *IDEA*, Part B, was *speech or language impairments* (44.7 percent). The next most common disability was *developmental delay* (37.2 percent), followed by *autism* (7.8 percent). The children ages 3 through 5 represented by the category "Other disabilities combined" accounted for the remaining 10.3 percent of children served under the *IDEA*, Part B. (p. xxiii)

Preschool services were not altered by the 2004 reauthorization of IDEA (see Chapter 2 for details).

Because children are still developing their language throughout preschool, delayed communication development can masquerade as simple immaturity. Children's communication skills are not yet stabilized, and many children may still be acquiring the last few complex sounds of their first or second languages. Researchers have repeatedly described the explosion of new vocabulary that a child acquires between the ages of 4 and 5 years, when school begins for most of them (Kaderavek, 2011; van Kleeck, 1998; Vygotsky, 1978). In the preschool setting, it is particularly important for speech–language pathologists to be thoroughly familiar with:

1. normal acquisition of speech and language, so that children are not overidentified, and
2. appropriate intervention models for this age group that are not merely scaled-down versions of similar services for school-age children.

Assessment and Eligibility for Preschoolers

Children ages 3 to 5 years with suspected communication disabilities must be assessed by speech–language pathologists. Preschoolers are referred by parents, community agencies, physicians, private preschool administrators, or others outside the school. There is no cost for the assessment. The assessment may take place at the neighborhood school or a central assessment center.

Young children should be assessed informally and formally using tools that are designed for their age group only. If a child's language or culture is different from that of the speech–language pathologist, the professional needs to be sensitive to the child-rearing practices of the family, be familiar with language development processes for Dual-Language Learners (Justice, 2006b), listen carefully to the family's concerns, and use an interpreter if needed (see also ASHA, n.d.-c, "Cultural Competence," and Chapter 3, "Timelines and Diversity"). For example, a speech–language pathologist must be careful not to mistake a 3-year-old's reluctance to engage while speaking to a stranger for a communication problem. Family members are often the best resource for the speech–language pathologist to learn about a child's typical performance.

Observation of children in their natural environments and in play, interacting with typical peers, is an important parameter. The use of dynamic assessment to see what children know and what they can learn if taught is a highly preferred method of assessing preschoolers. Speech–language pathologists must be conscious not to use assessment methods that are appropriate for older children and then consider a child disabled, when the reason he or she is not performing is a lack of experience or exposure. Criterion reference methods, such as language sampling and checklists, interviews with teachers and family or caretakers, and observation, are necessary to make appropriate determinations. RTI is also gaining increasing popularity for preschool-age children. RTI allows for assessors, educators, and parents to see what skills students truly have before making judgments based on limited interactions with a young child.

There are separate preschool eligibility criteria in most states because of the importance of early intervention and the difference between early development and school-age performance. The paucity of standardized tests at this level, the difficulty getting responses from a young child on demand, and the interplay of cognition and language at this age are accounted for in broader criteria at this level. Most criteria refer to developmental levels of children rather than test scores. States and school districts recognize the relatively short amount of time available to reach students during this critical stage of development and do not wish to delay or deny services by setting strict entrance criteria.

Speech–language pathologists and preschool assessment teams need to be cautious about identifying children as having a disability when experience, exposure, and cultural difference may interplay with the issues presented. This is a fine balancing act. Sometimes, preschool assessment teams may identify children as having a disability in order to allow them to access services (see "Conducting and Completing the Assessment Process" in Chapter 3). These efforts are attempting to provide these children, often students from low-socioeconomic backgrounds, with experiences they may not be receiving at home so that they can enter preschool ready to meet kindergarten standards and expectations. Sometimes the preschool assessment team may not identify a student as having a disability but may still wish to refer the child's family to other resources or opportunities for learning in the community (see "Developmentally Appropriate Early Childhood Programs and Services," later in this chapter).

Transitioning From Part C to Part B

Many young children with disabilities are served in the infant and toddler program, which is organized under Part C of the IDEA. Services to infants and toddlers are very different from services to preschool children. (See the section "Infants and Toddlers" in Chapter 7.) Both for families and for service providers, these transitions can sometimes be awkward and emotional. In many states, the agency responsible for providing services to infants and toddlers may not be the school district, and so notifications and coordination for transition assessments and meetings must be worked out between agencies. In addition, under Part C, services are identified through an Individualized Family Service Plan (IFSP); however, when a child becomes 3 years old, an IEP is developed. Transition assessments are required to determine eligibility and appropriate services. Families may wish to continue with the service delivery model offered under Part B, which may provide services in the family home, and families may wish to have the service providers who came to their home continue, because those individuals know their child and family. Despite these desires, when children become 3 years of age, the requirements and funding sources change, and typically the service delivery models and service providers change as well. Agencies need to work closely together for a smooth transition so that families understand the process and have all of their questions answered so they feel comfortable with these changes. Reassuring families that the preschool providers are also knowledgeable and caring will go a long way toward ensuring a smooth transition.

Caseloads and Scheduling

The models of service delivery and corresponding samples of speech–language pathologists' schedules discussed earlier in this chapter have some application for preschoolers. However, models and schedules for preschoolers often include a wider variety of settings and models. Service delivery locations may vary from either home-school, center-based, or, in rare situations, home-based programs. Caseloads and scheduling of services for preschoolers in any setting should follow effective evidence-based practice for this population.

Speech–language pathologists need to devote larger blocks of time to serve preschoolers, maintain close contact with caregivers and teachers, and allow for children's regular recharging through naps, snacks, and a mixture of fine- and gross-motor activities. Some preschoolers will have IEPs for phonological intervention and may have an IEP that calls for service only once or twice a week. Other children will have more intense services, in small-group settings or within a classroom program, depending on their needs. Speech–language pathologists may work directly and indirectly in the preschool classroom; meet with teachers and parents; use recess, snack time, and animal-petting time; and incorporate children's interests and friends to generalize new skills.

Preschoolers may have high energy one moment and be too tired to keep their eyes open 10 minutes later. Usually, mornings are better times for teaching new skills; however, afternoon preschools can be equally beneficial if time is used wisely. Center-based programs often run a morning class and an afternoon class. Some speech–language pathologists serve students in preschool classrooms, other preschool-age students are brought to centers for therapy only, and some students are served in inclusive neighborhood child or preschool programs. Some preschool classes are taught by speech–language pathologists, enabling these professionals to thread language activities throughout the curriculum.

Preschool Schedules

Preschool schedules need to incorporate some elements that differ from school schedules because of the children's young age, the role of families, and the types of services offered. Frequently, the following elements are on preschool schedules:

- Ten- to 15-minute individual treatment sessions
- Joint sessions with parent and child
- Group activities scheduled at the playground, art area, water table, clay sink, animal cages, and so on that integrate gross- and fine-motor skills with language
- Snack or nutrition time
- Bathroom schedules
- Parent meetings
- Home visits
- Nap or rest time if there is more than 1 hour of instruction
- Travel time to agency preschool sites, Head Start programs, or private facilities

Not all speech–language pathologists will need to schedule all these options. Some speech–language pathologists work exclusively with preschoolers; others work with preschoolers, infants, and toddlers; and others work with preschoolers and the school-age population.

Historically, ASHA (2000a) recommended a caseload of 24 preschoolers for a speech–language pathologist working exclusively in this setting. ASHA now does not provide a recommended caseload size but suggests working through a workload model to determine the appropriate balance for all workload activities. This is a guideline that many schools have followed; however, caseloads are determined by state agencies, so there are wide variations among states. ASHA's (2014a) "2014 Schools Survey" reported a median caseload size of 41 for preschool. Providing comprehensive preschool services to young children, their families, and other support personnel is a challenge. Keeping up to date on educational, therapeutic, and legal issues when dealing with families is equally important. Speech–language pathologists also need to be culturally competent (see "Students Who Are Culturally and Linguistically Diverse" in Chapter 7) and sensitive to families' interests and preferences and ensure that delays related to second-language acquisition or due to cultural differences are not identified as language disorders when children are young and do not have the same experiences as other children. (See the ASHA Web site on preschool language disorders: www.asha.org/public/speech/disorders/Preschool-Language-Disorders/.) For speech–language pathologists working with young children, working with families is the key to success.

Developmentally Appropriate Early Childhood Programs and Services

The topic of early intervention and programs for preschoolers has increasingly gathered the interest of parents and policy makers in this nation over the past decade. This interest is based on a variety of situations, including the increasing number of women in the workforce; research demonstrating the importance of providing early instruction and intervention to children who are at-risk for school failure because of environmental, socioeconomic, and developmental factors; and the increase in the identification of autism. Over the course of the past decade, competencies for early childhood educators and standards for early childhood programs have all become part of the fabric of services to these children. Increasingly, states have developed universal preschool programs and expanded opportunities for these children before they reach school age.

In the past, too many early intervention programs have been operated like school-age pull-out programs. It is inappropriate for a 3-year-old child to sit across a table from a speech–language pathologist in a room separate from a preschool environment and attempt to learn new skills through drill. This situation offers virtually no opportunity for the preschooler to incorporate speech–language acquisition into play, experimentation, or ongoing physical and cognitive trial-and-error efforts. Therefore, artificial "therapy" environments should be avoided.

The ASHA (2014a) "2014 Schools Survey" found that pull-out is still a commonly used service delivery model in preschools, with 14.2 hours a week spent in this service delivery model at preschool locations compared to 19.8 hours per week at elementary schools. Service delivery models in preschools are changing, just as they are in school-age locations. Bellini and Pina (2010) reported shifts to a more inclusive service delivery model in Rhode Island, which included a complete overhaul of eligibility and service delivery options, including an RTI-type model. Various models that seek to provide a longer diagnostic period and less reliance on standardized assessments are being used in districts and yielding positive results (Nishida, personal communication, September 28, 2016). Advantages to these models include greater relevancy, generalization, frequency of intervention, and opportunity to assist other children who are at risk but not receiving services. There were some advantages to having the expertise all in one place, but public policy and public pressure began to create a demand for programs that remained within the general education environment, including the natural environment for children not yet in formal schooling. The USDE (2014) reported the following in terms of location of services for children ages 3–5 years served under IDEA, Part B. Of the children served,

- 65% were served in regular early childhood programs for some part of their day;
- 37.2% attended at least 10 hours per week in typical early childhood programs;
- 23.6% attended a separate class;
- 4.9% were served in environments defined as separate school, residential school, or home; and
- 6.5% were served in service provider location or some other location.

Effects of Inclusive Practices

Inclusive practices for educating all children, including those younger than age 5 years, have not been defined in IDEA (1997, 2004) legislation. As long ago as the mid-1990s, ASHA (1996) produced a position statement on inclusive practices that, although it addressed all children, had a dramatic effect on the service provision for 3- to 5-year-olds with speech–language disabilities. Inclusive practices in preschools for children with communication disabilities set the tone for subsequent interventions in school. Speech–language pathologists played a vital role in integrating communication skill building into children's days—a big departure from pull-out sessions or therapy isolated from the normal activities of children's days.

The movement to provide greater inclusionary opportunities for preschool children is seen in several recent documents related to this issue. In February 2012, Dr. Melanie Musgrove, director of the Office of Special Education Programs (OSEP), wrote a "Dear Colleague" letter that provided guidance to the field that the mandate for least restrictive environment (LRE) applied to preschool children and school-age children. The OSEP director acknowledged that some local education agencies (e.g., school districts) do not have public preschools, which may lead to the need for funding of placements in private preschools or other options developed by the LEA. (See www2.ed.gov/policy/speced/guid/idea/memosdcltrs/preschoollre22912.pdf.) The California Statewide Special Education Task Force (2015) report cited both research in early childhood and brain-development research as calls for changes in the restrictive environments for preschool services found in that state. Extending and reinforcing the movements seen in Rhode Island and California and the guidance from OSEP and the Office of Special Education and Rehabilitative Services, the U.S. Departments of Education and Health and Human Services issued a "Draft Policy

Statement on Inclusion of Children With Disabilities" on May 15, 2015, which stated the following:

> Children with disabilities and their families continue to face significant barriers to accessing inclusive high-quality early childhood programs and too many preschool children with disabilities continue to receive special education services in separate settings. This lag in progress is troubling for many reasons:
>
> * Being meaningfully included as a member of society is the first step to equal opportunity, one of America's most cherished ideals, and is every person's right—a right supported by our laws.
> * A robust body of literature indicates that meaningful inclusion is beneficial to children with and without disabilities across a variety of developmental domains.
> * Preliminary research shows that operating inclusive early childhood programs is not more expensive than operating separate early childhood programs for children with disabilities.
> * Meaningful inclusion in high-quality early childhood programs can support children with disabilities in reaching their full potential resulting in societal benefits more broadly.
>
> It is the Departments' position that all young children with disabilities should have access to inclusive high-quality early childhood programs, where they are provided with appropriate support in meeting high expectations. (USDE, 2015)

These documents provide clear direction from state and federal levels and will affect the locations and services that will be provided to young children in the future. Because the majority of these young children have speech–language services due to speech, language, and communication issues, the trends and policy issues in this area will greatly affect speech–language pathologists providing these services.

Preliteracy and Literacy Acquisition

Preliteracy and literacy skills develop in preschool. Many children who exhibit later reading problems had speech–language disabilities identified in preschool (Justice, 2006a; Kaderavek, 2011; Kamhi & Catts, 2012). Speech–language pathologists need to know how reading is acquired and how children begin to acquire print meaning and print form between the ages of 3 and 5 years (van Kleeck, 1998). Phonological awareness skills are informally taught and reinforced by parents in this time period (e.g., nursery rhymes, poems, songs, word games) (Goldsworthy and Perretti, 2013; Torgeson, 1998). These are important precursors to reading and are frequently delayed in children who struggle with reading (Kaderavek, 2011). Speech–language pathologists have an important role to play in literacy development because it includes reading, writing, speaking, listening, and thinking skills. The breadth of print-related activities that young children need is staggering (van Kleeck, 2014), and literally all of these activities can be used by speech–language pathologists as language-based activities and objectives for preschoolers with communication disabilities. Models of reading that emphasize balanced reading and literacy instructional programs, such as those described by van Kleeck (1998), Adams (1999), and Justice and Skibbe (2005), are advocated by many state departments of education.

Typical preschools are often rich in the early auditory and visual patterning skills connected to reading, and children who have communication disabilities need to have the same opportunities to learn these patterns with their peers. They probably need even more exposure to and reinforcement of the patterns to be successful. Working with preschoolers requires speech–language pathologists to be constantly looking forward to the next stage of learning, no matter what the current performance level of a child might be. Low expectations at this early point can impede a child's ability to learn and grow in the mainstream of education. A disability or label does not indicate how much the child can achieve. Speech–language pathologists must be aware that diagnosis cannot be correlated with the child's ability, socialization, eventual employment, or motivation. Many professionals believe that preschool is the time to keep all future academic options open. All preschool children should be considered potential readers and writers, so speech–language pathologists who provide services to preschoolers must acknowledge and plan for this eventuality. Ensuring literacy-rich experiences is critical for all students with communication disabilities, regardless of their age, including students with significant cognitive disabilities and complex communication needs.

Feeding and Swallowing Problems in Preschool Populations

Children younger than 5 years of age who have feeding and swallowing problems may be eligible for services in preschool programs (Carbajal, Homer, Kelly, Priola, & Rizk, 2009; O'Toole, 2000; Whitmire, 2000) and usually present with fragile medical health, neurological disorders and syndromes, or related etiologies that place them at risk (Homer, 2008, 2009; Kurjan, 2000). An Individualized Family Service Plan or IEP may have goals and objectives that address a child's nutrition, eating habits, and skills at home and in a school program or center. Speech–language pathologists have been responsible for these specialized issues in preschools, using an interdisciplinary approach, including cross-training and cotreatment (Davis-McFarland, 2008; Homer, 2009; Kurjan, 2000). Homer, Bickerton, Hill, Parham, and Taylor (2000) found that a large suburban school district in Louisiana needed to have specially trained speech–language pathologists, called a swallowing action team (SWAT), to ensure that preschoolers and school-age students had safe nutrition and hydration during school hours. Preschool programs often require speech–language pathologists to have skills, such as working with swallowing problems, that extend beyond the education traditionally received in undergraduate or graduate programs plus an understanding of scope-of-practice statements for state licensure and ASHA certification (Carbajal et al., 2009; Homer, 2008, 2009; Kurjan, 2000; O'Toole, 2000; Whitmire, 2000). For a full description of the scope of practice for speech–language pathologists, go to www.asha.org/policy (ASHA, 2016c).

The Clock Is Ticking!

One of the troubling realities of working with preschoolers is the brief time available. All the assessment and intervention with children and families must be accomplished within a mere 24 months because, of course, the ages of 3 to 5 years have an established beginning and ending time. One cannot continue preschool services for just a few more weeks or months. The clock starts running immediately when children are at age 3 years and stops when children are old enough for kindergarten. From time to time, there may be a 5-year-old in preschool, but it is unusual and not encouraged. Speech–language pathologists must be cautious not to be misguided by thinking that another year of spending time with younger children would be beneficial for a 5-year-old. Such requests may be made by parents, but the professional team must understand the importance of children being with their same-age peers to have appropriate social and language models, as well as high expectations in grade-level curricula and developmentally appropriate practices. Assessment must be prompt and accurate, contacts with other service providers must be ongoing, and intervention must be targeted and results driven. It is clear that speech–language pathologists who wish to work in preschool settings will need to be familiar with all the service delivery models and intervention techniques, be well versed in the development of 3- to 5-year-olds, be innovative and flexible to meet family and child needs, and devote their energies to ensuring that a majority of the children who are served in preschool programs do not need continued communication services once they start school. Creating and maintaining preschool programs focused on maximum outcomes in 24 months or less is a major responsibility and an exciting area for speech–language pathologists.

Services for Secondary Students

IDEA 2004 mandates special education services for individuals from birth to age 21 years, but adolescents are "a population of students who have long been ignored," and few speech–language pathologists have attempted to support "the language they need to achieve academic and social success" (Apel, 1999, p. 229). Fortunately, since the time of the Apel quote, progress has been made in the knowledge base in the field about serving this unique population, as well as in the methods required to develop transition plans focusing on postsecondary goals for students with disabilities. Along with the increased focus on literacy came an increased national focus on adolescents, specifically in the area of reading (Biancarosa & Snow, 2004; Cassidy & Cassidy, 2007; Kamil, 2003). The National Joint Committee on Learning Disabilities (2008) provided an excellent discussion of the issues in its report "Adolescent Literacy and Older Students With Learning Disabilities" (see www.asha.org/policy/TR2008-00304.htm). A clinical forum of language, speech, and hearing services in schools (Joffe & Nippold, 2012) highlighted the progress that has been made in the field of understanding adolescent language disorders in the past 20 years. Interventions and service delivery considerations for adolescents have evolved in many positive ways. (See "Working With Adolescents" at www.asha.org/SLP/schools/prof-consult/Working-With-Adolescents/.)

Characteristics of Adolescents

As students move into adolescence, they spend greater amounts of time with their peers and often appear to dislike or avoid the company of adults. Intervention programs need to align with the consumer's interests, tastes, and motivation to be effective in any setting (Ehren, 2007, 2009; Larson & McKinley, 2003; Larson, McKinley, & Boley, 1993; National Joint Committee on Learning Disabilities, 2008; Nelson, 1992; Singer & Bashir, 1999). Students age 13 years and older frequently have well-defined interests and motivations. Their academic programs are typically departmentalized, including walking from class to class, working with many different teachers, and having increased personal responsibility for rules, regulations, homework, time schedules, and deadlines. They have more unscheduled time before and after school and are often exploring student groups, competitive athletics, clubs, service activities, and social time.

Apel and Swank (1999) reminded speech–language pathologists working with older students that "the self-concept and motivational level of these students must be recognized and addressed in their intervention program or success may be unattainable" (p. 239). Planning a service delivery program in middle school and high school must take these factors into account.

Adolescents with communication disabilities also experience related academic difficulties. Their language deficits may adversely affect their comprehension skills, attention, organization, and writing ability. Speech–language pathologists should recognize some of the unique characteristics of older students who have language disorders as described by Larson and McKinley (2007) in Table 6.5.

Academic-Centered Goals for Adolescents

Many students with communication disorders need continued assistance from speech–language pathologists and other special educators to be successful at the secondary level. The transition process (i.e., preparation for postsecondary employment or education) for students with special education needs must be carefully planned and implemented. Generally, a student age 13 years or older who is receiving services has been in speech–language programs for several years. The goals and objectives have changed for the student, but he or she continues to need support to be successful and access the curriculum. There is a close connection between intervention and academic achievement in middle school, and by high school, therapy is often completely integrated into academic standards. In secondary schools, students are no longer learning underlying skills; instead, they must apply strategies to increase their comprehension, retain needed information, and produce acceptable written work. Spelling, constructing sentences, expanding vocabulary, developing and describing ideas, and locating pertinent

TABLE 6.5. Characteristic Expectations and Problems of Older School-Age Students With Language Disorders

Category	Expectations	Problems
Cognition	• To be at the formal operational level • To observe, organize, and categorize data from an experience • To identify problems, suggest possible causes and solutions, and predict consequences • To place concepts into hierarchical order • To find, select, and utilize data on a given topic	• They often remain concrete operational thinkers. • They make chaos out of order. • They may not recognize the problem when it exists; if they do, they do not know how to develop alternative solutions. • They often cannot place concepts in a hierarchy. • They have limited strategies for finding, selecting, and utilizing data.
Meta-linguistics	• To demonstrate conscious awareness of linguistic knowledge • To talk about and reflect on various linguistic forms • To assess communication breakdowns and revise them	• They have difficulty bringing to awareness categories and relations in all aspects of language. • They do not know the labels for talking about language during formal education. • They do not have awareness of breakdowns, and, if they do, they lack repair strategies.
Compre-hension and pro-duction of linguistic features	• To comprehend all linguistic features and structures • To follow oral directions of three steps or more after listening to them one time • To use grammatically intact utterances • To have a vocabulary sufficient for expressing ideas and experiences • To give directions with clarity and accuracy • To get information or assistance by asking questions and to respond appropriately to questions asked of them • To comprehend and produce the slang and jargon of the hour	• They misunderstand advanced syntactical forms. • They may not realize that they are being given directions and/or have difficulty following them. • They often use sentences that are fragmented and that do not convey their messages. • They have word-retrieval problems and a high frequency of low-information words. • They often leave their listeners confused. • They may know what questions or answers to give, but they do not know how to do so tactfully. • They do not comprehend or produce slang or jargon, thus they are ostracized from the group to which they most desire to belong.
Discourse	• To produce language that is organized, coherent, and intelligible to their listeners • To follow adult conversational rules for speakers • To be effective listeners during conversation without displaying incorrect listening habits • To make a report, tell or retell a story, and explain a process in detail • To listen to lectures and to select main ideas and supporting details • To analyze critically other speakers • To express their own attitudes, moods, and feelings and to disagree appropriately	• They use many false starts and verbal mazes. • They consistently violate the rules (e.g., maintaining a topic, initiating a topic). • They often have poor listening skills. • They often leave their listeners confused. • They often do not grasp the essential message of a lecture. • Their judgments are arbitrary or illogical. • They have abrasive conversational speech.

TABLE 6.5. *(continued)*

Category	Expectations	Problems
Nonverbal communication	• To follow nonverbal rules for kinesics • To follow nonverbal rules for proxemics	• They violate the rules and misinterpret body movements and facial expressions. • They violate the rules for social distance.
Survival language	• To comprehend and produce situational phrases and vocabulary required for survival in our society • To comprehend and produce concepts and vocabulary required across daily living situations	• They do not have the necessary concepts and vocabulary needed in places such as banks, grocery stores, and employment agencies. • They do not have the necessary concepts and vocabulary needed across daily living situations such as telling time, using money, and understanding warning signs.
Written language	• To comprehend written language required in various academic, social, and vocational situations by organizing, planning, composing, and editing • To produce cohesive written language required in various academic, social, and vocational situations	• They do not consistently and/or efficiently process information obtained through reading. • They do not consistently and/or efficiently generate written language that conveys their messages.

Note. Adapted from *Communication Solutions for Older Students* (pp. 133–134), by V. L. Larson and N. L. McKinley, 2007, Austin, TX: PRO-ED. © 2007 by PRO-ED. Adapted with permission.

information and writing about it dominate the intervention process at this level. Remember, the main goal of most high school students is to earn a diploma and achieve academically. Supports from the speech–language pathologist will be addressing the skills needed so the student can attain a diploma. In addition, many students need assistance with pragmatics and social language to engage in the reciprocal friendships and working relationships so critical at the secondary level. Students with autism specifically experience higher levels of anxiety in adolescence and benefit from social communication strategies (Winner & Crooke, 2011), while many adolescents will also benefit from strategies in executive functioning (Trukstra & Byom, 2010).

Transition Plans

IDEA 2004 requires that for all students with disabilities, beginning at age 16 years (or younger, if appropriate), an IEP must include a statement about the transition service needs of a student that focuses on his or her course of study (34 C.F.R. § 300.320 [b][1]). Transition service is a coordinated set of activities that

> is designed to be within a results-oriented process, that is focused on improving the academic and functional achievement of the child with a disability to facilitate the child's movement from school to post-school activities, including postsecondary education, vocational education, integrated employment (including supported employment), continuing and adult education, adult services, independent living, or community participation. (34 C.F.R. § 300.43 [a][1])

Individualized Transition Plan (ITP) development is often a part of an IEP process but may be a separate assessment and meeting in a given school or district. The purpose of an ITP is to begin planning for a student's integration into the world of work and independent living. For many students, communication skills are critical to be successful in a job situation. Speech–language pathologists may find themselves designing role-plays of job interviews or working collaboratively with job coaches to help students achieve ITP goals. Functional outcomes are the best tool for evaluating adolescent services. The model chosen by speech–language pathologists and school teams is appropriate if students learn to function at a higher level on meaningful school-based or quality-of-life indicators. In middle school and high school, these indicators should be a part of an IEP and be observable beyond the speech room. Transition goals may help all educators focus on functional outcomes instead of limiting their efforts to helping students earn credits for graduation. Older students can help keep track of their own progress in many secondary school environments.

Making a Difference at the Secondary Level

Educational, social, ethical, and fiscal arguments are proposed for providing services to adolescents in unique and meaningful ways. Reversed patterns of failure and a refocus by previously undirected students on finishing high school and pursuing career or job opportunities become important functional outcomes for adolescents. Students, with the assistance of speech–language pathologists and other IEP team members, can develop highly practical, personally motivating IEPs for themselves. IDEA 2004 lists students as members of IEP teams, if appropriate. The law requires that students be invited to IEP meetings whenever transition services are considered, and if students do not participate in these meetings, the district must take other steps to ensure that students' preferences and interests are considered. It is hard to imagine that an effective IEP for an adolescent, transition related or not, could be written without that student's input.

Some students with significant disabilities will continue to receive speech–language services in middle school and high school if an IEP team agrees that improvement or progress is expected for a student within a year. Maintaining the student's functional level does not require intervention; it requires practice with the skill in an authentic setting. This type of practice may be carried out by other educators. All intervention should be directly tied to an observable improvement in the students' daily activities. An IEP for students in Grade 6 or higher should include one or more of the following goals written in measurable terms:

- Increased literacy (i.e., reading, spelling, and writing) skills
- Increased social language skills
- More appropriate peer interactions
- Progress on a transition plan
- Progress toward a vocational goal
- Improved organization, attention, or study skills

- Progress toward emotional control and stability
- Greater independence or interdependence than the previous year

With greater emphasis on accountability for all students' success (ESEA 2015; IDEA 2004), secondary schools have focused on their disabilities subgroup to determine why many of these students are not graduating. One such obstacle to graduation has been poorly developed written language skills (Montgomery & Kahn, 2005). Speech–language pathologists working with a team of secondary educators may instruct identified students to write both narrative and expository text to meet the grade-level standards needed for graduation (Montgomery & Kahn, 2007). This service may be effectively provided in pull-out or coteaching settings.

Models That Match Students and School Settings

Selecting one or more service delivery models to encourage these important outcomes will depend on the factors presented in Chapter 5, plus the adolescent's ages and interests. Larson and McKinley (2007) presented several models (see Figure 6.4) that speech–language pathologists use to structure service delivery at the secondary level. Of these, the prototype model (i.e., offering speech–language service as a course for credit) is often the most palatable to adolescents.

Older students are more likely to be grouped, seen for periods of time that mirror the academic schedule, and held accountable for their own progress. Some speech–language pathologists teach a class called Communication Skills, where students can

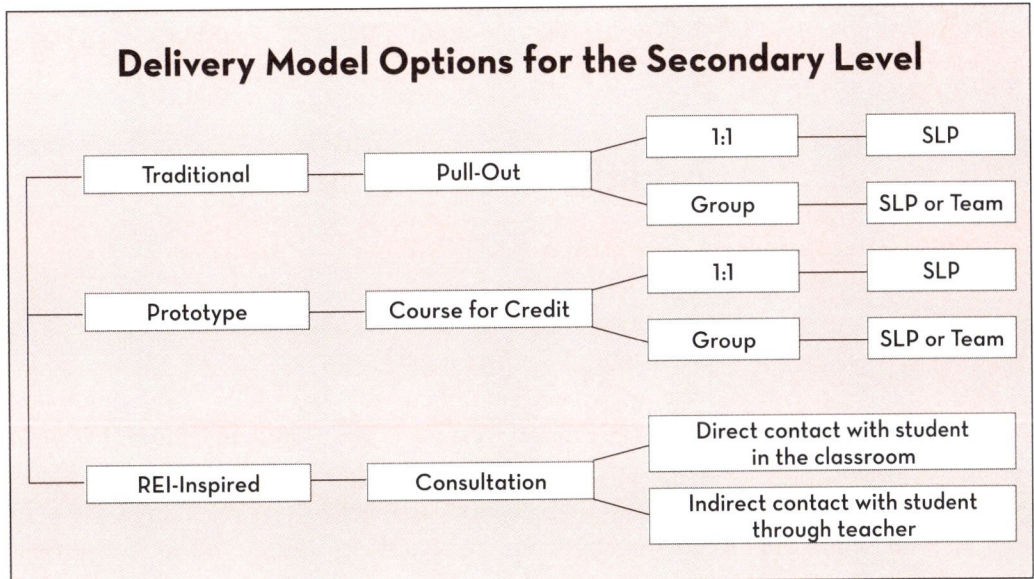

FIGURE 6.4. Delivery model options for the secondary level.

Note. Adapted from *Communication Solutions for Older Students* (p. 294), by V. L. Larson and N. L. McKinley, 2007, Austin, TX: PRO-ED. © 2007 by PRO-ED. Adapted with permission.

receive academic credit for working on IEP goals. Other speech–language pathologists award grades so student work can be figured into the grade point average. A school governing board must approve a class for students to receive credit. Other speech–language pathologists report that coteaching is the most effective way to support students in classes that have challenging subject matter and high student expectations.

Students with various types of special education needs will receive attention from a high-school IEP team. Service delivery models will need to be changed from time to time during the school year to accommodate students' changing needs or to intervene in, avert, or recover from a crisis situation (Montgomery & Moore, 2011; Sanger & Moore-Brown, 2000). Students who are fully included in high school may need speech–language pathologists' support. These students often fall into one of two categories: students with mild to moderate learning disabilities who require ongoing assistance to succeed or students with severe disabilities who require extensive supports—one-to-one aide, assistive technology (AT), modified physical environment, and other communication skills—to flourish in a general education placement. Students who are fully included do not automatically require speech–language intervention; however, adequate communication skills often determine whether students are successful socially and academically.

Students with disabilities are entitled to receive special education until they separate from the school district when they either receive a high-school diploma or age out at 22. Some students who are not on a diploma track may matriculate to an adult transition program, which is separate from the high-school program. Once students have completed a 4-year high-school program, generally when they are about 18 years old, their educational program should be focused on developing job and community skills. Speech–language pathologists may find themselves working with adults in these programs, helping these adult students learn communication skills and new vocabulary appropriate for community and job settings.

Additional Resources

Resources are available on the ASHA Web site that provide information on implementing the workload concept. (See www.asha.org/practice-portal/professional-issues/Caseload-and-Workload/.) The documents that accompany the position statement, including the technical report (ASHA, 2002b)and guidelines (ASHA, 2002a), and the implementation document, have subsequently provided additional documents and information on workload. The workload concept has been well received and also adopted by other professional organizations (e.g., National Association of School Psychologists, National Association of State Directors of Special Education, American Occupational Therapy Association [AOTA], and American Physical Therapy Association [APTA]). The joint statement by AOTA, APTA, and ASHA reflects the importance of this concept on improving student outcomes. (See "Workload Approach: A Paradigm Switch for Positive Impact on Student Outcomes" (2014) at www.asha.org/uploadedFiles/ASHA/Practice_Portal/Professional_ Issues/Caseload_and_Workload/APTA-ASHA-AOTA-Joint-Doc-Workload-Approach-Schools.pdf. See also the Speedy Speech Web site at www.speedy speechtherapy.com/.) Also see Mire and Montgomery (2009) for a description of another type of service delivery for speech-sound disorders.

For more information on integrated services in classrooms, see Vicker (2009), "The 21st Century Speech Language Pathologist and Integrated Services in Classrooms" (www.iidc.indiana.edu/?pageId=495).

Readers of this text are urged to expand their knowledge and skills in literacy instruction. Many excellent literacy Web sites are available. Periodic articles in Special Interest Division 1 and Division 16 newsletters from ASHA and ASHA's (2000b) *Roles and Responsibilities of Speech–Language Pathologists With Respect to Reading and Writing in Children and Adolescents* are also informative.

New publications related to reading and language are always available in the field. Recent publications that may be of interest include the following:

- Catts, H. W., Fey, M. E., Ellis Weismer, S., & Bridges, M. S. (2014). The relationship between language and reading abilities. In J. B. Tomblin & M. A. Nippold (Eds.), *Understanding individual differences in language development across the school years* (pp. 144–165). New York, NY: Psychology Press/Taylor & Francis.
- Kamhi, A., & Catts, H. (Eds.). (2012). *Language and reading disabilities.* Boston, MA: Allyn & Bacon.
- Stone, C. A., Silliman, E. R., Ehren, B. J., & Wallach, G. (Eds.). (2014). *Handbook of language and literacy: Development and disorders* (2nd ed.). New York, NY: Guilford.

CHAPTER 7

Specialized Service Delivery for Specialized Student Needs

● *In This Chapter*

Public schools are committed to educating all students. Many of these students bring unusual circumstances or special requirements with them. This chapter addresses students—both general education and special education—who may need the specialized services of speech-language pathologists because of these challenges. Some individuals will be English Learners, some will use assistive technology or augmentative and alternative communication, and still others may be infants or toddlers who were identified at birth, or soon after, with a hearing loss. Students with communication disorders may present characteristics on the autism spectrum. Some students must be temporarily educated at home or in hospitals, rehabilitation units, or detention facilities. Increasing numbers of these students with special needs are served in school-based programs, necessitating highly flexible service delivery models to accommodate their temporary location and/or unique needs. Speech-language pathologists must be prepared for expanded or specialized practice in the schools.

● *Chapter Questions*

1. Describe the important elements of working with the families of students with communication disorders whose culture or language is different from that of the speech-language pathologist. Contact a local school or look on the district's website to discover how many different languages their current students speak. Find out how English Learners are ensured access to the general education curriculum. What does this school do to prevent English Learners from being inappropriately referred for special education services?
2. Contact your state speech-language and hearing association or regional consortium and ask if it has a list of speech-language pathologists in the state who are able to assess and provide intervention in languages other than English. What languages are represented? How do speech-language pathologists qualify for this list?
3. Explain the difference between *accent* and *dialect* and how the speech-language pathologist can help other educators and administrators to differentiate both from communication disorders.

4. Why is it important to be familiar with the various definitions of autism spectrum disorder (ASD) to provide the services parents and administrators request in the schools? What role does the speech–language pathologist's professional judgment play in the decision-making process?

5. Compare and contrast assistive technology (AT) and augmentative and alternative communication (AAC). Arrange to meet and converse with a student who uses a communication system, as well as his or her speech–language pathologist. Discuss how the advancements in technology have made some AT easier to access for students.

6. Explain the universal newborn hearing screening (UNHS) mandated by law and how it affects the school service delivery programs for speech and language. Does your state have UNHS? Find out what hospitals in your area are doing to provide not only universal screening but also follow-up services for families. Interview an audiologist in the program if possible.

7. What are the educational rights of students who are adjudicated, sentenced, or detained during their school years? What impact does this have on the speech–language pathologist?

8. Locate a speech–language pathologist in the schools who has responsibilities as a lead speech–language pathologist. Interview this person about the advantages and disadvantages of this type of assignment. Examine his or her weekly and monthly schedules to appreciate the increased and varied responsibilities.

Students Who Are Culturally and Linguistically Diverse

Students whose culture or language differs from the mainstream English of public schools in this country are defined as *culturally and linguistically diverse* (CLD). Not all of these students are English Learners; however, typically over half of them are. When the culture of home and school are distinctly different, children may experience social and academic challenges. Students who are culturally and linguistically diverse may be having academic issues (due to cultural or second-language learning) that are affecting their mastery of the language needed to access the curriculum. Speech–language pathologists must be vigilant in ensuring that any assessments and involvement with these students reflect cultural competence and sensitivity. Service delivery for students with identified communication disabilities who are CLD has five distinct aspects: (a) using nonbiased assessment; (b) selecting the language of instruction, including special factors to consider from the Individuals With Disabilities Education Improvement Act of 2004 (IDEA 2004); (c) using interpreters in intervention; (d) being aware of accents and dialects; and (e) working with families who are culturally and linguistically different from the speech–language pathologist. (See also "Disproportionality" in Chapter 4.)

The National Center for Education Statistics (2016) reported that approximately 4.5 million students who are English Learners attended schools in the United States in the 2013–2014 school year, representing 9.3% of all students. Reports from the U.S. Department of Commerce predict that by the year 2044, minorities will constitute a majority in the United States but that the child population will achieve this plurality by 2020 (Colby & Ortman, 2015), and that by 2030, approximately 40% of school-aged children will speak a language other than English at home (Kramer et al., 2013; Lewis, Castilleja, Moore, & Rodríguez, 2010). These students represent the fastest growing population in our nation, and some of them will need special education, including speech–language services. Special education referrals of students who are English Learners have been reported to be inappropriately high in some parts of the country (IDEA 2004). Students learning English frequently struggle with academics until their English-language skills are more highly developed. (See the discussion on the increase in diverse populations in schools under "Children and Families in the 21st Century" in Chapter 1, "Disproportionality" and "Students Who Are English Learners or Dual-Language Learners" in Chapter 4, and "Trends in Students Previously Unseen or Unserved" in Chapter 10.) Prevention of school failure and early intervention for English Learners is the key to reducing the number of students who are inappropriately referred for special education. Ortiz and Yates (2002) identified three types of English Learners. Type I learners need a positive school climate, academically enriched curriculum, and effective instruction in the general education program to succeed. Type II learners need early intervention, clinical teaching, and teacher assistance teams to prosper. Type III students need culturally sensitive assessment, family involvement, and special education to experience success in schools.

To serve the needs of children who are CLD and have communication disabilities, assessment and intervention must incorporate culturally sensitive approaches (American Speech–Language–Hearing Association [ASHA], n.d.-c; Torres, 2013).

In the ASHA "2012 Schools Survey," 58% of the respondents reported that services were provided in English to English Learners on their caseloads. In a nationwide sample, almost a third of the children served in speech–language programs were CLD.

How to best serve students who struggle is an ongoing theme in schools. Students from diverse cultural and linguistic backgrounds pose significant challenges for schools that do not have the capacity or personnel to appropriately address this population (Fergus, 2010b; Garcia, Jensen, & Scribner, 2009; McLaughlin, Pullin, & Artiles, 2001). Because of the specific knowledge in language development and disorders that speech–language pathologists have, their role is important to ensure that they, along with other leaders in the school, appropriately serve English Learners with disabilities. This means that all educators, and especially those addressing language needs, must read and understand current research and thinking in the field in these matters.

One area of emerging research pertains to the linguistic development of second-language learners. Thordardottir (2006) reminded us that growing up bilingual is normal and positive and should not be treated as a problem. Research on bilingual language development is consistently demonstrating that bilingualism facilitates language development and vocabulary growth. Recommended intervention approaches, therefore, should promote the use of both languages and not be limited to one language. Similarly, code-switching (going back and forth between languages) is also typical in bilingual speakers and should not be discouraged. Code-switching, in fact, should be considered an emerging skill, because it occurs so frequently in the general bilingual population (Peña, 2012; Thordardottir, 2006).

Research in reading and language impairment is also gaining information from studying English Learners. In the past, much of the research in reading and English Learners has focused on phonological awareness, but research now points to how language development, the definition of language impairment, and reading all affect normal language and the development of disorders in reading. More importantly, the research provides new guidance in facilitating rather than harming through the therapeutic approaches chosen (August & Shanahan, 2006; Espinosa, 2013; Gerber & Durgunoglu, 2004; McCardle, Mele-McCarthy, Cutting, Leos, & D'Emilio, 2005; Peña, 2012; Shepard & Sheng, 2009; Silliman & Scott, 2006).

IDEA 2004 is highly concerned with appropriate services to minority students and students who are English Learners. Because of the tracking of the English Learners subgroup and the disability subgroup under the Elementary and Secondary Education Act, academic achievement is paramount. Implementing the current evidence base in the field is imperative for the student to experience success. The concern for English Learners is for both over- and underidentification. As referenced in Chapter 4, Peña (2012) explained that in preschool, Latino children are enrolled in special education at a lower rate than mainstream students are (3.21% vs. 2.03%), meaning that 26,000 children are not receiving services they need. However, when students reach school age, it is a different story. When students are school age, Latino children are enrolled in special education at higher rates than mainstream students are, including students identified as learning disabled more frequently (1.75% vs. 1.52%) and receiving speech–language therapy more frequently (4.69% vs. 3.98%). This means that 20,700 children are receiving learning disability services they do not need, and 63,900 children are receiving speech therapy they do not need. These data call for attention to and improvements in appropriate assessment and identification.

Nonbiased Assessment

Although it is beyond the scope of this chapter to discuss formal and informal assessment tools, important general principles are the following:

1. *Assess* English Learners in both English and their native language.
2. *Administer* equivalent procedures and instruments in English and the student's native language.
3. *Establish* the student's level of English proficiency and the amount of English instruction he or she receives in academic settings.
4. *Use* valid and reliable instruments with culturally and linguistically appropriate procedures to establish their norms.

5. *Seek* alternative assessments of academic and language skills.
6. *Seek* language assessment data (oral and written) that is no more than 6 months old.
7. *Obtain* culturally and linguistically sensitive assessment of intelligence and achievement.
8. *Rule out* all factors that may be causing the students' learning difficulties, using a team approach (Lewis et al., 2010; Ortiz & Yates, 2002).

Peña (2012) noted that practical considerations include determining the language of home, language of school, and demands across contexts. The experience of bilingual individuals is not that they "turn off" one language when they use another. Different languages are structured differently, so examining what communication abilities exist is the goal of assessment. Comprehensive school reform efforts are working to ensure that students in the process of learning English are not placed in special education if what they actually need is support in the general education classroom to be academically successful.

When assessing students who are from CLD backgrounds, speech–language pathologists are faced with two primary issues: first, the lack of standardized measures appropriate for this population, and second, issues of disproportionality (discussed in Chapter 4) (Kramer et al., 2013). A nonbiased approach, therefore, will require the use of nonstandardized measures, including (a) an in-depth caregiver interview, (b) dynamic assessment, (c) information processing tasks, (d) narrative skill assessment in each language, (e) review of portfolio data, and (f) use of trained and skilled interpreters and translators (Kramer et al., 2013).

Process is critical when assessing English Learners. Lewis and colleagues (2010) suggested the GRASP IT! process, which is illustrated in Figure 7.1.

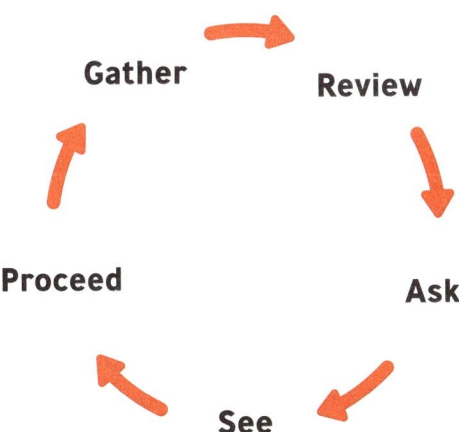

FIGURE 7.1. GRASP IT!, a panoramic framework for assessing English-language learners.

Note. From "Assessment 360: A Panoramic Framework for Assessing English Language Learners," by N. Lewis, N. Castilleja, B. J. Moore, and B. Rodríguez, 2010 July, *Perspectives on Communication Disorders and Sciences in Culturally and Linguistically Diverse Populations, 17*(2), pp. 35–56. Reprinted with permission.

According to these authors (Lewis et al., 2010, p. 42), *GRASP IT!* refers to the following procedures:

- *Gather.* Become a detective to gather the necessary information. This may take some digging, yet it is an essential component.
- *Review.* Continually examine what you find and determine what else is needed; you may decide to gather missing information.
- *Ask.* Interviewing teachers, family members, and/or members of the community will provide vital information that can help you determine the significance of assessment results.
- *See.* Observe the student in multiple settings with different partners to obtain information about the student as a communicator.
- *Proceed.* Determine the next step: Do you have the information you need to design effective instructional strategies? Does the student need additional support for English-language development? Is it appropriate to refer the student for a full and comprehensive evaluation?
- *Integrate.* Analyze the data you have gathered. Has the student had adequate support in acquiring English to ensure that the instructional material has been comprehensible? Have you conducted cultural due diligence to correctly interpret the data that you have? Are there aspects of the student's academic program that have not been investigated? Integrate all relevant data that have been gathered and reviewed. Once the need for assessment has been determined, the next obvious step is when formal testing begins.
- *Test.* Formal and informal assessment measures will complete the picture.

Nonbiased, nonstandardized measures using the GRASP IT! approach will match the ASHA recommendations for assessment and services to this population. (See also ASHA's English Learners in schools Web site at www.asha.org/practice/multicultural/ELL/. See Chapter 4 for a comprehensive discussion in "Disproportionality" and "Students Who Are English Learners or Dual-Language Learners.")

Choosing the Language of Instruction

When choosing the language of instruction and service delivery for a child, the Individualized Education Program (IEP) team must consider where on the continuum the student's language skills are within both his or her primary language and English. Speech–language pathologists play a role in this decision for the team and must consider the student's pragmatic, social, or interpersonal communication skills, not just the structural accuracy of the language. The key is to distinguish between errors made because of lack of exposure to the curriculum and errors made because of insufficient opportunity to master the language. Although English may be the language of instruction in the school, the child may have more advanced skills in a primary language used for social interaction. This would suggest that the home language should be used for instruction initially or concurrently.

Consideration of special factors is necessary for the assessment, eligibility, and IEP phases of the special education process. A communication limitation can make it very difficult to determine whether a student is struggling primarily with learning a second language or has one or more disabilities. Once eligibility is determined, the speech–language pathologist may work with the student because of communication disabilities related to a disorder or condition. Selecting the language for service delivery is based not on the skills the speech–language pathologist possesses but rather on the skills the student needs and in which language. The following questions may guide the IEP team in its decision making:

- What is the student's dominant language in various settings?
- What is the student's level of proficiency in both the primary language and English for social and academic language?
- What are the styles of verbal interaction used in the primary language and English?
- How much exposure has this student had to styles of verbal interaction in English?
- What is the extent and nature of exposure in each language (e.g., family, peers, TV, stories, etc.)?
- Are the student's language behaviors characteristic of second-language learners?
- What types of language intervention has this student already had and for how long?

"The literature in bilingual education of the last two decades suggests that children who are learning two languages may benefit from a bilingual approach in intervention" (Gutiérrez-Clellen, 1999, p. 299). Gutiérrez-Clellen (1999) emphasized that no studies were able to show that "English only" was a preferable intervention approach for students with communication disabilities. She stated that achievement and performance were maximized when the student's first language was used as an organizational framework. In addition, speech–language pathologists need to help students identified with special needs learn pragmatic and social–cultural aspects of language (e.g., eye contact, facial expression, nonverbal messages, tone) that will enable them to participate in the activities of the classroom (Kramer et al., 2013; Peña, 2012). Service delivery for children who are CLD must take the form of multidimensional, interspersing sessions in the therapy room, in the classroom, and in small interactive groups that encourage conversation. One of the primary findings in recent years about the experience of students who are English Learners is that these students must have rich experiences and opportunities to use oral language, make mistakes, and practice. Like any other skill, unless it is used, it will not grow or develop mastery. Creating these opportunities for children is vital to their success.

Using Interpreters and Translators in Intervention

When the child's primary language is not English, speech–language pathologists must either speak the child's language or use an interpreter or translator. (Note that *interpre-*

tation refers to oral language and *translation* refers to written language.) Less than 4% of the professionals belonging to ASHA report speaking a language in addition to English (ASHA, 1999). Some states have many more bilingual speech–language pathologists than others. In some large states and some border states (e.g., Florida, Texas, California, New Mexico, New Jersey, New York), bilingual speech–language pathologists are in great demand and can command salary bonuses and stipends.

Using an interpreter or translator is the method of choice for speech–language pathologists who are not fluent enough to provide therapy in both languages (ASHA, www.asha.org/practice/multicultural/issues/cb). Langdon (2002) and others pointed out both the cautions and the value of working with interpreters and translators when serving students. A resource titled *Collaborating With Interpreters and Translators* (Langdon & Cheng, 2002) describes effective service delivery and gives guidance specific to the speech–language pathology field.

Accents and Dialects

Accents and dialects, used both by speech–language pathologists and by students who speak languages in addition to English, have been controversial in the field of speech–language pathology. Although bilingual or multilingual speech–language pathologists have been in great demand in this country, many of them have reported facing bias in graduate education programs and in the job market (ASHA, 2011; Montgomery, 1999). Public school students with accents or dialects that are different from those of the mainstream culture of their school may be referred for special education services or speech services or viewed as low achievers. In the late 1990s, an effort to dispel these misguided concerns and avoid potential discriminatory behaviors resulted in a position statement and supporting technical report titled "Students and Professionals Who Speak English With Accents and Nonstandard Dialects: Issues and Recommendations" (ASHA, 1998a). In this statement, *accent* was defined as a phonetic trait from one's first language that was carried over to one's second language. The listener can hear some of the patterns of sound production found in the person's first spoken language that are not in the second language. Persons who use English as their second (or third or fourth) language may have accented English, depending on their age and the circumstances under which they learned English.

An ASHA (1993) position statement offered this definition of dialect:

> *Communication difference/dialect* is a variation of a symbol system used by a group of individuals that reflects and is determined by shared regional, social, or cultural/ethnic factors. A regional, social, or cultural/ethnic variation of a symbol system should not be considered a disorder of speech or language.

Each dialect has distinguishing linguistic characteristics (phonological, morphological, semantic, syntactic, and pragmatic), although the majority of linguistic features of the (American) English language are common to each of the varieties of (American) English (Montgomery, 1999).

The concluding sentence of ASHA's (1998a) position statement issues a clear directive:

> All individuals speak with an accent and/or dialect; thus, the nonacceptance of individuals into higher education programs or into the professions solely on the basis of the presence of an accent or dialect is discriminatory. Members of ASHA must not discriminate against persons who speak with an accent and/or dialect in educational programs, employment, or service delivery, and should encourage an understanding of linguistic differences among consumers and the general population. (p. 28)

As long ago as 1983, Cole stated, "No dialectal variety of English is a disorder or pathological form of speech or language. Each social dialect is adequate as a functional and effective variety of English" (p. 25). Dialects and accents are often called *language varieties* to emphasize that they are accepted differences in speech (Cole, 1983). The educational, emotional, political, and economic controversies related to these language varieties continue in many settings. Service delivery for students who are CLD must be grounded in what they need for academic success, not on accent or dialect differences falsely perceived as disabilities. School-based speech–language pathologists must provide appropriate service delivery options for these students, along with information for colleagues and families. Reasoned judgments based on current research should guide decision making and service delivery. Speech–language pathologists must model respect for the children who offer the richness and variety of their accented speech.

Working With Families

Families are often the basic social unit for students who are CLD, and they should be included in the context of the child's intervention program as much as possible for best results (Roseberry-McKibbin, 2007; Wyatt, 1999). For example, according to Wyatt and Weddington (2010), determining difference versus deficit in children's use of African American English is more accurate, and more appropriately treated, when there is family contact. Including the family in the intervention process shows respect, increases carryover, and knits the school and community together in the same cause.

Family literacy is a common school-related activity for children, parents, and extended families. The read-aloud aspect of family literacy has considerable appeal and effectiveness for families that are CLD. The speech–language pathologist may consider taking an active part in organizing such communication-related programs as Family Reading Night, Grandparents Read-Aloud Program, or Everybody Read Together. These activities are especially meaningful to families, encourage respect, and are extensions of the collaborative service delivery process described in Chapter 6.

Roseberry-McKibbin (2007, 2008) offered specific ways to include multiculturalism in speech and language intervention when the practitioner does not speak the student's native or dominant language. A few examples include showing interest in the student's home country, language, and culture and learning and using a few words of the student's first language.

The ASHA Web site contains innumerable resources on all of the topics discussed here. See the page for the Office of Multicultural Affairs at www.asha.org/practice/multicultural/.

Infants and Toddlers

IDEA 2004 and state special education programs provide early intervention for identified infants and toddlers in collaboration with developmental disability services, mental health agencies, or similar health-care entities. Programs for infants and toddlers in schools are covered in Part C of IDEA 2004, which attempts to link families, communities, and schools with a program for children from birth to 3 years of age that is qualitatively different from Part B. Section 631 describes an urgent and substantial need:

1. To enhance the development of infants and toddlers with disabilities and to minimize their potential for developmental delay
2. To reduce the educational costs to our society by minimizing the need for special education and related services after infants and toddlers with disabilities reach school age
3. To minimize the likelihood of institutionalization
4. To enhance the capacity of families to meet the special needs of their infants and toddlers with disabilities
5. To enhance the capacity of state and local agencies and service providers to identify, evaluate, and meet the needs of historically underrepresented populations, particularly minority, low-income, inner-city, and rural populations

Each state must have a statewide system for services to infants and toddlers that meets all the requirements of Section 635 of IDEA 2004. Each state has developed systems with different kinds and numbers of agencies involved, their own guidelines, and service delivery that matches that state's infrastructure. They all share the concept of the IFSP in place of the IEP for children younger than age 3 years. An IFSP may be also used for children ages 3 through 5 years if agreed to by the family and school, although this is rare.

Settings for Infant and Toddler Programs

An IFSP states all the services needed, the person responsible for each, the location of the services, and the specific roles and responsibilities parents or caretakers will have. Programs for infants and toddlers cannot be authentically discussed or treated outside the strong network of their families. Often parents have specific questions about how to communicate with their child that should be addressed in the assessment and the service plan. The IFSP is written for a year or less, whichever is appropriate for a particular child. Functional outcomes are incorporated into the planning, and accommodations for the language and culture of the family are integrated into the IFSP (see "Functional Outcomes and the School-Based Speech–Language Pathologist" in Chapter 5 for a discussion on functional outcomes). Some of these are family outcomes rather than direct child outcomes. The use of lay language rather than professional jargon is a marker of a family-responsive plan (Polmanteer & Turbiville, 2000; Woods, 2008).

One of the qualitatively different aspects of serving infants and toddlers is the setting; they are typically served in their homes or child-care settings. Speech–language pathologists and other specialists work directly with families in these settings, showing them methods to encourage speech and language development, and coaching families as they work with their infants.

To be effective, speech–language pathologists need special training to work with infants, toddlers, and families. This training is available from some graduate education programs, many state personnel development grants, some employers, and every major annual state speech–language association conference or ASHA convention. Journals that focus on the communication needs of infants and toddlers are available (e.g., the National Association for the Education of Young Children publishes *Young Children*, and the Council for Exceptional Children, Division for Early Childhood, publishes *Journal of Early Intervention* and *Young Exceptional Children*), as are online continuing education courses and teleconferences offered by experts in the field.

Speech–language pathologists work closely with medical staff, counselors, other therapists, and families when infants have multiple health and medical needs in the first 2 years of life. This is facilitated in center-based rather than home-based programs. Although some school districts hire speech–language pathologists for these positions, others contract with county agencies, state Early Start or Even Start programs, or university clinical programs. Because smaller districts have fewer families and reduced resources overall, they often assign the speech–language pathologists at K–12 schools responsibility for the infants and toddlers in their own communities. Although not ideal, this arrangement is financially feasible and helps the school staff prepare for some children's needs years before the children enter school.

If babies are served in a center, the family members, who must come with them for training, support one another and get new ideas from professionals. Direct therapy with a baby for prespeech development is highly unusual and not a preferred practice. Paul and Roth (2011) presented an excellent compilation of recommended practices from the research, including reporting that several factors are noted to be "red flag" indications that toddlers should be evaluated for needed services. These factors include the following:

- the presence of significant delays (>6 months) in comprehension as well as production
- limited response to name and language
- few vocalizations
- limited number of consonants in babble

- few spontaneous imitations
- lack of object or symbolic play
- few communicative gestures or vocalizations
- reduced rate of nonverbal communication
- communicative intents limited to requesting
- difficulty gaining access to peer interactions
- preference for adults over peers
- family history of language delays or reading problems

See also ASHA's (2008b) document "Roles and Responsiblities of Speech–Language Pathologists in Early Intervention."

Unique Aspects of Infant and Toddler Programs

A program conducted in natural environments, generally an infant's home with the family, is the most common service delivery model and is recommended by the professional organizations for all service providers of early intervention, including ASHA. The practice statements, literature, position statements, and/or resources of professional organizations who engage in early intervention are compiled in an excellent document: "Key Principles of Early Intervention and Effective Practices: A Crosswalk With Statements From Discipline Specific Literature" (Wipple, 2014). The principles are as follows:

1. Infants and toddlers learn best through everyday experiences and interactions with familiar people in familiar contexts.
2. All families, with the necessary supports, can enhance their children's learning and development.
3. The primary role of the service provider in early intervention is to work with and support the family members and caregivers in a child's life.
4. The early intervention process, from initial contacts through transition, must be dynamic and individualized to reflect the child's and family members' preferences, learning styles, and cultural beliefs.
5. IFSP outcomes must be functional and based on children's and families' needs and priorities.
6. The families' needs and interests are addressed most appropriately by a primary provider who represents and receives team and community support.
7. Interventions with young children and family members must be based on explicit principles, validated practices, best available research, and relevant laws and regulations.

Speech–language pathologists travel to the home weekly or monthly, often followed up by an assistant or support person for a later visit. The family is taught communication support techniques and encouraged to integrate them into their daily routines. The speech–language pathologist has the responsibility to be culturally competent, recognize and appreciate the child-rearing approaches the family uses, include all the relevant family members, and not present information or techniques that may offend care providers or make them feel uncomfortable (ASHA, 2008b; Woods, 2008).

When assessing infants, speech–language pathologists first consider readiness for communication, including the concept of reciprocity, which will indicate whether the child is ready for communicative interaction. In addition, the speech–language pathologist will need to assess parent communication and family functioning (Woods, 2008). The speech–language pathologist recognizes that the child is a product of how the parents have raised him or her and the way the baby has influenced the parents. It is a constant give-and-take relationship. Each time that parents interact with babies, the baby learns; babies in turn shape the parents' responses. The speech–language pathologist goes into the home to help the baby develop communication skills with the parents but also to help the parents develop a communication system with their child. Each must change and react to the other.

Assessment of Infants and Toddlers

Speech–language pathologists use vastly different measures to assess for communication delays in infants and toddlers compared to what they use for school-age or even preschool children. There are a few standardized tests, but most are rating scales, family inventories, structured observations, caregiver reports, and medical histories. In the hands of competent and experienced speech–language pathologists, these are fine tools. The speech–language pathologist who has not worked extensively with infants, toddlers, and families; who has not taken appropriate course work; or who has not been mentored by an experienced professional team is advised to seek out the many excellent resources in the communication field before performing assessments. They should also be guided by ASHA's Practice Portal for assessment.

ASHA's (2008b) position statement on the "Roles and Responsibilities of Speech–Language Pathologists in Early Intervention" defined the expectations for speech–language pathologists working with this population:

> It is the position of the American Speech–Language–Hearing Association (ASHA) that speech–language pathologists have a central role in providing services and supports for families and their infants or toddlers with disabilities as members of the early intervention team. Furthermore, the appropriately certified and licensed (as applicable) speech–language pathologist is qualified to address delays and disabilities in communication, language, speech, emergent literacy, and feeding/swallowing. Effective communication is fundamental to all aspects of human functioning, particularly learning and social interaction. The development of communication skills begins at birth. Families with infants and toddlers (birth–36 months) who are at risk for or have disabilities should receive developmentally supportive care that addresses a broad spectrum of priorities

and concerns (Individuals With Disabilities Education Improvement Act, 2004; National Association for the Education of Young Children, 2005; National Research Council & Institute of Medicine, 2000; Sandall, Hemmeter, Smith, & McLean, 2005).

Speech–language pathologists, as autonomous professionals, assume various roles in addressing the concerns and priorities of families and their infants or toddlers and should be included on any early intervention team for children who are at risk for or have communication, language, speech, emergent literacy, or feeding or swallowing impairments. These roles are implemented in collaboration with families, caregivers, and other professionals and include but are not limited to (a) prevention; (b) screening, evaluation, and assessment; (c) planning, implementing, and monitoring intervention; (d) consultation with and education for team members, including families and other professionals; (e) service coordination; (f) transition planning; (g) advocacy; and (h) awareness and advancement of the knowledge base in early intervention. These roles should be implemented in accord with the following guiding principles:

1. Services are family centered and culturally and linguistically responsive.
2. Services are developmentally supportive and promote children's participation in their natural environments.
3. Services are comprehensive, coordinated, and team based.
4. Services are based on the highest quality evidence that is available.

Extensive information and references about these guiding principles and roles and responsibilities of speech–language pathologists in early intervention can be found in the companion ASHA (2008a, 2008b, 2008c) technical report, guidelines, and knowledge and skills documents.

Increasingly, assessment of infants and toddlers is conducted through arena assessment using a dynamic assessment approach (see the discussion on dynamic assessment in Chapter 3 in the section "Dynamic Measures"). One of the primary assessment measures for this population is to find the category of risk for a condition evident at birth. Assessment might begin at any of these risk categories and may or may not lead to a diagnosis of a disability that requires special education support from the speech–language pathologist. The condition of "at risk" does not immediately translate into identification or services.

Whenever intervention is planned for babies and young children, the speech–language pathologist will be working closely with a variety of individuals who care for and are a part of the child's life besides the parents. Those involved in a child's care, and therefore the intervention plan, can include grandparents, aunts, uncles, siblings, partners of parents, babysitters, nannies, and neighbors. Any one of these individuals may serve as the caregiver in a center-based program or participate in the assessment or intervention activity. They must all be taught to facilitate the child's development. Rather than being frustrated or annoyed at having many different family members involved, the speech–language pathologist appreciates the richness that numerous care providers can bring to the child's program.

Impact of Universal Newborn Hearing Screening on Infant and Toddler Programs

Screening babies at birth is a long-established method of identifying risk conditions as soon as possible, which allows medical or other intervention to begin before the baby starts to develop. Disabilities that would have materialized later may be prevented at birth. Infants have been screened for phenylketonuria (PKU), Tay-Sachs disease, and Rh incompatibility for many years. Hearing loss was typically not discovered in children until age 2.5 to 3 years, an age when auditory behavioral testing was more dependable. Hearing loss in babies could go undetected during the critical first years of their lives, sharply reducing their language skills (Herer, 2015).

This wait-and-see situation changed dramatically in 1993, when the National Institutes of Health Consensus Development conference recommended that all newborns in this country should have their hearing screened prior to hospital discharge (National Institutes of Health, 1993). As of 2000, early hearing detection programs became the standard of care in essentially all states within the United States. The format of these programs includes (a) hearing screenings that use a physiologic measure by 1 month of age (preferably before birthing hospital discharge), (b) audiological and medical evaluations for those not passing the initial screen to confirm hearing loss by no later than 3 months of age, and (c) early intervention services for all infants with permanent hearing loss as soon as possible but no later than 6 months of age. (See ASHA Web site on Early Detection Hearing and Intervention, www.asha.org/advocacy/federal/ehdi/.)

Now, screening a baby's hearing can occur as early as 9 hours after birth (Herer, 2015). A relatively new technology, called *otoacoustic emissions* (OAE), has allowed sleeping babies to be tested in about 3 minutes using a small ear probe to record the "echo" of the cochlea's response on a computer. The OAE procedure is often used in newborn hearing screening programs in conjunction with a screening version of auditory brain stem response technology. Data from 7 years of screening indicate that these technologies are reliable and relatively inexpensive and can identify babies with hearing loss at birth (Herer, 2015).

Most children with hearing loss at birth are otherwise healthy and are discharged from a birthing hospital's well-baby nursery. Some babies, however, have serious health challenges at birth requiring hospitalization for a period of time (even as long as 3 months) in the newborn intensive care unit (NICU). These health problems and the lifesaving treatments required in the NICU can affect babies' central nervous system. For example, the prevalence of sensorineural hearing loss among well babies is 1.2 per 1,000 births. By contrast, the rate for those hospitalized in the NICU is three times greater (Herer, 2015). Any collateral central nervous system problems affecting babies with hearing loss from the NICU could affect their response to intervention. It is recommended, therefore, that speech–language pathologists providing intervention services to young children with hearing loss examine their case histories. If NICU hospitalization at birth is reported, the speech–language pathologist should maintain a heightened awareness for variations in responses to intervention. Changes may be necessary. There may be undiagnosed early hearing loss that affected speech and language development. Recognizing a NICU history for a child with a sensorineural hearing loss should also raise the speech–language pathologist's "alert factor" for a progressive loss. Perhaps it was not picked up earlier because it has been slowly progressing until it has become a communication disability. Such an outcome has been reported in the literature for babies with a NICU history (Delaney, Meyers, Ruth, Faust, & Talavera, 2014).

The potential for progressive loss necessitates hearing testing on a regular basis (likely semiannually) and should be in the speech–language pathologist's protocol of care for those children. This may occur in the infant, early intervention, or even school-age population. Changes in hearing aid amplification, modifications of speech–language intervention, and consideration of cochlear implant use may be necessary depending on the extent of the progressive hearing loss. The speech–language pathologist is a major player in each of these scenarios, as social language development, articulation acquisition, and access to the curriculum are at stake.

Infant hearing screening has had a profound effect on families, early intervention programs, and school-based infant and toddler programs. Speech–language pathologists develop the skills to work with 3-month-old babies using hearing aids, teach parents multiple communication systems, and help families choose educational interventions for their child during the critical early years when speech and language skills are acquired. Early intervention services play a unique role supporting families during a child's first 3 years. Hopefully, the child will not have to catch up or receive services later. There is great potential for these children to be in fully inclusive settings, working at grade level with appropriate supports by the time they enter the school system (Herer, 2015; Yoshinaga-Itano, 2014). Prevention is the essence of IDEA 2004 philosophy. Communication disorders may be one of the first disciplines to demonstrate the value of preventive intervention.

A universal newborn hearing screening (UNHS) program, designed and supervised by an audiologist, is implemented by trained technicians in a birthing hospital. Protocols for universal programs do not screen only at-risk babies or those with familial histories of deafness or hearing loss. Rather, a UNHS program screens all newborns—hence, universal. Babies who are not screened face the potential of reduced auditory input as their speech, language, and cognition develop (Herer, Knightly, & Steinberg, 2007).

Herer (2007) reported results based on 47,920 newborns tested in a UNHS program from 1997 to 2004. He showed that (a) the prevalence rate for hearing loss in newborns from the well-baby nursery is 1.8 per 1,000 but significantly greater, 7.4 per 1,000, for those in the NICU; (b) babies with conductive hearing losses can also be identified early for medical interventions; (c) almost half of the babies identified with a hearing loss, 47.7%, did not have risk factors and would not have been reported to a high-risk registry; and (d) if only infants from the NICU had been screened, as some have suggested, 72% of the babies with hearing loss born during the 7 years of the study would have been missed. (See Table 7.1 for more information.)

TABLE 7.1. Overall Prevalence Rates of Hearing Loss for 47,920 Newborns, 1997–2004

Type of hearing loss	Well-baby nursery[a]	Newborn intensive care unit[b]
Bilateral sensorineural	0.731	2.158
Bilateral conductive	0.343	1.918
Unilateral sensorineural	0.503	1.678
Unilateral conductive	0.251	1.678
Total incidence rate per 1,000	1.828	7.432

Note. Adapted from *Early Detection and Intervention*, by G. R. Herer, 2015. Seminar at Chapman University, Orange, CA.
[a]Well-baby nursery: 80 of 43,749 newborns, 1.8 per 1,000. [b]Newborn intensive care unit: 31 of 4,171 babies, 7.4 per 1,000.

Herer (2015) also noted the following:

> NICU infants discovered to have hearing loss could have other deleterious outcomes involving their central nervous system (CNS) that interfere with normal processing of auditory information and thus effect language–speech acquisition. Such outcomes arise from reasons that require hospitalization in the NICU such as very low birth weight; or, life-saving treatments while in the NICU such as the use of drugs having toxic effects. Children with hearing loss who experienced hospitalization in a NICU at birth should be considered at-risk for language–speech development beyond that expected from hearing loss alone. Therefore, early intervention professionals serving children with hearing loss need to explore the children's histories for NICU hospitalization. If such a history is noted, the child should be carefully followed for any signs of language–speech learning difficulties and appropriate intervention methods initiated as needed.

The impact on services that speech–language pathologists provide in school districts is under way. Audiologists and speech–language pathologists work with their school districts to develop appropriate IFSPs for toddlers who were identified at birth with moderate to severe sensorineural hearing losses. Many of these babies use hearing aids or have a cochlear implant and are developing speech and language skills within normal limits (Yogashani-Otani, 2014). The toddlers use hearing aids, attend typical preschools, and receive family-centered therapy from their local school districts. There are real changes ahead in these programs as audiologists, teachers of the deaf, and speech–language pathologists work closely with families of infants and toddlers with hearing loss identified at birth. Services for infants typically take place in the home, and speech–language pathologists visit families weekly or monthly, with related professionals, to provide consultation and direct therapy. States have reported declining numbers of students in schools for the deaf and far fewer classes in public schools for children with severe hearing loss. These children have not left the system; it is quite the opposite. They are in the general education classrooms, accessing the core curriculum (Miller, 2015)! Student outcome data have confirmed that evaluation requires a number of different strategies to examine overall effectiveness of early intervention (Mullen, 2000). Although changes in babies' communication can be measured, effectiveness is often judged most authentically by families, the consumers of services for infants and toddlers. Perhaps the most cogent source of evaluation is family satisfaction with the program. If families feel that they have been supported in their efforts to provide the best possible environment for child development, the program has had a positive impact.

Children With Autism Spectrum Disorder

One of the most challenging areas of school-based speech–language service delivery is meeting the needs of students identified with autism spectrum disorder (ASD). The awareness of ASD as an educational concern has skyrocketed in recent years, with research indicating that it is being diagnosed in 1 in 68 children (Centers for Disease Control and Prevention, n.d.-a). Communication is a primary issue for children with ASD, and speech–language pathologists play a prominent role in programming for these students. School districts in every state have added comprehensive professional development courses for their special education staff, and many districts have identified and trained speech–language pathologists and other team members as experts in the ASD field. Most school districts have comprehensive programming for children with ASD, including services that are unique to this population. With the increase in incidence, professional development is increasingly provided to administrators and general education staff, as well.

The focus on services and specialized programming for children with ASD has dominated special education services since the mid-1990s. Specialized services vary from placements in private or state-administered schools, to 40-hour-a-week intensive behavior modification discrete trial training sessions, to general education placements with pull-out sessions with the speech–language pathologist, to full inclusion programs with one-to-one aide support in the general education classroom. Perhaps educational and therapeutic programming for children with ASD is so diverse because ASD is so diverse, presenting in so many different forms and degrees of ability. Autism is truly a spectrum disorder, with many variations in its manifestation and consequently variations in treatment programs. Autism, however, requires a true multidisciplinary or transdisciplinary approach, with the collective expertise of specialists, teachers, education specialists, administrators, parents, and medical personnel managing and developing programs.

The National Research Council's (2001) addressed the question of what are considered appropriate educational services for young children with ASD:

> At the root of questions about the most appropriate educational interventions for autistic spectrum disorders are differences in assumptions about what is possible and what is important to give students with these disorders through education. The appropriate goals for educational services for children with autistic spectrum disorders are the same as those for other children: personal independence and social responsibility. These goals imply progress in social and cognitive abilities, verbal and nonverbal communication skills, and adaptive skills, reduction of behavioral difficulties, and generalization of abilities across multiple environments. (p. 5)

Speech–language pathologists need to be well informed on this topic through course work, independent study, recent literature, and experience working with children who present with ASD. Speech–language pathologists and their multidisciplinary colleagues in school programs are well versed in several methodologies specific to this population and seek to know what combination of services are best for a child and then make continual adjustments for age and progress (Bevilacqua & Norlin, 2004; Diehl, 2016; National Autism Center, 2015; National Research Council, 2001; Prizant, 2015). Speech–language pathologists in the schools must be well acquainted with ASD and the wide range of service delivery options that schools and parents request. In a school-based intervention program, a comprehensive approach to treatment is expected. Approaches that are both developmental and behavioral will intersect to build a program that will provide functional, developmental, behavioral, and academic improvement. In recent years, deficits in social communication skills and anxiety resulting from these deficits have come to the forefront of treatments for students with autism. While behavioral challenges may present as the most apparent need, because of safety concerns and disruptions at home and school, ultimately communication is frequently the underlying issue. Serving students with autism always requires an integrated team approach. Speech–language pathologists will find that they learn useful information from behavior specialists, occupational therapists, education specialists, early intervention specialists, school psychologists, and others in this work.

Defining Autism Spectrum Disorder

ASHA's Web site defines *autism* in the following way, which is consistent with the latest definition in the *Diagnostic and Statistical Manual of Mental Disorders* (DSM-5; American Psychiatric Association, 2013):

> Autism spectrum disorder (ASD) is a neurodevelopmental disorder characterized by deficits in social communication and social interaction and the presence of restricted, repetitive behaviors. Social communication deficits include impairments in aspects of joint attention and social reciprocity, as well as challenges

in the use of verbal and nonverbal communicative behaviors for social interaction. Restricted, repetitive behaviors, interests, or activities are manifested by stereotyped, repetitive speech, motor movement, or use of objects; inflexible adherence to routines; restricted interests; and hyper- and/or hypo-sensitivity to sensory input. (ASHA, n.d.-h)

Autism is a spectrum disorder, which means that each person is affected in a different way. The degree of impact can be from mild to severe and may vary across the life span. According to the Centers for Disease Control and Prevention (CDC, n.d.-a), the range of symptoms can be analyzed across the following domains: measured intelligence, social interaction, communication, behaviors, sensory, and motor (see Figure 7.2).

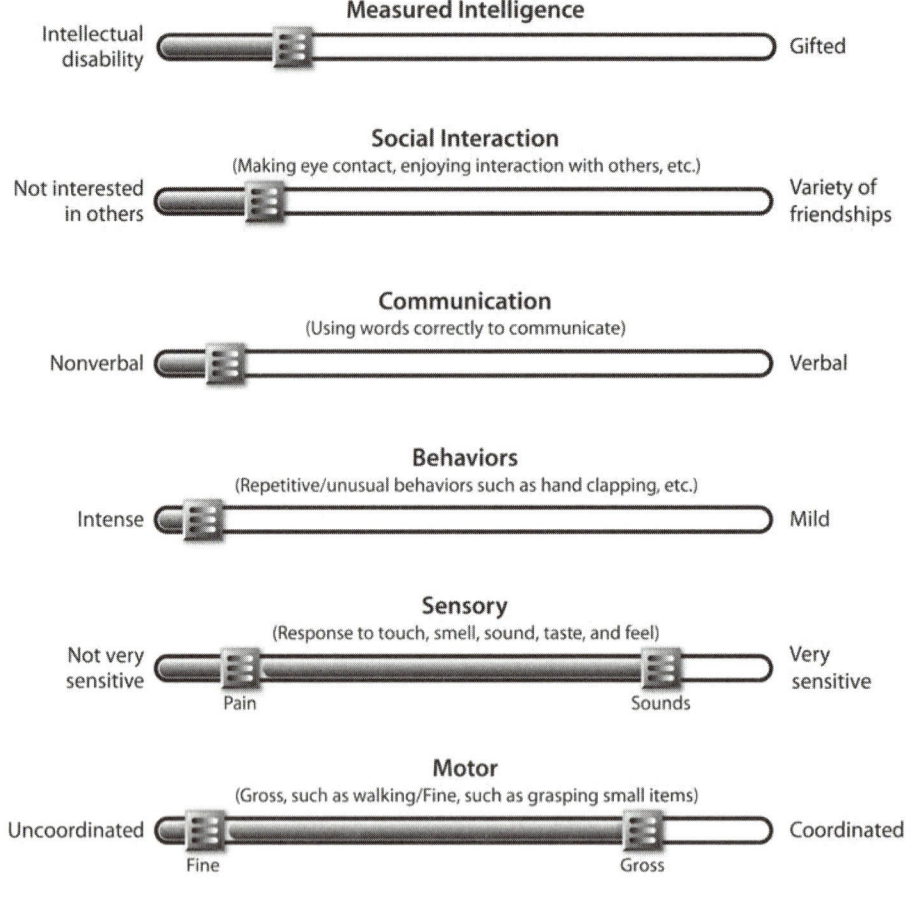

FIGURE 7.2. Autism symptom domains.

Note. Adapted from "Autism Spectrum Disorder (ASD) Data and Statistics," by Centers for Disease Control and Prevention, n.d.-a. Retrieved from http://www.cdc.gov/ncbddd/autism/data.html.

The IDEA 2004 definition (34 C.F.R. § 300.8) is as follows:

(c)(1)(i) Autism means a developmental disability significantly affecting verbal and nonverbal communication and social interaction, generally evident before age three, which adversely affects a child's educational performance. Other characteristics often associated with autism are engagement in repetitive activities and stereotyped movements, resistance to environmental change or change in daily routines, and unusual responses to sensory experiences.

(ii) Autism does not apply if a child's educational performance is adversely affected primarily because the child has an emotional disturbance, as defined in paragraph (c)(4) of this section.

(iii) A child who manifests the characteristics of "autism" after age three could be diagnosed as having autism if the criteria in paragraph (c)(1)(i) of this section are satisfied.

Assessment of ASD

Assessment of children with ASD requires a highly skilled multidisciplinary team because of the complexities and pervasiveness of the condition (ASHA, n.d.-h; National Research Council, 2001; Prelock, Beatson, Bitner, Broder, & Drucker, 2003; Richard, 2008). The National Research Council (2001) indicated, "Difficulties in communication are a central feature of autism, and they interact in complex ways with social deficits and restricted patterns of behavior and interests in a given individual. Accurate assessment and understanding of levels of communicative functioning is critical for effective program planning and intervention" (p. 29). The following recommendations are made in terms of communication assessment (National Research Council, 2001):

- Communication skills should be viewed in the broad context of overall development and documented in a natural context.
- Standardized tests should constitute only one component of the assessment.
- It is important to assess language comprehension skills in addition to expressive skills; communicative intent and the functions of delayed and immediate echolalia, if present, should be noted.
- Oral-motor difficulties should be noted.
- Checklists and parent interviews can be used.

Prelock (2001) offered the following diagnostic parameters that are particularly relevant to speech–language pathologists:

- Examination of family prevalence and patterns of decreased cognitive skills, specifically verbal and adaptive function
- Observation of verbal and nonverbal communication, and specific deficits in speech and language

ASHA has an extensive Web site related to many aspects of diagnosing, treating, and serving students with autism (ASHA, n.d.-h). The reader is strongly encouraged to use this resource, particularly the Practice Portal for emerging information on this area of practice. The site has specific information on the roles and responsibilities of speech–language pathologists related to the diagnosis and assessment of children with autism. Appropriate roles for speech–language pathologists, include providing information to individuals and groups known to be at risk for ASD, to their family members, and to individuals working with those at risk (see www.asha.org/PRPSpecificTopic .aspx?folderid=8589935303&section=Roles_and_Responsibilities for complete information).

Planning for Long-Term Services

Because ASD and pervasive developmental disorders include specific speech–language characteristics, the speech–language pathologist is always involved in the assessment, planning, and intervention for students who are so identified. The condition is pervasive, long lasting, and disruptive to learning, requiring professionals to consider many service delivery approaches over time to be sure that the programming remains suited to the student. It is important to weigh program options, work closely with families, collaborate with team members, and be exceptionally creative, while also being mindful of the student's unique individual needs, ensuring that the treatment selected has evidence-based outcomes for children with similar conditions. Parents of children with autism often come to IEP meetings with their own ideas about treatment regimens they want utilized for their children. The IEP team and/or the speech–language pathologist may or may not consider what the parent is seeking as appropriate for the student. Being knowledgeable in the literature and evidence base in this practice area is critical for these discussions (see Chapter 8, "Working With Families").

Again, the readers of this text are highly encouraged to visit the ASHA Practice Portal and the evidence-based map on autism spectrum disorder to gain the most current information about assessment and treatment in this area (see www.asha.org/Practice-Portal/Clinical-Topics/Autism/).

Intervention Approaches

Intervention for ASD generally falls within either a behavioral (e.g., functional) approach or a social communication (e.g., developmental) approach. The approach that works best for the child with ASD is the one that is the most specific to a given child's needs. Children with ASD demonstrate highly individualized learning styles (ASHA, n.d.-h; Diehl, 2016; National Autism Center, 2009, 2015; Prelock et al., 2003; Prizant, 2015).

Functional or behavioral approaches and developmental or social communication approaches need not be mutually exclusive or competitive. Behavioral techniques include applied behavioral analysis (ABA), discreet trial training (DTT), and positive behavioral supports. Some children may respond best to applied behavior analysis methods, which are highly structured teaching and speech–language intervention in a controlled environment. More currently, the blending of these methods has combined functional communication and positive behavioral supports to examine and intervene in social contexts while considering the communicative function of the behavior. Because challenging behavior is a hallmark of ASD, educators, interventionists, and speech–language pathologists should be well versed in positive behavioral supports (Prizant, 2015).

Some children with ASD benefit from play therapy using sociodrama, peer interaction, and child-led interactions. Still others chiefly have pragmatic language disorders and respond well to social scripts. Most often, intervention related to social communication establishes goals for joint attention, gaze regulation, gestural communication, and communicative function. Language goals are mapped onto this social communication approach.

Social skills intervention for students with ASD, and in particular for students who are older, is highly requested by parents and teachers and recommended by speech–language pathologists. Related to this area is consideration of a construct called *Theory of Mind*, or perspective taking, which is typically absent or impaired in the individual with ASD. Social skills training and groups are increasingly being incorporated into intervention approaches for this population. Because some students have higher cognitive skills but also have greater anxiety and are affected with severe pragmatic and social communication deficits, speech–language pathologists have a direct and critical role in providing intervention in the following areas: conversational skills, narrative skills, speech and voice (e.g., prosody), academics, self-regulation, and understanding the hidden curriculum of school. Although this area of practice has increased, clear evidence leading to evidence-based practice in this area is still lacking and needs to be developed. Social communication deficits are known as the hallmark of communication issues in autism. Social Thinking (see www.socialthinking.com) intervention is popular with students of all ages who have social communication issues. These intervention methods are highly sought by parents and speech–language pathologists in schools. Video modeling has also received increasing attention as an effective approach for building social and friendship skills. Although a 2007 systematic review (Delano, 2007) was cautious in reporting the positive effects, more research has been conducted since that time, and this approach has been reported to be successful (Thrasher, Burke, Klaer, & Schaller, 2012).

The obvious deficits in behavior and social skills can often overshadow the actual language impairment experienced by children with ASD. Some children experiencing ASD may exhibit some of the same deficits as children with speech–language impairment. Narrative abilities have been found to be deficit in individuals with ASD (Diehl, 2016). This language skill is essential to learning, and the speech–language pathologist's role in intervention is evident in this area. Language intervention methods, such as social stories (Gray & White, 2002), priming, and pivotal response treatment, occurring in natural language contexts can support language and learning development and also help in controlling challenging behavior. These and other treatment strategies can be useful for a child's specific needs (see also www.asha.org/PRPSpecificTopic.aspx?folderid=8589935303&section=Treatment). Diehl (2016) reported that the deficits related to autism (e.g., lack of central coherence, inability to suppress irrelevant information) will also lead to difficulties in reading comprehension.

The National Autism Center (2015) reported on the evidence base in treatments for autism, finding 14 effective treatments. These established treatments for children, adolescents, and young adults (younger than 22 years of age) are as follows:

- Behavioral interventions
- Cognitive–behavioral intervention package
- Comprehensive behavioral treatment for young children
- Language training (production)
- Modeling
- Natural teaching strategies
- Parent training
- Peer training package
- Pivotal response training
- Schedules
- Scripting
- Self-management
- Social skills package
- Story-based intervention

The speech–language pathologist's professional philosophy regarding therapy for children with ASD may or may not coincide with the team's or parents' ideas. Because intensive speech–language intervention with the child and training for the family may be viewed as the core of the program when children are younger than 3 years of age, the way communication services are provided is a critical decision. Several approaches that school-based speech–language pathologists have used successfully in different circumstances are summarized in Table 7.2. Speech–language pathologists must have knowledge of the entire range of choices parents may be considering, enabling different approaches to be introduced, advocated, or discontinued when progress is slow or change is needed. In addition, knowing when to change approaches because of a child's developmental level, age, and educational needs is important. It is tempting to continue to use an approach that has been successful but may not be appropriate for advancing to the next skill level. Continuing with an approach such as discrete trial training may be appropriate for a younger child in order to establish some behavior controls but can actually limit skill development in other areas such as social communication and generalization of skills to other environments as the child gets older. As more research is conducted, and more is known about autism, new methodologies and treatments will become available, and our approach will continue to evolve (National Autism Center, 2015; National Research Council, 2001; Prizant, 2015).

TABLE 7.2. Intervention Methods for Students With Autism Spectrum Disorder

Method	Description and examples
Applied behavior analysis (ABA) is based on principles of operant learning theory. These techniques use positive reinforcement and are often used with children with autism to introduce new and replacement behaviors and academic learning. ABA techniques are often used with very young children who present with noncompliant or challenging behaviors. The intention is to increase attention so that children will be available for learning.	*Discrete trial training* (DTT) breaks down skills in teaching attempts, known as *discrete trials* (see www.educateautism.com/applied-behaviour-analysis/discrete-trial-training.html).
	Intense behavior intervention (IBI) involves 1 to 5 years of structured learning opportunities for 37 to 40 hours per week and addresses all significant behaviors in all of the child's environments by all significant persons. It emphasizes speech and language in the early years, and one-to-one training sessions are most effective. This method requires specialized training.
	Pivotal response training (PRT) is based on the IBI approach and teaches a cluster of stimulus cues that will trigger simple or complex behaviors (like speech). It increases children's motivation, broadens opportunities for children to respond, and increases generalization (Koegel, Robinson, & Koegel, 2009) (see also http://education.ucsb.edu/autism/pivotal-response-treatment).
Visual supports (see Harris, n.d.)	*Visual schedules* use symbols, pictures, images, or graphics to illustrate a daily or weekly schedule. They may be combined with other signaling techniques, such as bells or countdowns for alerts to timing. They provide organization and predictability.
	With *visual modeling* the student watches a video of someone using a targeted behavior or skill to learn the skill (Bellini & Akullian, 2007).
	A small, systematic review demonstrated gains in social communication, functional language skills, and perspective taking (Delano, 2007).
	Treatment and Education of Autistic and Related Communication Handicapped Children (TEACCH) involves highly structured teaching and accommodations in the learning environment and includes parents as teaching assistants. Picture schedules are posted for children, and visual cuing is used in instruction. It applies to many settings (Mesibov & Shea, 2009) (see also http://teacch.com/).
	Picture Exchange Communication System (PECS) is an augmentative communication system designed to provide children a functional communication system. PECS teaches children to initiate communication in a social context by giving pictures for requesting (Bondy & Frost, 1994; Flippin, Reszka, & Watson, 2010).
Social Stories™ (Gray & Garand, 1993)	A Social Story identifies a context, skill, achievement, or concept according to 10 defining criteria. The Social Story is used to teach the expected behavior and communication for a specific situation that may be a challenge to the child (Reynhout & Carter, 2006) (see http://carolgraysocialstories.com/social-stories/what-is-it/).
Social Thinking® is a language and cognitive-based *methodology* that focuses on the dynamic and synergistic nature of social interpretation and social communication skills, both of which require social problem solving (Crooke, Olswang, & Winner, 2016).	Social Thinking interventions teach social competencies addressing core deficits of individuals with autism. The methodology utilizes a strategy-based framework and incorporates aspects of cognitive–behavioral theory (Crooke & Winner, 2015) (see www.socialthinking.com/Articles?name=Research to Frameworks to Practice Social Thinking's Layer of Evidence)

(continues)

TABLE 7.2. *(continued)*

Method	Description and examples
Social relationship models	*Greenspan's DIR/Floortime Approach*, a developmental, individual-difference, relationship-based approach model, is a framework using feelings and ideas to build relationships. The Floortime intervention process operationalizes these constructs through joint attention, problem solving, and gestures (Wieder & Greenspan, 2003). *Relationship development intervention* (RDI) is a family-based behavioral therapy that is based on dynamic intelligence and teaches strategies for flexible thinking to take different perspectives, respond to various stimuli, and cope with change (Gutstein, Burgess, & Montfrot, 2007). *Social Communication, Emotional Regulation, Transactional Support* (SCERTS) is an educational model that provides assessment and guidelines for intervention focusing on authentic progress in the identified domains, including behavior and communication. Through the model, other intervention practices can be incorporated (Prizant, Wetherby, Rubin, Laurent, & Rydell, 2006).
See also *ASHA Autism Treatment* (www.asha.org/PRP-SpecificTopic.aspx?folderid=8589935303&section=Treatment) and *Autism Speaks Treatment* (www.autismspeaks.org/what-autism/treatment)	

ASHA (n.d.-h) reports that treatment for individuals with ASD typically includes

- setting goals based on assessment data that target the core deficits in ASD and focus on initiating spontaneous communication in functional activities, engaging in reciprocal communication interactions, and generalizing gains across activities, environments, and communication partners;
- using a multimodal communication system (e.g., spoken language, gestures, sign language, picture communication, speech-generating devices, written language) that is individualized according to the individual's abilities and the contexts of communication;
- considering family priorities when selecting intervention goals—meaningful outcomes are strongly correlated with communication competence across functional social contexts (e.g., home, school, vocational, and community settings);
- incorporating cultural, linguistic, and personal values and attributes unique to each individual into therapeutic activities;
- using a range of approaches for enhancing communication skills along a continuum from behavioral to developmental;
- using developmental sequences and processes of language development to provide a framework for determining baselines and implications for intervention goals; and

- measuring progress using systematic methods to determine whether an individual with ASD is benefiting from a particular treatment program or strategy.

Intervention approaches for children with ASD stress the functionality of language for these students. In addition to balancing the providers, activities, and contexts of service delivery decisions, the speech–language pathologist will need to consider the belief system of the educational team and parents and the availability of comprehensive training for all service providers (Crais, 2000). Because of the nature of ASD, and its overwhelming impact on language and social development, these students will need comprehensive communication intervention (National Autism Center, 2009, 2015; National Research Council, 2001; Scott et al., 2000).

Information on effective intervention for students with ASD continues to develop (ASHA, n.d.-h; Diehl, 2003, 2016; National Autism Center, 2009, 2015; Wetherby, 2000). Screening for ASD should routinely be part of "well-child" checkups, according to the Centers for Disease Control and Prevention (n.d.-b.). There are many speculations regarding what is responsible for the increase in ASD, which are typically centered on genetic factors, neurobiological factors, or environmental factors (ASHA, n.d.-h). Regardless of the cause, improved public and professional awareness will continue to improve health and education for children, because the "epidemic" of ASD is a national crisis that severely taxes families and the health-care and education systems. There is no doubt that continued research and resources will need to be directed to this area.

Appropriate Benefit

Parents and teachers of students with ASD are brought into contact with many medical and educational professionals. Some are brief encounters, whereas others are ongoing. Speech–language pathologists must be aware of the ongoing controversy when schools serve students with ASD. School programs can provide effective interventions for students; however, their underlying treatment premise can vary at times from that in the private sector. Families and school teams can disagree heartily on what the school can or should do for students with ASD. Speech–language pathologists need to understand why service delivery recommendations appear to clash.

Because *appropriate* (not best or maximally feasible) benefit remains the federal standard for students with disabilities, the expectations of the IEP team may be different from those of the parent. This frequently comes into conflict with the culture of ASD. Many parents of children with ASD are well aware of what they should expect in the way of the "best" education and best related services. The pervasiveness of ASD often drives parents to seek popularized interventions, believing those will benefit their child. As is mentioned in Chapter 8, cases regarding free appropriate public education (FAPE) dealing with autism have been on the rise in the past decade (Zirkel, 2011). School personnel may feel like parents are asking them to extend beyond the FAPE standard, but parents feel they need to advocate for whatever they believe will benefit their child. Terms such as *best, maximum,* and *minimum* become points of contention in these cases. (See the discussion related to the *Endrew F.* decision in Chapter 2.) However, this culture also means that schools and school personnel, including speech–language pathologists, need to always be informed and implementing current, effective, and defensible practices in order to be able to explain and justify why they are doing what they are doing.

Professionals in communication disorders play a very active role with the treatment of ASD. In the 1990s, treatment selection was often polarized; however, more recently, approaches that integrate methodologies and focus more on the interaction of the domains seen in Figure 7.2 are more common and certainly yield greater benefit to the student. The Interdisciplinary Council on Developmental and Learning Disorders (2000) presented interdisciplinary clinical guidelines. In addition, the Interdisciplinary Council on Development and Learning (see www.icdl.com) offers an approach that uses a cross-disciplinary, comprehensive, and functional developmental intervention system for students and families. The *d*evelopmental, *i*ndividual-difference, *r*elationship-based (DIR) approach is designed to meet the unique needs of children and families. The model is built on research that shows that although students with ASD have common characteristics, they are not all alike. Their interventions must be matched to personal characteristics, interests, and family strengths. The speech–language pathologist is required to build a relationship with the student and experience the world the way he or she does (Greenspan & Wielder, 1999).

Another comprehensive model for treatment of children with autism is SCERTS (Prizant, Wetherby, Rubin, & Laurent, 2010). SCERTS stands for Social Communication (SC), Emotional Regulation (ER), and Transactional Support (TS) (see www.scerts.com). What is important about models such as SCERTS and DIR is that these approaches reflect both specific therapeutic approaches and the importance of a cohesive integration of professionals and families in treating autism, including approaches both at home and school. These methods will provide consistency and a foundation for the child. The SCERTS model provides an evolution in the focus of autism treatment on social communication and emotional regulation. Prizant's (2015) latest work, *Uniquely Human*, also provides an evolving perspective about behavior connected to emotional regulation and communication issues in individuals with autism, and the authors highly recommend this resource.

Contrasting Perspectives

Some interventions for students with ASD that were considered highly controversial in the 1990s continue to be the focus of carefully constructed and appropriately controlled research. Facilitated communication, auditory integration training, sensory integration therapy, and intensive, computer-assisted auditory temporal processing programs have all been interventions difficult to validate using conventional procedures. (See the ASHA references indicated in this chapter for additional information on these approaches.) Parents and advocates may request nonvalidated approaches, and it is important that speech–language pathologists know the positions of ASHA on these methods. Systematic reviews such as those from the National Autism Center (2009, 2015) contribute greatly to the evidence on appropriate approaches that will hopefully provide clear professional direction and prevent hope and emotion from driving the choices of intervention. The speech–language pathologist has the educational background and the professional resources to make valid communication intervention decisions for students with ASD.

Communication is a core deficit of autism, so speech–language pathologists in schools should expect to be highly involved with all students with this condition, as well as in program development and interventions for this student population. Many specialized programs have been developed at all grade levels for students with ASD. Because these students have such a wide range of skills, abilities, and needs, creative programming is necessary. School personnel can expect that students with ASD will be served across the continuum from general education classes to highly restrictive settings. Support and services will need to be developed to meet their individualized, unique needs. However, what is now known about successful intervention for children with ASDs across the life span will help to build supports for these students. Speech–language pathologists and all educators should embrace this opportunity to think in an evidence-based manner about what students need and then help to design these programs.

Students Who Use Assistive Technology and Augmentative and Alternative Communication

In 1992, Congress recognized the importance of assistive technology (AT) devices and services as tools to help students with disabilities lead more independent and productive lives (Rehabilitation Act Amendments). AT was used in schools before this time (ASHA, 1991), but use was sporadic and often overlooked by busy school special education teams. At times, knowledge about AT was minimal, and staff did not feel confident about what equipment was available, how it was used, and how it could augment the communication and education of a child. Concerns about cost and lack of funds also caused teams to avoid the AT discussion. Speech–language pathologists and others lobbied Congress heavily to include specific wording in the IDEA Amendments of 1997 to ensure that these service delivery problems would be addressed and resolved. Many students with severe physical and neurological disabilities could not communicate with speech, and they needed alternative, often technological, methods to communicate and learn. The addition to the law in 1992 was crucial to the field, and further refinements occurred in the reauthorization of IDEA in 1997: "Assistive technology device means any item, piece of equipment, or product system, whether acquired commercially off the shelf, modified, or customized, that is used to increase, maintain, or improve functional capabilities of a child with a disability" (34 C.F.R. § 300.5).

AT service encompasses any service that directly assists a child with a disability in the selection, acquisition, or use of an AT, including the following:

(a) The evaluation of the needs of a child, including a functional evaluation of the child in the child's customary environment

(b) Purchasing, leasing, or otherwise providing for the acquisition of assistive technology devices by children with disabilities

(c) Selecting, designing, fitting, customizing, adapting, applying, maintaining, repairing, or replacing assistive technology devices

(d) Coordinating and using other therapies, interventions, or services with assistive technology devices, such as those associated with existing education and rehabilitation plans and programs

(e) Training or technical assistance for a child with a disability, or, if appropriate, that child's family

(f) Training or technical assistance for professionals (including individuals providing education or rehabilitation services), employers, or other individuals who provide services to, employ, or are otherwise substantially involved in the major life functions of that child. (34 C.F.R. § 300.6)

The IDEA Amendments of 1997 required that technology be considered at every IEP meeting. Schools must consider, on a case-by-case basis, the use of school-purchased AT devices in the child's home or other settings if the IEP team determines a device is needed to ensure FAPE. To comply with IDEA requirements, many school districts have hired or trained personnel to be AT specialists and provided in-service education for special education staff. Some professionals embraced the concept easily, whereas others have remained somewhat intimidated by technology and reliant on other team members to handle this part of special education. IDEA 2004 revised the definition of AT to exclude a medical device that is surgically implanted or the replacement of such device (§ 614 [d][3][B][v]).

Audiology continues to be a related service, and as a result, cochlear implant mapping done by an audiologist could still be provided under IDEA. In addition,

> medically implanted devices are excluded from the definition, but Sec. 614 (d)(3)(B)(v) requires that every IEP team consider whether a child requires assistive technology and states that each public agency must provide the necessary technology if necessary as part of the child's special education. Additionally, funds may be used to improve the use and support of technology in the classroom to "maximize accessibility to general education curriculum for children with disabilities" (§ 611 (e)(2)(C)(iv) & (v)). (Golden, n.d.)

Recent advances in technology have led to a boom in the availability of devices and equipment, which are now much more easily available to students than they were even a few years ago. It is nothing to see iPads, iPods, or other tablets or devices in classrooms now. Access to these devices has made all the difference for many students, but their providers still need to know how to obtain and use this equipment for communication purposes. Many speech–language pathologists are well equipped by education and experience to become AT specialists in their districts. Some have been using AT systems for many years and are able to "think outside the box" to support a student who struggles with the motoric aspects of reading, writing, speaking, and listening. Technology has changed every aspect of our daily life, but the focus of AT in schools needs to be driven by the communication needs of the student and not simply having equipment for motivation or enjoyment. The role of the speech–language pathologist is quickly evolving into a role where AT is no longer the exclusive domain of an AT specialist but rather is within the scope of more and more speech–language pathologists, who find this role exciting and interesting.

AT and augmentative and alternative communication (AAC), though closely related, are not the same. AT can be used to support students with many types of disabilities. AAC may be a type of AT for students who need to have their communication supported so they can access the curriculum and take part in their daily life activities. AT and AAC can be either low tech or high tech.

IDEA 2004 requires IEP teams to consider the student's need for AT. The law divides this into the consideration for AT devices and AT services (§ 602, Definitions; 20 U.S.C. § 1402, P.L. 108-446, December 3, 2004):

> Assistive Technology Device means any item, piece of equipment or product system, whether acquired commercially off the shelf, modified, or customized, that is used to increase, maintain, or improve the functional capabilities of a child with a disability.
>
> Assistive Technology Service means any service that directly assists a child with a disability in the selection, acquisition, or use of an assistive technology device. Including:
>
> - The evaluation of the needs of the child, including a functional evaluation of the child in the child's customary environment
> - Purchasing, leasing, or otherwise providing for the acquisition of assistive technology devices by such child
> - Selecting, designing, fitting, customizing, adapting, applying, maintaining, repairing, or replacing assistive technology devices
> - Coordinating and using other therapies, interventions or services with AT devices, such as those associated with existing education and rehabilitation plans and programs
> - Training or technical assistance for such child, or, where appropriate, the family of such child
> - Training or technical assistance for professionals, employers, or other individuals who provide services to, employ, or are otherwise substantially involved in the major life functions of a child
>
> Assistive Technology is different from Educational Technology:
>
> - Assistive Technology: Increases, maintains or improves the functional capabilities of an individual. It doesn't teach a skill.
> - Educational and Instructional Technology: Increases, maintains or improves learning outcomes. It teaches a skill such as reading, math, or typing.

Adapted textbooks are available through the National Instructional Materials Accessibility Standard (NIMAS), which is a federally funded, national electronic file repository that makes NIMAS files available for the production of core print instructional materials in specialized formats. Created under IDEA 2004, NIMAS receives source files in NIMAS format from textbook publishers and makes these files available for download to authorized users in the United States and its territories through an online database. Once downloaded, the files can be used to create a variety of specialized formats, such as braille, audio, or digital text, on behalf of qualifying students who are blind, visually impaired, or print disabled in elementary or secondary school.

According to ASHA (n.d.-i),

> augmentative and alternative communication (AAC) includes all forms of communication (other than oral speech) that are used to express thoughts, needs, wants, and ideas. We all use AAC when we make facial expressions or gestures, use symbols or pictures, or write.

People with severe speech or language limitations rely on AAC to supplement existing speech or to replace speech that is not functional. Special augmentative aids, such as picture and symbol communication boards and electronic devices, are available to help these individuals express themselves. This may increase social interaction, school performance, and feelings of self-worth. AAC users should not stop using speech if they are able to do so. The AAC aids and devices are used to enhance their communication (ASHA, n.d.-i).

Low-tech examples include equipment and other supports readily available in schools, including off-the-shelf items to accommodate the needs of students that can be provided by general or special education through the student study team or IEP process. Low-tech items also include calculators, tape recorders, pencil grips, school-constructed language boards, and TV captioning.

High-tech examples encompass specialized equipment and support services beyond basic AT and require more in-depth assessment and customizing. These are often needed by students with low-incidence or severe disabilities. Examples of high-tech items include closed-circuit television, FM systems, augmentative communication devices, sound field systems, computer access devices, and specialized software (see Table 7.3).

When considering AT, teams should begin by considering low-tech adaptations that may be appropriate for the student and easily obtained. The term *technology* suggests highly sophisticated equipment, but that was not the intent of the law. A team needs to be sure the student needs it and will use it. AAC is listed under the activity of speaking; however, there is considerable overlap with writing, reading, and other curriculum-based school tasks because communication intersects with so many daily activities. For medical insurance coverage, the term *speech-generating device* is often used to denote high-end AAC equipment that produces simulated speech.

The increased awareness and use of technology in the general population in the past few years have made it easier for the necessary technology to reach students in schools. Computers are an expected part of every classroom and school. A student's curriculum and learning strategies incorporate computers as learning tools, providing better access for students with severe speech disabilities to use AT for literally all of their communication. In some cases, a student with learning disabilities may use AT

TABLE 7.3. Tech Range Examples of Assistive Technology Tools

Low-tech tools (do not require electricity to function)	Mid-tech tools (use batteries or some basic circuitry to function)	High-tech tools (have advanced circuitry)
Slant boards	Lights	Computers
Chalk	Buzzers	Software
Highlighters	Vibrating switches	Dynamic display communica-
Pencil grips	Touch windows	tion devices
Schedules	Basic environmental control	Electronic portable desktop
Calendars	units	assistants
Pictures	Portable word processors	iPad, iPhone, iPod Touch
Symbols	Static display communication	
Index cards	devices	
Footrests		
Sticky notes		

Note. Adapted from *Assistive Technology*, by C. Krueger, 2012, May 1, lecture given at California State University Long Beach, CSD 481A.

for writing (spell-checker, speech-to-text, word prediction) or mathematics (calculator) unrelated to his or her communication skills, and the speech–language pathologist will simply incorporate this technology into speech services if needed. In other cases, communication will be such a critical component of the child's needs that the AAC will dictate all the other parts of the education program. Training teachers, family members, peers, and communication partners to use the AAC with the child is also the responsibility of the speech–language pathologist and is listed on the IEP as a related service necessary for the child to benefit from special education. Such activities may also be listed in the accommodations sections and/or in the section on support to the teacher provided to enable the student to access the general curriculum (see the following box).

Frequently Asked Questions About AT and AAC

Q. Are schools required to pay for AT and AAC devices?

A. Yes. School districts have the responsibility under IDEA 2004 to provide equipment, services, training, and programs for students with an IEP who need AT to increase, maintain, or improve their functional capabilities. Other funding resources may include insurance companies, foundations, fraternal organizations, businesses, and individuals.

Q. Do students have access to AT or AAC if they are eligible for extended-year services?

A. Yes, if the IEP team decides that the student needs AT to access the curriculum in summer school or extended-year programs.

Q. Is a school district required to provide state-of-the-art equipment for a student?

A. No. The equipment needs to be appropriate for the student's needs to ensure FAPE. The IEP is guided by the assessment and is under no obligation to select a more or less expensive or sophisticated device.

Q. Under what conditions can AT or AAC be considered a related service?

A. AT equipment is a related service if it is a complementary service necessary for the student to benefit from his or her special education. Instruction or technical assistance for family members or staff to communicate with a student using AAC is also an example of a related service. The legal citation for assistive technology is as follows:

> Sec. 300.105 Assistive technology.
>
> (a) Each public agency must ensure that assistive technology devices or assistive technology services, or both, as those terms are defined in Sec. 300.5 and 300.6, respectively, are made available to a child with a disability if required as a part of the child's—
>
> (1) Special education under Sec. 300.36;
>
> (2) Related services under Sec. 300.34; or
>
> (3) Supplementary aids and services under Sec. 300.38 and 300.114(a)(2)(ii).
>
> (b) On a case-by-case basis, the use of school-purchased assistive technology devices in a child's home or in other settings is required if the child's IEP Team determines that the child needs access to those devices in order to receive FAPE.
>
> *Source.* 20 U.S.C. § 1412(a)(1), 1412(a)(12)(B)(i).

Q. How can school districts use Medicaid funds to purchase AT or AAC?

A. Medicaid regulations vary in each state, but the parent must always give permission to access the funds. Funds can be used according to Medicaid regulations that are based on medical necessity.

Q. How can school personnel locate AT and AAC resources?

A. Working with AAC resources requires more than the usual materials and supply catalogs. Many states have technology centers that may also function as assessment centers in some regions. AAC is available in every state and many countries around the world. Local manufacturing representatives have been known to visit schools, join planning teams if requested, or bring loaner equipment for students to try.

For both AT and AAC, the evaluation is critical. The needs of the student, especially in terms of cognitive, communicative (speech and language), physical, motor, vision, hearing, and social needs, must to be taken into consideration. In addition, the types of environment and supports needed or available must be considered. AAC system considerations should include the following:

- Ease of use and programming
- Accessibility
- Size
- Portability
- Voice output

- Language demands
- Static or dynamic display
- Reliability
- Expense

Intervention using AAC is a big task that speech–language pathologists should not do alone. It is always more successful when the full team is involved (Blackstone, 2000; Dodd, Schaefer, & Rothbart, 2015), widening the circle of potential communication partners for the student and vastly increasing the number of daily opportunities for practice and reinforcement.

Successful AT and AAC services in schools can generally be examined by using five critical elements. Speech–language pathologists are not responsible for all the elements, but they frequently play a large role in the coordination of this effort and the linkage with parents and other agencies. If the AT is an AAC system, the speech–language pathologist usually functions as the team leader or case manager and will likely be involved in the following five elements:

1. Assistive technology evaluation
2. Training and technical assistance
3. Acquisition and use of devices
4. Maintenance of devices
5. Coordination of services

The following sections describe each element as it relates to an AAC device, being mindful that the same would be true of any other AT device. Use of low-tech devices may take less time to implement, because they are easier to obtain and their effectiveness can be evaluated more quickly. Training and technical assistance are important, even for low-tech devices, as an appropriate tool can be rejected if the professionals do not know how to implement the technology or if the student's use is inconsistent. High-tech devices require a slower pace for decision making and have greater consequences for the student and the school's resources if they are later found to be unsuccessful. Assessments do not have to entail long test batteries or trips to a distant rehabilitation center. Teams who are willing to work with AT and learn what to do will become accomplished at making all low-tech decisions. Some teams can also handle high-tech decisions or make them in conjunction with another agency or regional support center that has access to equipment for trials.

Assistive Technology Evaluation

States have regulations and procedures for assessment, and districts may have selected resources to use for this purpose. The assessment must be both developmental and functional and at least partially conducted in the student's customary environment. A series of questions may be asked at the IEP meeting to determine what types of technology would be helpful. A speech–language pathologist within the district, an

AT specialist in the district or consortium, or a technology center outside the district could be used. Technology centers may be set up by nonprofit agencies, or even within educational agencies, to enable families to try out various systems, which are often too expensive to rent or buy outright. Usually an occupational or physical therapist assists with seating and positioning if that is an issue. There should be a written report and recommendations based on the student's trial with a device or devices. A student has changing needs, so the evaluation may need to be updated from time to time, either by the educational team or by an outside team. Newer technology is constantly becoming available, so reevaluation will allow the team to focus on better interventions as they become available.

Training and Technical Assistance

Training is critical to success with all AT. Training is an organized, scheduled event with specific goals and topics for the participants (e.g., educators, the AAC user, parents, peers). Technical assistance, on the other hand, is more informal, involving an ongoing relationship between the persons on the team and the family, including troubleshooting, discussions, and moral support.

The speech–language pathologist typically provides student instruction during therapy or collaborative sessions in the classroom. The speech–language pathology assistant (SLPA) often continues this instruction until the next level of skills is needed. The classroom teacher may assist with AT instruction that is connected to the curriculum. All three of these people may need training to be proficient enough on a device to teach the student. Sometimes, the classroom aide or an instructional assistant assigned by the school will help to encode new vocabulary to expand a device, teach new access skills, or practice an oral or written report with a child. When more people are involved in the instruction phase, the AAC user will have more skilled communication partners such as the teacher, peers, and paraprofessionals (Blackstone, 2000; Dodd & Gorey, 2014).

Technical assistance for the speech–language pathologist will likely be needed if the device malfunctions or if adjustments or modifications need to be made. Some of these can be done by the speech–language pathologist or assistants, but many are time-consuming or require special tools. The technical support person must be a part of the team and easy to reach. Technical assistance may be listed on the IEP as a support for either the trainer or the trainee.

Both training and technical assistance need to be set up ahead of time so that the student can begin using the communication system without long delays or interruptions. There are some costs involved here, and the speech–language pathologist needs to be sensitive to how they are handled. IDEA 2004 requires that a member of the IEP team, called the local education agency (LEA) representative, be a person who is authorized to commit the district's resources as needed to carry out the IEP. If an AAC device is written into the IEP, the costs for training and technical assistance are absorbed by the school district. In some cases, the family or another agency will step in to assist with costs. Teams should discuss these training and technical assistance requirements at the IEP so that all team members are aware of them. Technical support may be included in the purchase of a device, or it may involve an additional fee. The speech–language pathologist should encourage the team to arrange for such services to make the AT choice successful. Increasingly, especially with the use of more common devices, such as iPads or iPods, the school district information technology staff may be able to support some needs when devices malfunction.

Several years ago, prior to the ready availability of technology, school districts would limit the student in taking the device home. This, of course, does not make sense if the device is designed to serve as the student's communication system. However, if the device is provided as part of the student's FAPE in the IEP, then when the device is damaged, the school system would be responsible for paying for the repairs. This is true even if the damage occurs at home and even if an accident at home due to negligence causes the damage. Some districts may attempt to have the family members sign a form indicating they are responsible for the device in the event it is damaged or broken at home. However, the enforceability of such agreements is questionable. This is sometimes frustrating for school systems that are strapped for money. Repairs or replacement of these devices can be expensive. In addition, there is typically a delay when the device is being repaired or replaced. In these cases, a loaner device may be obtained through the company or a loan center.

Acquisition and Use of Devices

An AAC device is used by students to communicate, and thereby participate in and benefit from, their educational program. This condition of educational benefit is necessary for AT to be identified on the IEP as a related service. The AAC device often enables a student to engage in academics for the first time, have increased control of his or her school environment, and have access to more personal choices. All of these lend themselves to a less restrictive environment, greater access to the general education curriculum, and improved academic progress and functional outcomes. AAC must be tied to these educational expectancies, or the family becomes responsible for providing AAC through other funding sources.

Devices can be purchased, leased, loaned, or received as a gift or donation. They are listed either generically or specifically on the IEP with other related services. When school systems are responsible for acquiring the AAC system, devices purchased by the LEA remain the property of the school. At times, the family may choose to purchase the device so the student has sole access to the device in all settings. Regulations state that the equipment must be procured in a timely manner and not delay the implementation of the signed IEP. Insurance companies and Medicaid may also purchase equipment if it is found medically necessary for the student. In some states, there may be other agencies that may purchase equipment for students. For example, in California, California Children's Services (CCS) or the Department of Rehabilitation (DOR) will purchase equipment for students who meet certain criteria for such support. The school IEP team makes AAC decisions based on what is educationally beneficial for the student. Different agencies have various obligations and can be in conflict at times in terms of funding, and the speech–language pathologist may be the only team member who can differentiate between health-care requirements, vocational requirements, and educational standards.

Students use their AAC device in school, but the IEP team may also determine that it can be taken home for educational purposes that allow the child to receive FAPE. As mentioned previously, some school districts have developed a form for when equipment goes back and forth to home, with some liability provisions for the parent to sign. Although whether these provisions are enforceable is unclear, at least parents are being advised that the equipment is the property of the school district and that there is an expectation of care for the device. A device may be used by more than one student at school, as long as it is available to each student whenever it is needed according to each student's IEP.

When students move from school to school or from school to postschool environments, the ideal situation is for customized AAC equipment to follow them. As noted previously, the equipment is often the property of the school district. Ownership of a customized piece of equipment must be addressed in state and local policies, but the issue is often neglected at the local level until the student relocates. The U.S. Department of Education issued a policy guidance statement on June 28, 1998, encouraging this transfer of devices to the person's new setting, but this guidance was not stated in the IDEA Amendments of 1997 or IDEA 2004. The speech–language pathologist is in a pivotal position to be sensitive to the user's need for a personal communication system yet recognize the financial commitments of the school district. The policy guidance statement may be helpful to avoid the public relations disaster that is likely if a school attempts to reclaim its device from a graduating student with disabilities. With the rapid turnover in high technology, most AAC systems have extremely limited resale value. Speech–language pathologists should seek advice from their supervisor early in the process to ensure that an equipment transition will be smooth. Some school districts and some states have manuals to provide guidance in these matters. An excellent example is from the Montana Office of Public Instruction (2004), *Assistive Technology: A Special Education Guide to Assistive Technology.*

Maintenance of Devices

AAC devices are rarely ready for use right out of the box. They must be designed, fitted, programmed, customized, adapted, maintained, repaired, and replaced. The school may need to use technical assistance for fitting or customizing. The speech–language pathologist, teacher, and student may personalize the AAC system with identification, photos, taped messages using a friend's voice, and so on. The school district is responsible for maintenance and repairs of student-owned equipment if it is used at school.

A list of approved repair vendors is invaluable. The speech–language pathologist may be the person who arranges for a substitute AAC device while the main one is being repaired. Substitute devices must allow students to maintain their communication skills and not jeopardize their educational activities or grades during a lengthy repair period. Though few states have specific qualifications for those who repair AAC equipment, the repair person should be knowledgeable and experienced with that equipment. The speech–language pathologist is rarely qualified to be the repair person. In most cases, the speech–language pathologist will work with the district specialists, the special education office, and/or the information technology department to make these arrangements. This process is widely variable within districts according to their resources and processes.

Coordination of Services

AT needs to be coordinated with all other interventions or services the student receives. For example, typically, one team member works directly with the student and AAC device, knows the technology well, and has contact with all the other members of the team, including the parents. This coordinator is usually not the AT specialist who is responsible for AT support for the entire district or region. The AT specialist serves the team better in technical assistance than in day-to-day coordination of services for each AT or AAC user.

Occupational therapists, physical therapists, or teachers may coordinate a student's IEP, but experience has shown that it is often speech–language pathologists who coordinate the AAC user's overall program because of their education and skills and also because communication is so central to these students' school lives. The entire team will contribute to any brainstorming or problem solving necessary for the AAC user, but one team member has to see that the plan is completed, that each person follows through, and that parents and students have an informed role in the process. Misunderstandings between team members are common while a program is being implemented.

The IEP should identify roles and persons to carry out these tasks. When AAC is coordinated, the IEP goals and objectives will reflect how the technology serves as a support to the student's education program.

Has Technology Been Considered?

Figure 7.3 illustrates the steps a school district could take to select an AT service or AAC device when the team responds affirmatively to the IEP question "Has technology been considered?" and determines that AT or AAC is appropriate for the student. Notice how each step leads to one of the five elements of AT. Selection of functional outcomes and writing of goals and short-term objectives or benchmarks lead to the expected progress. If the student shows lack of progress, the team returns to the decision-making process and tries again. All AAC decisions are complex and have many possible results, largely because communication is a very personal act and because any method of communication must take multiple factors into account.

Working with AT can be an exciting and challenging part of the speech–language pathologist's job that requires use of many diagnostic, negotiation, prediction, therapeutic, educational intervention, and coordination skills. Because speech–language

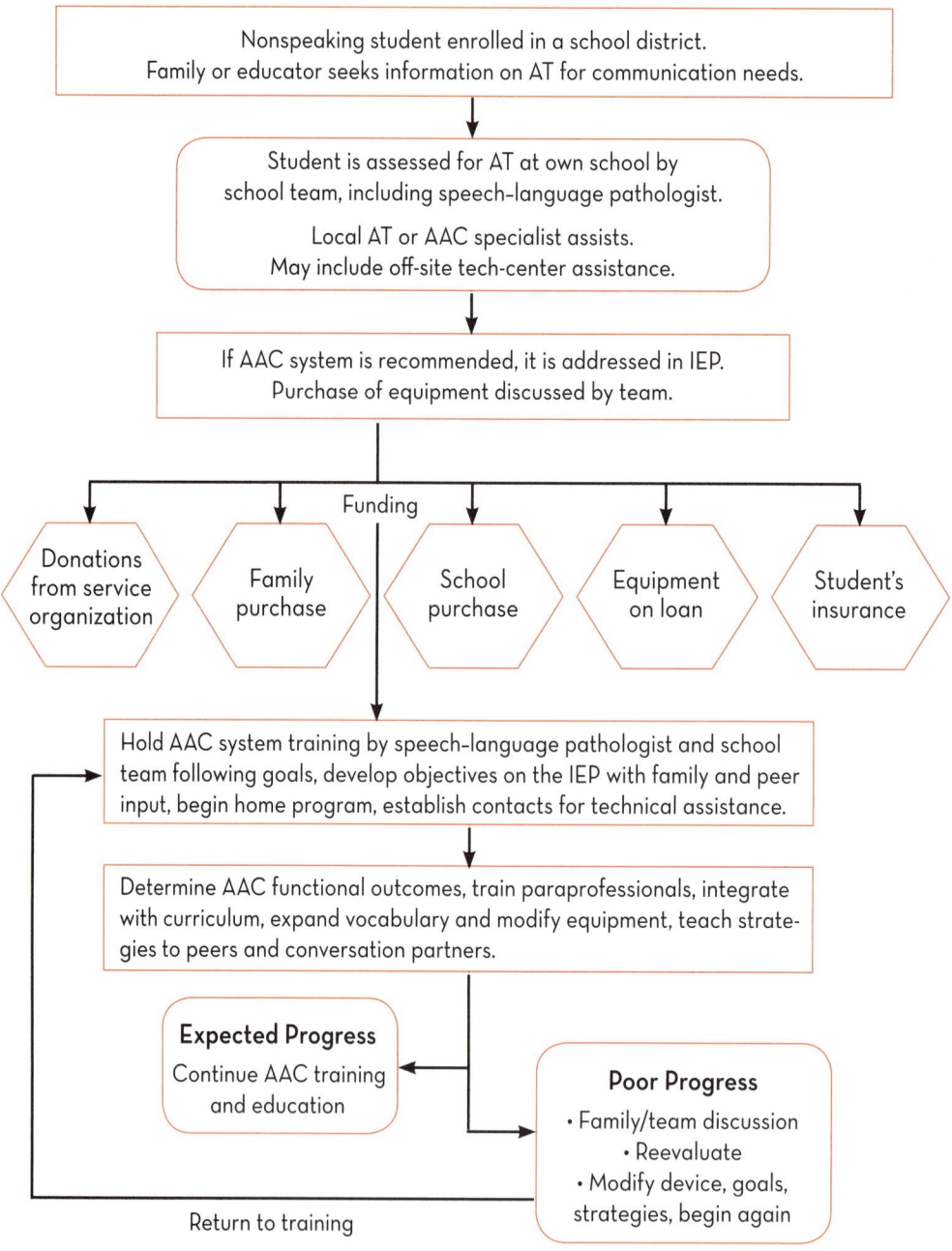

FIGURE 7.3. Augmentative and alternative communication (AAC) as a part of assistive technology (AT).

pathologists are often key IEP team members for AAC, they must learn techniques for working with students with significant communication needs, coordinating large numbers of people, obtaining and maintaining a relatively costly intervention device, and directing ever-changing sets of student skills and emerging technologies.

Student Head Injuries or Athletes With Sports-Related Concussions

A concussion was once thought to be a very mild head injury with a short recovery period and no long-term cognitive effects. Speech–language pathologists in schools were rarely involved with assessment or intervention for students who were injured in a high-school football game on the weekend or in bicycle or car accident after normal school hours. However, recent research has shown that even mild concussions, especially after three or more occur, may result in long-term fatigue, dizziness, memory loss, poor judgment, and other cognitive impairments (Mealings, Douglas, & Olver, 2012). Combined with lengthy school absences, depression, mood swings, disrupted reading performance, and inability to take tests, the student soon displays chronic academic problems (Kennedy, Krause, & O'Brien, 2014). The speech–language pathologist is one of the team members who identifies, assesses, and helps to rehabilitate the student with mild head injury. Various programs have been developed to bring the student back into the busy school environment slowly, with the goal of gradually adding more cognitive tasks, guiding decision making, catching up with content area work missed, and learning new grade-level work that was introduced while the student was unable to attend or was there but could not focus on academics.

Sometimes coaching approaches are used to help the student select and relearn executive functioning techniques to monitor daily tasks and responsibilities (Kennedy, 2017). Both boys and girls experience these sports-related injuries, and there is a tendency to downplay their importance and impact on the adolescent brain. This is an area of increasing concern in schools, with the potential for individuals to have cumulative effects that occur 10 to 20 years later in adulthood. Several university programs are now conducting research and building these clinical experiences into their curriculum (e.g., Chapman University, Orange, CA; University of Texas, El Paso) (see also Duff & Stuck, 2012; Elbin, Covassion, Gallion, & Kontos, 2015; Fjodbak, 2011; Manasse-Cohick, 2011).

Homebound, Homeschooled, Hospital-Bound, Suspended or Expelled, or Incarcerated Children and Youth

Students who are eligible for special education services, including speech–language services, may need to receive such support in locations other than the school for periods of time. This can occur for various reasons.

A student may be restricted to home because of a medical condition, such as severe allergies, autoimmune disorders, cancer, or diabetes, and may need to have his or her education provided by a home-based teacher assigned by the school district. Students hospitalized for a period of time (the amount of time varies from state to state) may receive general and special education services from either their home district or the school district in which the hospital or rehabilitation facility is located. If students were eligible for speech–language services before the protracted hospitalization, they are entitled to continued services if they are physically able to participate. This is usually coordinated with the provision of academic instruction. Speech–language pathologists who are employees of the hospital or rehabilitation facility may provide services, but there are often complicated fiscal issues to resolve between the school district, other funding sources, and service providers.

In the previously described cases, the school speech–language pathologist would provide speech–language services according to the specifications on the IEP. The IEP may be revised, however, to accommodate the student's medical situation. IEPs for students who are off-site are written to provide adequate progress in the curriculum. Students typically spend much less time with a teacher providing homebound services than they would spend at school, because they are receiving intensive one-to-one support. Some districts require the speech–language pathologist from the student's school to travel to the home or hospital. Others have a home or hospital special education team that serves all students at temporary home or medical sites.

Students with an IEP for speech–language services who are suspended for more than 10 days or expelled from school may need to receive these services at home until another school can be found, although such a delay may also be a violation of the student's FAPE. Even after expulsion, students retain their right to FAPE, and the IEP goals must be pursued. Other students may receive special education services at a neutral site, usually due to safety or discipline concerns present at the school site. Special educators are expected to carry out such assignments, with adequate safety precautions provided.

Students who are incarcerated during their school years typically receive their special education at the youth detention site. The assessment and appropriate intervention for speech–language services can be done by the home district, but more densely populated areas or larger penal institutions usually have speech–language pathologists employed by the state's corrections agency, or these services may be the responsibility of a county or regional agency. Incarcerated persons 21 years of age and younger are entitled to special education services if they were identified with a disability, had an IEP prior to their incarceration, and have not yet received a regular high school diploma.

IDEA 2004 requires that all school-age children who reside in a district must be included in Child Find activities. This includes children who are homeschooled or who are enrolled in private education facilities. Schools must make parents and professionals aware of the availability of special education services and how children may be referred for evaluation. Speech–language services, as one of those programs, are frequently requested.

Under IDEA 2004, students who are enrolled by their parents in private school are entitled to evaluation for suspected disabilities, but they may not be entitled to the full continuum of special education services provided to children in public schools. Speech–language pathologists should inquire how their school district deals with this regulation.

Schools may provide special education services to some of these children in a variety of locations. If the child is transported to a special location for services, including the public school, the school district is responsible for the transportation cost. From time to time, school-based speech–language pathologists may need to travel to a distant site to serve a student or have a student transported for services. Working in a school may require the practitioner to negotiate the best way to offer services or create a delivery model that includes an adjusted compensation for time or travel. Telepractice is also an increasingly viable option to provide access to services to students who are not in a typical school setting. (See Chapter 5 for more discussion on telepractice.)

All children in the United States must develop communication skills, as they are vital to their success in life. Through the models described in this chapter, school-based speech–language pathologists have added several new dimensions to their work that have been well received by educators and communities.

Additional Resources

The following are excellent Web sites for early intervention and services to infants and toddlers:

- "Roles and Responsibilities of Speech–Language Pathologists in Early Intervention: Technical Report" (www.asha.org/policy/TR2008-00290/)
- "Roles and Responsibilities of Speech–Language Pathologists in Early Intervention: Position Statement" (www.asha.org/policy/PS2008-00291/)
- "Knowledge and Skills Needed by Speech–Language Pathologists Providing Service to Infants and Families in the NICU Environment" (www.asha.org/policy/KS2004-00080/)

The ASHA Web site on augmentative and alternative communication (www.asha.org/slp/clinical/aac/) provides access to the following instructive practice documents:

- "Roles and Responsibilities of Speech–Language Pathologists With Respect to Augmentative and Alternative Communication: Position Statement"
- "Roles and Responsibilities of Speech–Language Pathologists With Respect to Augmentative and Alternative Communication: Technical Report"
- "Augmentative and Alternative Communication: Knowledge and Skills for Service Delivery"

CHAPTER 8

Procedural Safeguards, Legal Protections, and Appeal Procedures

In This Chapter

This chapter focuses on the procedural safeguards afforded to parents and children under the Individuals With Disabilities Education Improvement Act of 2004 (IDEA 2004). In addition, the processes of resolution sessions, mediation, due process hearings, and complaint procedures will be discussed. These processes are designed to ensure the due process rights of individuals with exceptional needs. Legal requirements are an important component of working within special education. The chapter also addresses strategies for working with families to increase parent involvement and for dealing with difficult situations, including student discipline, which has specialized regulations for students with exceptional needs.

Chapter Questions

1. Review the rights and protections outlined in this chapter. Why do you think these specific rights were developed? What are the implications of implementing these rights? (Recall that Chapter 2 discussed the foundations of due process in the development of the Education for All Handicapped Children Act [EAHCA].)
2. Why is it important for speech–language pathologists to be familiar with student discipline codes?
3. What role might speech–language pathologists take in dealing with the prevention of student violence? How might this role assist students on a speech–language caseload?
4. Locate and review a parental-rights (e.g., procedural safeguards) document. Discuss the presentation of the rights. Is it understandable to the general reader? Would the reader know what to do if a disagreement develops? Where would the reader go for help in understanding these rights?
5. What procedures would a school-based speech–language pathologist want in place to ensure proper preparation in the event a case goes to mediation or a due process hearing?

6. Reflect on how you handle conflict. How might your reactions help or hinder a contentious interaction with a family? What skills might you need to learn?

7. Discuss how the mandate for positive behavior supports affects speech-language pathologists in their practice as members of the Individualized Education Program (IEP) team and as service providers. What skills will the speech-language pathologist need outside of those learned in training programs for communication sciences and disorders?

Parental Notification and Involvement

Special education laws, including the Education for All Handicapped Children Act (EAHCA) of 1975 and the Individuals With Disabilities Education Improvement Act (IDEA 2004), are considered civil rights laws (see Chapter 2). Congress enacted legislation in 1975 that prevented situations in which parents were left out of the educational decision-making process for their child. Subsequently, the rights and protections afforded to parents and children through special education laws have been strengthened. Parental participation, or lack thereof or allegations of denial of involvement, in the Individualized Education Program (IEP) process is a major issue that comes forth in due process challenges. Procedural safeguards that are written into these laws are the means by which parent involvement is ensured and defined. These safeguards are designed under constitutional principles known as *due process of law*. The requirements for due process of law are also applied in school discipline requirements for all students, with specialized requirements for students receiving special education. Over 20 years ago, Turnbull (1993) explained due process passionately in his work *Free Appropriate Public Education: The Law and Children With Disabilities*:

> For those who pioneered the right-to-education doctrine, the procedures for implementing the right were as crucial as the right itself. Procedural due process is a means of challenging the multitude of discriminatory practices that the schools had habitually followed. . . . Without due process, the children would have found that their right to be included in an educational program and to be treated non-discriminatorily (to receive a free appropriate education) would have a hollow ring. Procedural due process—the right to protest—is a necessary educational ingredient in enforcing every phase of the disabled child's right to an education.
>
> Procedural due process is also a constitutional requisite under the requirement of the Fifth and Fourteenth Amendments that no person shall be deprived of life, liberty, or property without due process of law. In terms of the education of disabled children, this means that no disabled child can be deprived of an education without the opportunity of exercising the right to protest what happens to him or her. (p. 207)

The legal requirements under IDEA 2004 may seem overwhelming to educators. Knowing the ramifications of these legal requirements is critical to the practice of special education and to the assurance of free appropriate public education for students. Violations can result in serious consequences for public agencies and the individuals whom IDEA 2004 was designed to protect.

Procedural compliance questions have historically focused only on whether procedures had been followed correctly. Although the focus of special education is now on educational results, procedural compliance and the assurance of due process of law remains an essential cornerstone of IDEA 2004.

IDEA 2004 describes the processes and procedures that agencies and staff must follow to protect the rights of parents and children when delivering special education programs. Procedural safeguards are found in Title 20 § 1415 of the *United States Code* (U.S.C.) and in Title 34, Subpart E, "Procedural Safeguards Due Process Procedures for Parents and Children" of the *Code of Federal Regulations* (C.F.R.). These regulations include the following due process procedures: records examination and participation in meetings, Independent Educational Evaluation (IEE), notice requirements, and parental consent.

Records Examination and Parent Participation in Meetings

All documents related to a student's educational information are considered student records and are governed under the Family Education Rights and Protection Act (FERPA). This law specifically outlines who has access to student records, the types of student records, and how long an educational agency is required to maintain the different types of records (Moore, 2010, 2013). The confidentiality provisions of special education and restrictions regarding who has access to different types of records is tied to the regulations given by FERPA.

Types of Student Records

There are three major types of pupil records: mandatory permanent, mandatory interim, and permitted student records (Moore, 2010, 2013):

- *Mandatory permanent pupil records* are required by state law, which usually includes identifying information about the pupil, when the student attended the schools in the district, and records of subjects taken, grades, immunizations, and date of graduation or exit.
- *Mandatory interim pupil records* are held for a stipulated period of time, including health information, special education information, language training records, progress reports, parental restrictions, parent or pupil challenges to records, parent authorizations or prohibitions for student participation in certain programs, and results of standardized tests.

- *Permitted pupil records* include counselor or teacher rating scales, standardized tests older than 3 years, routine discipline, behavioral reports, discipline notices, and attendance records.

Parents have a right to review all educational records and participate in all meetings that relate to their child's identification, evaluation, educational placement, and FAPE provision. However, Title 34 C.F.R. § 300.501 (b)(23) stated the following:

> A meeting does not include informal or unscheduled conversations involving public agency personnel and conversations on issues such as teaching methodology, lesson plans, or coordination of service provision if those issues are not addressed in the child's IEP. A meeting also does not include preparatory activities that public agency personnel engage in to develop a proposal or response to a parent proposal that will be discussed at a later meeting.

Parents must be involved in special education placement decisions about their child. Educators must understand the provisions of this requirement and all that it entails in both the spirit and the regulatory provisions of the law. Many legal challenges (i.e., *Doug C. v. Hawaii* and *R.B. v. Napa*) involve parent participation as a basis of the due process action. If parents are unable to participate in IEP meetings, "the public agency must use other methods to ensure their participation, including individual or conference telephone calls or video conferencing" (34 C.F.R. § 300.501 [c][3]). An IEP team can make placement decisions about a student without the parents only after several attempts have been made to involve the parents. These attempts must be documented according to standards set in 34 C.F.R. § 300.322 (d):

1. Detailed records of telephone calls made or attempted and the results of those calls
2. Copies of correspondence sent to the parents and any responses received
3. Detailed records of visits made to the parent's home or place of employment and the results of those visits

IEP teams are advised to never hold an IEP meeting without a parent unless these actions have been taken and unless an administrator has knowledge of the situation.

Independent Educational Evaluation

The parents of a child with a disability have the right to obtain an IEE at public expense if they disagree with an evaluation obtained from a public agency (34 C.F.R. § 300.502 [b][1]). If parents request that the school pay for the IEE, the district must inform them of the criteria for an acceptable evaluation and recommended service providers (34 C.F.R. § 300.502 [e]). If parents obtain a private evaluation that meets agency criteria and submit results to the school, an IEP team must consider the results of the evaluation as part of the IEP (34 C.F.R. § 300.502 [c][1]). If parents submit a report from an evaluation they obtained at their own expense, an IEP team meeting should be called to consider this information.

All educators must be familiar with the regulations regarding an IEE. Oftentimes, it is the general education classroom teacher, school administrator, or counselor who is the person given such information by parents. If parents request an IEE, educators must be careful not to give any impression that such a request might not be honored. Learning the appropriate protocol for the local education agency is necessary in the event that such a request is made. When parents request an IEE, notification of a supervisor, administrator, or program manager is highly advisable. Procedures will vary among school districts regarding the approval of and payment for an IEE. In some states, the law requires districts to "Fund or File," meaning either fund the requested IEE or file for due process to defend the district's evaluation. (See also Chapter 3, "Independent Educational Evaluation.")

Prior Written Notice Requirements

The process whereby public agencies notify parents about proposed actions or refusals to act is highly regulated. Every time an action is being considered by IEP team members, written notice must be given to parents, including the items described in 34 C.F.R. § 300.503:

1. Parents must receive prior written notice whenever an agency proposes, refuses, or initiates a change regarding
   - Identification
   - Evaluation
   - Educational placement
   - Provision of FAPE
2. The prior written notice must
   - Be in language understandable to the general public
   - Be in the native language of the parents or translated orally for them
   - Describe the action proposed or refused
   - Explain why the agency is proposing or refusing the action
   - Describe other options considered and the reasons why those options were rejected
   - Describe the information used as a basis for the action
   - Include any other relevant factors used in making the decision
   - Include a statement that the parents have protection under the procedural safeguards of IDEA 2004 and, if the notice is not an initial referral for evaluation, include how a copy of the procedural safeguards can be obtained
   - Include sources of information to assist parents in understanding IDEA

Usually, LEAs have booklets for parents or have the notice of rights written on the back of an IEP document. Under IDEA 2004, LEAs are allowed to post copies of the procedural rights on their agency's Web site (34 C.F.R. § 300.504 [4][b]). The list of procedural safeguards is very long and complex under IDEA 2004 and may be daunting to parents attempting to understand it. Speech–language pathologists and other educators must be aware of their responsibilities under school policies for notifying parents of their rights, and may be called on by parents to help explain the notice.

IDEA 2004 requires that parents be given notice (i.e., provided with written documentation and a verbal explanation) of their rights at each of the following times: when a student is initially referred for evaluation to determine eligibility for special education, when a student is reevaluated, upon receipt by the public agency of a state complaint or filing of a due process action, when a student is being considered for removal that constitutes a change of placement because of a disciplinary incident according to the discipline procedures of the *Code of Federal Regulations* (34 C.F.R. § 300.530 [h]), or upon request by the parent. Responsibility for preparing the notice documents (i.e., parental-rights booklets or notice-of-meeting forms) belongs to educational agencies; however, under school policy, it may be the responsibility of special education service providers to ensure that parents receive and understand these rights and protections.

Speech–language pathologists who are new to public agencies should ask for assistance to learn how their employers want procedural safeguards to be explained to parents. Speech–language pathologists should review the procedural-safeguards-notice document, ask for clarification on questions they may have from administration in their agency, and be able to explain the document to families. Some LEAs may require that copies of procedural safeguards be given to parents other than at the mandated times outlined in the *Code of Federal Regulations*. Local agency policies should always be followed and documented in this regard.

Parental Consent

Congress intended that decisions or actions never be taken regarding a child's education without parent involvement. IDEA 2004 requires that parental consent be obtained before conducting an initial evaluation or a reevaluation. To comply with this requirement, most agencies have a "consent to assess" form, also known as an assessment plan or something similar. (See Chapter 3 for a discussion about when an assessment plan is needed.) The requirements for parental consent do not apply to reviews of files or data as part of an initial evaluation or a reevaluation (34 C.F.R. § 300.300 [c][2][i]) or to the administration of testing done with all students in the school, such as group tests, unless consent is required from all parents (34 C.F.R. § 300.300 [a][2][ii]).

If parents refuse to sign an assessment plan (i.e., decline to have their child assessed to determine whether the child has special needs), a public agency may choose to or may be required to pursue a due process action to proceed with an evaluation, depending on state law (34 C.F.R. § 300.300 [3][i]). (See "The Mediation Process" and "Impartial Due Process Hearings" later in this chapter for a discussion on mediation and due process.) Reevaluations may proceed if parents do not respond to requests for consent, but only after documentation of numerous attempts to secure the consent (34 C.F.R. 300.300 §

[c][ii]). Again, these regulations may vary from state to state. This section of the C.F.R. now gives the public agency the ability to conduct a reevaluation without parental consent if reasonable steps to obtain consent have been taken and the parents have not responded. As state law will vary in procedures to be taken under these circumstances, speech–language pathologists should never make a decision to conduct an evaluation in the absence of consent without first consulting with their special education administrator and seeking direction in such a matter. Documentation of such contacts and conversations with school officials is also advised.

IDEA 2004 prohibits denial of other services to a student based on parental refusal to consent (34 C.F.R. § 300.300 [c][ii][3]). An example of this would be a student who is receiving specialized academic instruction in addition to speech–language services. At the time of the triennial evaluation, the parents may agree to give access to the speech–language pathologist but not to the education specialist. In such a situation, all services to the child must continue, but the team should consult the supervisor or administrator for guidance on how to proceed.

Resolution Sessions, Mediation, Due Process Hearings, and State IDEA Complaints

Due process of law is an element in both the Fifth and Fourteenth Amendments of the U.S. Constitution. Due process guarantees civil rights through procedural safeguards designed to protect individual rights. *Due process* tends to be a phrase that is used in a variety of contexts in special education. Due process procedures include mediation, impartial due process hearings, and state IDEA complaints. Procedural safeguards are intended to ensure that due process of law is provided to families and students. *Due process* also refers to the hearing process available when parents and LEAs disagree on issues related to a student's identification, evaluation, educational placement, or receipt of FAPE. Table 8.1 compares the procedures for resolving procedural complaints.

Resolution sessions, mediation, and due process hearings are used for disputes related to a student's special education; that is, anything that deals with evaluation, goals and objectives, programs, placement, and services. The complaint process is designed for violations of procedural safeguards, such as timeline or implementation violations. These processes are available to parents and public agencies.

Although requests for hearings or investigations through the complaint process are most often actions taken by the parents, states hold school districts accountable for ensuring a child's FAPE when there is a disagreement with parents. School district personnel are often reminded by attorneys that FAPE belongs to the child, not the parent. As part of its affirmative duty to provide a student with FAPE, an LEA may be held responsible for compensatory education for the student if a hearing officer finds that the school district failed to aggressively pursue the student's FAPE despite the disagreement on the part of the student's parents. As part of their practice, therefore, speech–language pathologists and other special educators must be very cautious when there

TABLE 8.1. Individuals With Disabilities Education Improvement Act of 2004 Dispute Resolution Processes Comparison Chart

Topic	Mediation	Due process complaint	Resolution process	State complaint
Who can initiate the process?	Parent or local education agency (LEA) or public agency but must be voluntary for both	Parent or LEA or public agency	The LEA schedules the resolution meeting upon receipt of a due process complaint unless the parties agree to waive or use mediation.	Any individual or organization, including those from out of state
What is the time limit for filing?	None specified	Two years of when the party knew or should have known of the problem (or a timeline specified by state law) with limited exceptions	The process is triggered by a parent's due process complaint.	One year from the date of the alleged violation
What issues can be resolved?	Any matter under Part 300, including matters arising prior to the filing of a due process complaint (there are exceptions)	Any matter relating to the identification, evaluation or educational placement, or provision of a free appropriate public education (there are exceptions)	The issues raised are the same as in the parent's due process complaint.	Alleged violations of Part B of IDEA or Part 300
What is the timeline for resolving the issues?	None specified	Forty-five days from the end of the resolution period unless specific extensions to the timeline are granted	LEA must convene a resolution session within 15 days of receipt of the parent's due process complaint unless the parties agree in writing to waive the meeting or agree to use mediation. The resolution period is 30 days from receipt of the parent's due process complaint unless the parties agree otherwise or the parent or LEA fails to participate in the resolution meeting or the LEA fails to convene the resolution meeting within 15 days of receipt of the parent's due process complaint.	Sixty days from receipt of the complaint unless an extension is permitted
Who resolves the issues?	Parent and LEA or public agency with a mediator (the process is voluntary and both parties must agree to any resolution)	Hearing officer	Both parties (parent and LEA or public agency) must agree to any resolution.	State education agency

Note. Adapted from *IDEA Dispute Resolution Processes Comparison Chart*, by Office of Special Education Programs, n.d. Retrieved from www.directionservice.org/pdf/IDEA%20DR%20 Process%20 Comparison%20Chart.pdf.

are disagreements with parents regarding the recommendations and implementation of IEP procedures. Although disagreements and challenging situations may be difficult, IEP teams are advised that they need to design their offer of FAPE around what the student needs and not simply relent to parent requests because of the pressure being brought to bear. Defending such action is very difficult. This does not mean that a parent's requests and suggestions are not considered, but it does mean that the offer of FAPE needs to be reasoned and defensible.

The Resolution Session

IDEA 2004 added an additional step in the due process procedures to allow local education agencies and parents one more opportunity to resolve differences outside of the constraints of an IEP meeting. This step is known as a *resolution session process* (34 C.F.R. § 300.510). Under this section, the LEA arranges a meeting with the parent within 15 days of receiving the notice of a due process complaint. The resolution session should include a representative of the LEA (i.e., typically a district-level administrator) who has decision-making authority, significant members of the IEP team (which means that not all members of the IEP team need to be present), and the parent (34 C.F.R. § 300.510 [a][i]). Attorneys for the school district are prohibited from attending these meetings unless the parent brings an attorney (34 C.F.R. § 300.510 [a][ii]). The C.F.R. outlined the following:

> The purpose of the meeting is for the parent of the child to discuss the due process complaint and the facts that form the basis of the due process complaint, so that the LEA has the opportunity to resolve the dispute that is the basis for the due process complaint. (34 C.F.R. § 300.510 [a][ii][2])

The resolution session process is intended to give parents and school districts one more opportunity to resolve the disputes between them. A binding written settlement agreement is developed if an agreement is made during this session (34 C.F.R. § 300.510 [d]). Often these sessions can be productive in not only resolving the disputes but also allowing families and districts to work together in a nonadversarial manner and preserve the relationships between them. Depending on his or her role in the case, the speech–language pathologist may or may not be part of the resolution session and may or may not be involved in implementing an agreement reached in the session.

Litigation and Legal Ramifications

Procedural safeguards afforded to parents and students under IDEA 2004 provide for a system to resolve disputes arising from special education evaluation or the contents of the IEP. Collectively, the dispute processes are referred to as due process, which generally implies actions and processes that occur following a filing on behalf of one party requesting a due process hearing. Litigation in special education, often referred to as due process, is of ongoing concern to public school personnel.

IDEA 2004 encourages dispute resolution and mediation processes prior to actual hearings. Due process hearings are held if agreement cannot be reached during dispute resolution or mediation. Each state has a somewhat different system for managing due process hearings. Because IDEA 2004 is a federal law, any appeals of a due process hearing decision are made to a federal trial court at the U.S. District Court for that judicial region. There are 94 judicial districts in the U.S. District Court system. Appeals from the U.S. District Court are reviewed in one of 12 regional U.S. Courts of Appeals (or circuit courts) as shown in Figure 8.1. Any appeal from the U.S. Court of Appeals system is reviewed by the U.S. Supreme Court. Understanding the appeal system in the U.S. judicial system is necessary, first because trends can be seen in the rulings, and second, because decisions made at the U.S. Court of Appeals level apply to all school districts in that region, and, of course, decisions made at the U.S. Supreme Court level apply to all districts in the country.

The Mediation Process

Under IDEA 2004, mediation is a voluntary process that at a minimum must be available whenever a hearing is requested (34 C.F.R. § 300.506). Mediation is a process of formal discussion with a neutral third party to resolve differences. At the point that due process procedures are being used, emotions may be running high on either side of the case, and the mediator should help parties refocus on the issues. Many states had mediation available prior to 1997, but the reauthorization of IDEA (IDEA Amendments of 1997) made the availability of this process mandatory, and this process continued in the reauthorization of IDEA 2004.

The U.S. Circuit Courts of Appeals

1st	Maine, Massachusetts, New Hampshire, Puerto Rico, Rhode Island
2nd	Connecticut, New York, Vermont
3rd	Delaware, New Jersey, Pennsylvania, U.S. Virgin Islands
4th	Maryland, North Carolina, South Carolina, Virginia, West Virginia
5th	Louisiana, Mississippi, Texas
6th	Kentucky, Michigan, Ohio, Tennessee
7th	Illinois, Indiana, Wisconsin
8th	Arkansas, Iowa, Missouri, Nebraska, North Dakota, South Dakota
9th	Alaska, Arizona, California, Guam, Hawaii, Idaho, Montana, Nevada, Northern Mariana Islands, Oregon, Washington
10th	Colorado, Kansas, New Mexico, Oklahoma, Utah, Wyoming
11th	Alabama, Florida, Georgia
12th	District of Columbia

FIGURE 8.1. The U.S. Courts of Appeals.

Mediation is a state-level process. Through the agency responsible for handling special education due process requests, each state has a process for assigning mediators to these matters. LEAs may establish procedures to encourage mediation for parents who elect not to participate in a resolution session after requesting a due process hearing. Such procedures might include arranging a meeting for parents with a neutral party so that the benefits of mediation are explained, and parents are encouraged to use the process. Most states now have information regarding due process procedures available on their state department of education's Web site, which is easily available to parents and educators.

To attempt to resolve issues prior to entering into a mediation process, some regional and local agencies provide *alternative dispute resolution* (ADR). This follows a win–win type of process, acknowledging desires and limitations on both sides. This is a local-level process that occurs before a state-level mediation agency is involved. Mediation and ADR procedures may never be used to delay or deny the right to a due process hearing. Useful information about ADR and other dispute resolution processes may be found on the Center for Appropriate Dispute Resolution in Special Education (CADRE) Web site (www.directionservice.org/cadre/).

The mediation process involves parties from the school district and parties from the family meeting with a mediator. Depending on the agency's procedures and the case, a speech–language pathologist may or may not be involved in the mediation process. Discussions occurring during the process must be confidential and cannot be used in a due process hearing (34 C.F.R. § 300.506 [b][7]). Both sides have an opportunity to tell the mediator their perspective of the dispute and what it would take to solve the dispute. If a solution cannot be reached with both parties in the same room, the parties caucus separately with the mediator. The mediator moves back and forth between the two parties, attempting to reach a mediation or settlement agreement. Such an agreement must be put in writing (34 C.F.R. § 300.506 [b][6]). The agreement may resolve all of the issues being brought forward, or it may resolve only some of the issues. If issues are not resolved, either of the parties may choose to proceed to a due process hearing.

Speech–language pathologists, and other educators, should understand that mediation may result in agreements that are highly unusual. These agreements should be considered individualized in all cases and are not precedent setting. For example, a speech–language pathologist may be required to make up missed therapy sessions or give extra therapy sessions over and above what was previously agreed to in the IEP. Although not precedent setting, the agreement may change the way services are offered or documented district-wide to prevent problems in the future. Implementation of a specialized program might lead to others deducing the outcomes of an agreement, but all mediation agreements are confidential.

Impartial Due Process Hearings

With or without voluntary mediation, parents, students who have reached the age of majority (age 18 years in most states), and school districts are able to request an impartial due process hearing. Issues that can be resolved in a due process hearing are limited to issues involving the IEP process: identification, evaluation, educational placement,

FAPE, and placement of a student in an interim alternative educational setting as a result of a disciplinary matter. School districts and parents should always work with each other to avoid going to a hearing, which is expensive and time-consuming and often contributes to agitation on both sides. In a small percentage of cases, however, a hearing will be held to decide the dispute.

A due process hearing is a formal procedure with a hearing officer who presides and considers evidence presented by both sides. Typically, legal counsel represents each side. Unlike the mediation process, where parties have a neutral third party attempting to assist in developing a compromise, a due process hearing is a quasi-judicial proceeding where testimony is taken, evidence is presented, and, ultimately, one side prevails.

School districts are typically reluctant to use their power to file for (i.e., request) a due process hearing against parents. In California, the education code (56346) dictates a school district's affirmative duty to file for a due process hearing if the district believes that the parents' actions are resulting in the denial of FAPE to students. As explained previously, the right to FAPE belongs to students, not parents, and cannot be denied by the school district based on parental wishes. In California, a district's failure to file a request for a due process hearing in such a case may result in the district later being ordered to provide compensatory education to the student. This can happen if a student files for due process once he or she reaches the age of majority and prevails in a claim that FAPE was withheld. Other states may have similar requirements.

Attorneys often become involved in cases that could lead to a hearing. All state education agencies (SEAs) and LEAs are required to provide parents with information about low-cost legal services and other relevant services when parents request a due process hearing (34 C.F.R. § 300.507 [b]). This is the responsibility of an administrator, not a speech–language pathologist. In any situation where parents mention an intent to seek counsel from an attorney or advocate, the speech–language pathologist should notify a supervisor. Such a comment is considered a red flag, indicating that parents are unhappy about something. Hopefully, the speech–language pathologist is aware of the specific concerns of the parent and can inform the administrator about the situation. In that way, once the administration is notified, attempts to resolve the issues can begin prior to the situation escalating.

Under IDEA 2004, parents cannot seek reimbursement from a school district for their attorney's fees for attendance at an IEP meeting unless the meeting is ordered by a hearing officer or administrative law judge. A court may award attorney fees to parents when the parents are the prevailing party in a due process proceeding, meaning that one or more of their issues are upheld. In such a situation, the school district will be responsible for the cost of attorneys on both sides (if both sides have attorneys), in addition to any costs involved (e.g., the costs of equipment, staff, or training that is found to be necessary) in the parents' educational request (34 C.F.R. § 300.517).

Depending on agency procedures and the case, a speech–language pathologist may be involved in a mediation process leading up to the hearing. If a case goes to a due process hearing, the speech–language pathologist may be required to testify. The situation is much like testifying in court. When school personnel are called to testify, most attorneys for the school district will prepare them prior to the hearing. This means that the speech–language pathologist testifying will know what to expect to the best of the attorney's knowledge. Statements of training and evidentiary information about education, background, documentation on student progress, and the like will probably be a part of the testimony. This is one reason why speech–language pathologists, and all special educators, should be sure that they keep detailed records about student progress and build treatment plans that are grounded in research-based protocols. (See Table 8.2 for helpful tips on testifying.) The speech–language pathologist should rely on ASHA's (2004c) "Practice Portal" as a rationale for assessment and intervention methods.

Every time a due process hearing is requested by either side, the procedural safeguard known as *stay put* goes into effect. "Stay put" means that a student will remain in the educational placement he or she was in when the due process hearing request was filed unless the parties agree otherwise (34 C.F.R. § 300.518). For example, if an IEP calls for speech–language services twice a week for 40 minutes per session and the parents request a due process hearing, the amount of service remains the same (i.e., at present educational placement) until the matter is settled unless both parties agree otherwise through a mediation agreement. IDEA 2004 regulations for "stay put" clarify that when a child transitions from Part C (infant services) to Part B (preschool and school-age services), the LEA is not required to provide Part C services if there is a dispute regarding services (34 C.F.R. § 300.518 [c]).

Timelines apply when due process is initiated. States are required by IDEA 2004 to ensure that due process decisions are reached within 45 days of receipt of a request (34 C.F.R. § 300.515 [a]). If mediation is used, the parties may agree to an extension. The

TABLE 8.2. Dos and Don'ts of Testifying

Do	Toot your own horn (be willing to talk about your accomplishments and expertise). Be affirmative. Answer direct questions. Answer "I don't know" if you don't know. Ask for a break if you are feeling anxious. Take your time so you can answer accurately. Set your own pace. Tell the hearing officer or judge if you are feeling hassled. Check the clock and remember that it will eventually be over.
Don't	Be modest. Be tentative. Volunteer information that you weren't asked about. Guess if you don't know. FREAK (become too stressed to function)! Rush. Let the family's attorney set a rapid pace of questioning. Be defensive.

decision of the hearing officer is final unless appealed. In some states, the first appeal is to the SEA; in others, the appeal is directly to a state court of competent jurisdiction or federal court.

Ultimately, due process hearing decisions, and those cases that are appealed to state and federal jurisdictions, create what is known as *case law*. These key cases set the court's interpretation of disputes that arise in special education. Both districts and parents monitor the court's decisions in these matters, and this lays out arguments for future disputes and gives guidance to the field in terms of legal interpretation. Chapter 2 presented a listing of cases that have given practice guidance for speech–language pathologists and other special educators. Table 2.4 reviews additional important cases that set case law and interpretation on common issues of concerns to special educators. These decisions affect how school districts, parents, and IEP teams conduct their business.

State IDEA Complaint Procedures

Complaint procedures can be used by families, staff, organizations, or individuals when violations of special education law occur (34 C.F.R. § 300.151–153). Examples of common reasons complaints are filed include failure to provide records when requested and failure to implement an IEP. When parents are advised of their procedural due process rights, they must also be advised of the state complaint procedures (34 C.F.R. § 300.504 [c]). This information is typically preprinted on parental-rights forms and may be available on the state agency Web site. To file a complaint, the party filing it must send a written letter to the SEA outlining the alleged violation. The SEA is required to respond, investigate, and issue a written decision within 60 days of receipt of the complaint. The time limit may be extended only if an exceptional circumstance exists in respect to a particular complaint (34 C.F.R. § 300.152).

Positive Behavior Supports and Student Discipline

Positive Behavior Supports

School safety has been one of the top concerns of American citizens following the tragedies on school campuses that have become all too familiar news stories. Positive behavioral supports (PBS) reflect a philosophy and behavior management systems that encourage the use of proactive teaching of positive behavior and decrease or eliminate the use of punishment as methods of behavior management. PBS systems can be used for schools or individuals. In these systems, data are used to analyze environmental variables that can be used to create positive intervention for students and teach prosocial skills (Cohn, 2001).

Positive behavioral intervention and support (PBIS) is a systems-change process that reflects school-wide efforts to teach behavioral expectations in the same way that curriculum is taught. Advocates of PBIS often suggest that although teachers, parents, schools, and society understand that reading, writing, and math are skills that need to be taught, we sometimes think that children "just know" how to behave. When schools engage in a school-wide PBIS program, every individual in the school becomes involved in the program (see www.pbis.org). Many states promote the use of PBIS programs and approaches, especially to address the behavioral side of the response to intervention (RTI) pyramid.

Teaching students behavioral expectations and having school-wide systems that both are clear about behavioral expectations and provide reinforcement when students follow expectations have been shown to be very successful. For students who have greater needs due to disability or other issues, such as mental health or home-related issues, the behavioral pyramid allows for more intense intervention. The use of PBS is required for students with disabilities who receive special education under IDEA (Cohn, 2001). When behavioral challenges present themselves, a functional behavioral assessment (FBA) is required. IDEA requires (*Positive Behavioral Interventions and Supports*, n.d.)

- the IEP team to consider the use of PBIS for any student whose behavior impedes his or her learning or the learning of others (20 U.S.C. §1414[d][3][B][i]),
- an FBA when a child who does not have a behavior intervention plan is removed from his or her current placement for more than 10 school days (e.g., suspension) for behavior that turns out to be a manifestation of the child's disability (20 U.S.C. §1415[k][1][F][i]), and
- an FBA when appropriate to address any behavior that results in a long-term removal (20 U.S.C. §1415[k][1][D]).

Challenging behavior may manifest across disability areas. Speech–language pathologists will likely work with students who have challenging behavior. Understanding behavior and how to intervene according to PBS principles is very important. In addition, it is critical that all educators understand that dealing with students' behavioral difficulties is part of their responsibilities in both general education and special education. Most specifically, speech–language pathologists must learn how to be a part of designing interventions that will assist students in learning appropriate prosocial skills.

Discipline Procedures

Guidelines regarding the discipline of all students in a school setting are founded on the principle of due process of law.

Goss v. Lopez, 419 U.S. 565 (1975) was the U.S. Supreme Court ruling that put into law the necessary components of due process for all student discipline. *Honig v. Doe* (1988) was a later Supreme Court ruling that required a manifestation determination for students receiving special education prior to expulsion or long-term suspension. This means that before a student in special education is subject to a district's regular discipline procedures, an IEP team must determine whether the behavior for which the student is being disciplined was a manifestation of the student's disability and whether the student's placement was appropriate.

All schools, school districts, and states have a code of conduct for their students. Consequences for inappropriate actions are administered at the classroom level, with consequences of increasing severity for more significant violations under the educational code or policy of a district. The goal is to shape students' behavior, encouraging them to learn appropriate behavior that allows them and those around them to learn.

Two types of disciplinary removals are typically common in schools: suspension and expulsion. Suspension is the removal of a student from a classroom or a school for a limited period of time, usually 1 to 5 days. Expulsion refers to the removal of a student from the educational programs of a school district for a lengthy period of time, usually two semesters or longer, and is imposed by a school board or other governing body. Suspensions can be imposed by teachers and school principals and require a minimum of due process. However, the number of days a child with a disability may be suspended without any educational services is limited to 10 cumulative days in a school year (34 C.F.R. § 300.530 [b][2]). Therefore, cumulative suspensions over 10 days require an IEP team meeting to respond to the change in placement and consider changes to the behavioral intervention plan (BIP). Expulsion can be imposed by a school board only and requires more extensive disciplinary due process procedures, including an expulsion hearing where evidence is heard. Children with disabilities who are expelled from school must continue to receive FAPE (34 C.F.R. § 300.530 [d]). (See "Homebound, Homeschooled, Hospital-Bound, Suspended or Expelled, or Incarcerated Children and Youth" in Chapter 7 for further discussion of how to serve students who have been suspended or expelled.)

Manifestation Determination

For students receiving special education, IDEA 2004 provides protections designed to ensure that students are not penalized for behavior that is manifested as part of their disability. Discipline procedures were specifically addressed in IDEA 2004 to make clear that all special educators have responsibilities in these matters. This includes conducting a functional behavioral assessment (FBA) and implementing a behavioral intervention plan (BIP), required components of IEP meetings when a student is experiencing behavioral or discipline problems.

Functional Behavioral Assessment and Behavior Intervention Plan

IDEA 2004 contains specific requirements to guarantee that IEP teams and school-based personnel work to remediate problematic behavior in students with disabilities (34 C.F.R. § 300.530). Speech–language pathologists must be aware of requirements for conducting a functional behavioral assessment and implementing a behavioral intervention plan, which are necessary components of the IEP when a student is experiencing behavioral and/or discipline problems. FBA is a systematic method of analyzing a student's behavior, examining when a student acts inappropriately and what circumstances precipitate the behavior. Most often, a school psychologist or behavior specialist conducts the FBA, but the multidisciplinary team is involved, especially those members who work with the student on a regular basis. The purpose of the FBA is to reveal patterns that predict the student's misbehavior. The FBA will consist of observations in a variety of settings, as well as interviews with staff, the parent(s) of the child, and, if appropriate, the student. One of the goals of the FBA is to discover situations or conditions that are reinforcing for the student. These situations or conditions will eventually become part of the BIP. When the BIP is developed, the team will identify skills and strategies that need to be learned by the student. Speech–language pathologists may feel that their training did not encompass strategies for dealing with difficult behavior. In fact, communication strategies are frequently needed by students with challenging behavior.

The IEP team should conduct an FBA whenever a student's challenging behavior is persistent despite implementation of generally successful behavior management techniques. In addition, an FBA should be conducted whenever a student's behavior is harming himself or herself or others and if the behavior is placing him or her at risk of, or subject to, disciplinary action, such as repeated suspensions or expulsion. Once a BIP is developed, consistent implementation is critical, especially to ensure student success (Browning-Wright & Cafferata, 2013).

Although FBAs and BIPs are intended for use with a student who is presenting behavioral issues, specific regulations apply for a student involved in disciplinary matters. If the student has been suspended for up to 10 days, manifestation determination provisions of IDEA go into effect. Under these circumstances, the C.F.R. directs teams to conduct an FBA and develop a BIP if one is not already in place for the student or to review the BIP if one is in place and determine whether modifications are necessary (34 C.F.R. § 300.530).

In situations when expulsion is recommended or required (e.g., carrying a weapon into school or to a school function, possessing or selling illegal drugs or controlled substances), a manifestation determination review must be conducted immediately, if possible, or no later than 10 school days after the decision to take disciplinary action. (See local regulations and practice for timelines and procedures.) The purpose of the review is to determine

(i)   if the conduct in question was caused by, or had a direct and substantial relationship to, the child's disability; or

(ii)   if the conduct in question was the direct result of the LEA's failure to implement the IEP. (34 C.F.R. § 300.530 [e][1][i][ii])

An IEP team and other qualified persons must consider relevant evaluative and observational data, the student's IEP, teacher observations, and information provided by the parent that is relevant. The team must use this information to make the determinations laid out in 34 C.F.R. § 300.530 (e)(1)(i) and (ii). If the answer to the questions posed under these two criteria is "yes" (e.g., the conduct was caused by or had a direct and substantial relationship to the child's disability; the conduct in question was the direct result of the LEA's failure to implement the IEP), then the student may not be processed for general disciplinary actions. If, however, the answer to these questions is "no," then the student can be subject to the same disciplinary procedures as are general education students. Educators who are called to be a part of a manifestation determination review must consider what they know about the student and what could have been predicted about his or her behavior.

If the IEP team makes a determination that the action was a manifestation of the student's disability, it must take the following additional steps:

1. If a functional behavioral analysis had not been conducted before the incident and a behavioral intervention plan did not exist, the IEP team must develop an assessment plan with the goal of developing a behavioral intervention plan (34 C.F.R. § 300.530 [b][1][i]).

2. If a behavioral intervention plan was in place at the time of a serious incident, an IEP team must review the plan and decide if adjustments are needed (34 C.F.R. § 300.530 [b][1][ii]).

A common complaint about special education is that students cannot be disciplined—this is not true. However, procedural violations on the part of staff will stand out glaringly when a determination is made that a student's IEP was not being implemented, and therefore the student will not be disciplined accordingly. In all situations involving student discipline, the speech–language pathologist must work closely with administrators to ensure that laws are followed. The manifestation determination review process is summarized in the box that follows. Speech–language pathologists might be involved in discipline cases because of the relationship between communication and violence (Sanger, Moore-Brown, & Alt, 2000). The current focus on bullying across the nation applies to children with disabilities in a concerning way, as these students not only run the risk of being the perpetrators of misbehavior and violence but also may be victims, especially students with cognitive impairments, learning disabilities, and emotional disturbances.

Manifestation Determination Reviews

When are manifestation determination reviews conducted? A manifestation determination review is conducted when a student receiving special education is subject to the following disciplinary actions:

- Has been suspended for 10 school days (consecutive)
- Has been suspended for 10 school days (cumulative)
- Is recommended for expulsion

Who conducts a manifestation determination review? The IEP team members and other qualified personnel (34 C.F.R. § 300.530[e]).

What is the timeline for conducting a manifestation determination review? Within 10 school days of any decision to change the placement of a child with a disability (34 C.F.R. § 300.530[e]).

What does the review consist of? [It] ... must review all relevant information in the student's file, including the child's IEP, any teacher observations, and any relevant information provided to the parent to determine

(i)   If the conduct in question was caused by, or had a direct and substantial relationship to, the child's disability; or

(ii)   If the conduct in question was the direct result of the LEA's failure to implement the IEP.

What if the IEP team meets and determines that the behavior was related to the student's disability, or that the placement was inappropriate, or that the student was unable to determine right from wrong? If any of the review standards are not met, the behavior is determined to be a manifestation of the disability. The student cannot be subject to the relevant disciplinary procedure. If the public agency has identified deficiencies in the child's IEP or placement, it must remedy them immediately.

What if the IEP team determines that the behavior is not a manifestation of the student's disability and that placement was appropriate and the student was able to determine the consequences of his or her behavior? Then the student can be disciplined in the same manner as nondisabled students with the exception that FAPE must continue to be provided.

What other requirements exist? If a behavioral intervention plan was in place at the time of the incident, then the IEP team must convene a meeting to review the plan. If a functional behavioral analysis had not been conducted prior to the incident and a behavioral intervention plan did not exist, the IEP team must develop an assessment plan toward the goal of developing such a plan.

Source. 34 C.F.R. § 300.530.

Working With Families

IDEA 2004 put specific emphasis on the importance of and requirements for working with families. Speech–language pathologists will find that the experience of working with families can vary greatly. No one will argue that parents are a critical part of the special program design and implementation of an IEP. Certain realities provide perspective and may be helpful when dealing with challenging situations. One reality is that parents and children have rights; school districts and school district personnel have legal obligations to ensure those rights. Another reality is that children do not choose the circumstances into which they are born. This applies to any circumstance, including economic, physical, and familial. A third reality is that a positive partnership with families can be rewarding personally and professionally and will benefit the student greatly. Most educators and parents desire this type of relationship with families, although it is not always realized.

Speech–language pathologists will encounter a multitude of family situations. Communication impairments affect the entire family constellation. When working with children, considering the impact of their disability on their home lives, in addition to their school lives, helps speech–language pathologists understand the big picture of the impact of the disability. The role of school-based intervention is to improve educationally related difficulties. However, because communication is at the heart of relationships and learning, both at school and at home, expanded understandings can promote effective interventions.

Working with families can put speech–language pathologists in some trying situations, such as being the person who confirms the presence of a disability or having to share data with parents that present a child as being more impaired than the family may be prepared to accept. When specialists are dealing with parents, the circumstances can be sensitive. Children are the most precious connection to a parent's being.

Dealing with difficult issues regarding children can be rewarding and challenging at the same time. A reality of the entire IEP process, including assessment, identification, eligibility determination, and intervention, is that educators participate in IEPs as a part of the professional team. For parents, this is a part of their personal life. Participation in this process is new, frequently confusing, and even intrusive. As a school professional, speech–language pathologists have the job to work with parents in designing and carrying out an educational program for their child.

Speech–language pathologists may believe that the given circumstances in a particular home are not conducive to supporting education. There may be no one available to help a child with homework or books, or other printed materials may not be available, or the parents may be illiterate or experience a disability themselves. A child's linguistic development may be adversely affected in a home where the primary language is other than English or where cultural differences exist that are dramatically different from those of the school culture or classroom expectations. These issues can be difficult for typically developing children and may be either more or less difficult for children with disabilities. Low-socioeconomic-status homes often also have limited or poor access to health care. This may mean that medical situations that might lead to learning disabilities or communication impairments are not treated, exacerbating the situation. These examples do not mean that all children from low socioeconomic or culturally diverse situations are at risk of developing communication disorders, but when evaluating such children, educators must distinguish between *difference* and *disorder* and *delay* and also consider all aspects of the child's and family's situation. In addition, referrals to the instructional support team (IST) or problem-solving team may be helpful to secure assistance from community support or social service agencies. (See Chapter 3 for a discussion of ISTs dynamic assessment, and Chapter 7 for further information on students who are culturally and linguistically diverse [CLD].)

Parent Involvement

Children have a wide range of family constellations; *family* can mean any number and relationship of people who are involved with taking care of a child. Regardless of the circumstances, speech–language pathologists must remember that only parents or legal guardians assigned educational rights can sign for permission to assess or consent to placement in an IEP. Even when children have been removed from parental custody, parents may still retain educational rights. This is regulated differently in each state, so speech–language pathologists should check state laws for clarification.

If children do not have a custodial parent, LEAs will assign a surrogate parent. Surrogate parents are individuals who have received specialized training and are assigned by the school district to represent children in all matters relating to children's identification, evaluation, placement, and provision of FAPE (34 C.F.R. § 300.519). When children are placed through court action in a licensed child-care institution (e.g., a group home) or a foster home, birth parents may still have educational rights, even if children do not live with these parents. These situations can become very complex for care providers, educators, children, and birth parents. In addition, the dynamics of these situations can be trying. Speech–language pathologists should enlist the assistance of a supervisor when questions arise regarding parental status. These situations, however, do not need to be difficult. If the approach taken by the school is that the student has many adults who care, then positive results can happen. Many states have also increased and improved laws surrounding children who are foster youth. Knowing how these laws affect IEP consents and other issues in special education is very important for the students, especially so that services are not delayed or inadvertently denied.

Parents may react in any variety of ways when asked to be involved in educational planning for their children. Speech–language pathologists may work with parents in any of the following situations:

- *Parents who do not respond to phone calls or do not come to appointments or IEP meetings.* These parents may seem not to care but may also have other demands that prevent active participation. IDEA 2004 requires holding meetings at a mutually agreed-on time when parents can attend but does not require undue hardship of staff. Teleconferencing is allowed if that is the only way that parents can participate in their child's IEP.
- *Parents who are grateful for the help and appreciative of the assistance of the specialists involved with their child.* These parents may even be too passive in their acceptance of the information shared. The goal in all situations is to make parents partners in evaluation, planning, and treatment. Parents of this type may at first seem to be the most cooperative with which to work but then may not follow through at home or recognize their role in their child's education.
- *Parents who are active team members and bring ideas and suggestions to planning sessions.* These parents are usually actively involved in home programs established for their child.
- *Parents who are active team members and bring ideas and suggestions to planning sessions but may bring ideas that are contrary to those brought forward by professionals.* This type of situation may be more challenging for professionals. This can lead to a situation that may be on the path to mediation or a due process hearing. Under no circumstances should ideas brought forth by parents be

dismissed or not discussed. Seek assistance as soon as a situation appears to be adversarial or one that will create dissent. In all cases, professionals should listen closely, seek more information, and document what parents are requesting.

- *Parents who are adversarial or mistrustful of the IEP process and may be confrontational or uncooperative.* These types of people are challenging in any walk of life; however, in special education, a federal law requires that parents and school personnel work together. The next section gives some suggestions on strategies to use in difficult situations.

These generalities are likely exaggerations of any situation but do represent differing types of situations that speech–language pathologists should be prepared to encounter. In any of these situations, strategies that focus a group on children's needs can help to improve the situation.

Strategies for Avoiding or Managing Conflict

Training programs and literature in the field often do not prepare speech–language pathologists; they may feel unprepared for work situations that involve conflict. Working in special education can, at times, be sensitive and perhaps even contentious because of the trying nature of the work. Parents are struggling to adjust to the circumstances of their children's disabilities while maintaining jobs, families, and other personal situations; general educators are attempting to work with these children as students in their classrooms while attending to the needs of the other students and demands for improved student performance; and special educators are grappling with increased student needs, demands for accountability and outcomes, and paperwork that can seem overwhelming. Administrators are trying to balance all of these needs and be fiscally accountable. Stressors exist at every level.

In training programs, speech–language pathologists learn how to use a scientific method to approach the disabilities presented by students. In many ways, approaching difficult situations should be viewed in much the same manner while adding heart, understanding, and patience. IDEA 2004 provides for a team approach to planning for and working with children. In the best of all possible worlds, all people come to their roles in the team equally prepared to work together and use solid, up-to-date information and research-based methods to help students. In such a scenario, the team acknowledges the importance of each person's role, including the valuable role that parents play.

IEP teams, like any other team, are made up of individuals who each bring differing backgrounds and experiences to their responsibilities. In such circumstances, difficulties can arise. Some of these are unique to the situation of special education, others are unique to education in general, and some are characteristic of working with difficult people. For the latter circumstance, speech–language pathologists may find it useful to take a workshop on working with difficult situations. For the other circumstances, speech–language pathologists might be wise to watch and learn from those who have successfully worked under such situations for several years (e.g., fellow speech–language pathologists, mentor teachers, principals or other administrators). These people have developed skills and abilities that can be learned and applied when necessary.

Chapter 4 described the IEP as a process. Involving all parties as part of the process can help to achieve a win–win situation. All parties have a stake in the agreement reached with the IEP document. In an ideal scenario, all parties come to the process with something to contribute and respect the input of others, and the process goes well. However, in some situations, this scenario does not occur. In these less-than-ideal cases, team members should examine issues that might confound successful teamwork and decide how to approach the process.

The number one way to avoid problems with parents or colleagues, however, is to be sure that the IEPs are done correctly. Many problems that districts have with IEPs are because of mistakes that could have been avoided. Fagan, Friedman, and Fulfrost (2007) identified the following 10 most common IEP mistakes that can be avoided:

1. *Mistake:* No placement offer
   What to do: The placement offer should be stated clearly.
2. *Mistake:* More than one placement offer
   What to do: The district's offer must be clear and not give parents options from which to choose.
3. *Mistake:* Absence of key teachers
   What to do: Reschedule the meeting if necessary, but teachers must be at the meeting that works directly with the student.
4. *Mistake:* No transition plan
   What to do: There needs to be transition plans for any school movement, from nonpublic school to a self-contained classroom, from Part C to preschool, from preschool to school age, from high school to postsecondary, and so on. Failure to provide an appropriate transition plan can result in the need to provide the student with compensatory education, despite the fact that the student has earned a diploma. Also, transition plans are needed for students moving from feeder elementary districts to high school districts.
5. *Mistake:* Missing important assessment information
   What to do: There needs to be adequate assessment information to lay the foundation for the IEP.
6. *Mistake:* No review of prior goals
   What to do: If the student has not made progress or has made limited progress, the goals should not be continued but be changed.
7. *Mistake:* Needs without goals
   What to do: For each area of need, there should be goals, which then drive service. Follow the process.
8. *Mistake:* Unclear service levels
   What to do: Everyone needs to have a clear understanding of the services the IEP offers.

9. *Mistake:* Extended school year (ESY) services: not specified, not enough, not offered

   What to do: ESY services are needed for students who may regress during long breaks and will not be able to recoup their prior levels in a short period of time. Consider ESY individually according to student need.

10. *Mistake:* Lack of professional judgment

    What to do: Professional behavior should be used at all times. This enhances relationships with parents and colleagues.

When working through difficult IEP processes, speech–language pathologists and IEP teams may find the following strategies useful:

- Always check with participants about what is being documented. For example, if parents and school staff see a behavior differently, then document both points of view (e.g., "School staff report that Sally does not speak at school. She uses gestures to express her wants and needs. Parents report that Sally uses one- and two-word phrases at home to express her wants and needs").
- Be sure that recommended goals and objectives or benchmarks are founded on research-based practices so the rationale for their recommendation can be explained to other IEP team members.
- When team members disagree on recommended services or goals, attempt to agree on a short-term solution (e.g., agree to small-group services three times per week for 3 months rather than a full year).
- Set a meeting time for 2 to 3 months in the future to address or readdress sensitive issues.
- Keep meeting notes for all IEPs. Always document parental comments and requests.
- Always begin meetings by identifying what issues are to be discussed and what process will be used. Always ask parents what issues they would like discussed at the meeting.
- Be sure everyone is comfortable with the language used (English or other), or have interpreter services available.
- Use a flip chart or whiteboard to write issues and illustrate discussion items. This is particularly helpful when drafting goals, illustrating students' schedules, and writing topics that need to be covered.
- Make every attempt to resolve disagreements between professionals prior to a meeting. In other words, do not engage in professional debates in front of parents.
- Begin with one or two items everyone can agree on to set a positive tone.
- Offer to have weekly or bimonthly (i.e., every other week) meetings of one or more members of the school team to check progress. Such meetings are not IEP meetings but collaboration or team meetings.

- If there is a time constraint for the meeting, identify it at the beginning. Keep track of the time throughout the meeting, as well as what still needs to be addressed.
- Set time limits for meetings. Check with local administration on this. In general, lengthy IEP meetings just make people more positional and do not contribute to building relationships. If multiple meetings need to be scheduled to work through the tough issues of the IEP, then do it. This approach is preferred to holding an IEP that lasts for a full day. We believe that IEPs should not last any longer than 3 hours at a time. If there are so many issues that the meeting cannot be completed within this time frame, then it is wise to reconvene. This is actually respectful of people's time. Appropriate management of the time is important at all meetings, but it is especially so when a meeting is contentious.
- Write all decisions into the IEP document.
- If emotions run very high, suggest a 5-minute break for fresh air, a drink of water, or a quick change of scene.
- Always thank everyone for being in attendance at the meeting.
- Remember that everyone has the student's best interests at heart. There just may be different versions of how to achieve them.
- Smile, use a sense of humor (as appropriate), and shake hands.

Additional Resources

- "The BIP Desk Reference" (www.pent.ca.gov/dsk/BIPdeskreference2013 .pdf)

- "Bullying and Youth With Disabilities and Special Health Needs" (www.stopbullying.gov/at-risk/groups/special-needs/)

The Work World of Speech–Language Pathologists in Public Schools

● *In This Chapter*

The purpose of this chapter is to consider some of the practical and professional issues that affect school-based speech–language pathologists, to develop an understanding of the school environment, and to describe how to work effectively in a school environment. Topics include how to obtain a position; the roles and responsibilities of speech–language pathologists, audiologists, and speech–language pathology assistants; where to go for assistance; and a variety of professional and organizational issues that are characteristic of a public education system. This chapter is also intended to provide a school-based perspective to the speech–language pathologist exploring a career as an educational professional working in the child's natural environment.

● *Chapter Questions*

1. Discuss why providing private paid therapy for students from your school caseload on Saturdays would be unethical. What policies would be violated, and which speech–language pathologist certifications could be endangered?

2. What does it mean to receive Medicaid payment for speech–language and hearing services in schools? If this is a practice in your area, invite a school-based speech–language pathologist to share the way the program works and how it can be structured as a benefit for children with disabilities and for the speech–language staff in a district.

3. Review the credentialing and licensing requirements for speech–language pathologists for your state. What do you need to know about your state credential or license to practice in the schools?

4. Do your state's licensure rules address assistants or support personnel? Why or why not? What value might they provide to a school setting? How would you use their skills?

5. Why should school-based practitioners belong to more than one professional organization?

6. Does your state have labor unions in the schools? Why or why not? How are the school-based speech–language pathologists that you know represented in negotiations for salary and working conditions?

7. Practice answering the interview questions discussed in the section "The Interview" in this chapter.

8. Interview a speech–language pathologist from a local school system. Discuss the organizational structures in that school system. Who evaluates the speech–language pathologist? Where does the speech–language pathologist find help and support? Report your findings.

9. Review the list of roles and responsibilities of school-based speech–language pathologists and discuss your impression of this list. What roles do you consider particularly interesting? Are there any that seem less familiar to you?

10. Discuss why the prudent professional carries liability insurance.

Certification and Licensing

The world of schools requires a specialized understanding of how "the system" works and what it means to be an employee in a public school system. To work in an educational setting, speech–language pathologists and speech–language pathology assistants (SL-PAs) must be licensed or credentialed according to the regulations of their state. There is a relationship between the requirements set at national, state, and local levels. Being familiar with these regulations is important. The American Speech–Language–Hearing Association (ASHA) Web site has a complete listing of the requirements for each state. Before applying for a job (see the section "Securing a Position" later in this chapter), a candidate must make certain he or she has completed all the necessary requirements and paperwork for certification, licensing, or both, if required. With the mandates for highly qualified staff under the Elementary and Secondary Education Act (ESEA) and the Individuals With Disabilities Education Improvement Act of 2004 (IDEA 2004), all of these requirements are given serious attention by the human resources departments of educational agencies. The licensing and certification requirements of the profession are sometimes confusing for individuals new to the field and even to those in the field. The following will describe the differences between the three credential levels. School-based personnel should always check with their potential employer to verify what certificates and licenses are required for employment in various settings and states.

National Certification

The Certificate of Clinical Competence (CCC) was established in 1952 by ASHA. See Table 9.1 for a comparison of certification and licensing requirements for speech–language pathologists. ASHA certification is a professional certification that may or may not be required in a school setting, depending on the state. Although ASHA certification is voluntary, it is recommended, because holding the CCC indicates to potential employers that speech–language pathologists have met the standards of excellence established by this national organization. In addition, national certification demonstrates to parents, advocates and attorneys that the bearer can match credentials from outside private providers in the event of a challenge. ASHA certification is typically required in health care, private practice, and other settings that receive third-party reimbursement, because Medicare and Medicaid require ASHA certification for reimbursement. In a school setting, depending on the state, ASHA certification may also be required for third-party billing. At the national level, the CCC permits its holders to provide independent clinical services and to supervise the clinical practice of students studying speech–language pathology and uncertified clinicians. States have the option to require the speech–language pathologist to have the CCC to supervise SLPAs, monitor a student intern, participate in ASHA data collection projects, or oversee a colleague completing a clinical fellowship (CF). In addition, those who have earned the CCC in speech–language pathology have the verified knowledge and skills to work in many settings worldwide, including American schools and military schools abroad.

On a professional level, the concept of national certification has received heightened attention with a recognized system for national teacher certification established by the National Board for Professional Teaching Standards (NBPTS or the National Board). As this movement emerged, holders of the CCC asserted that they have held such national recognition for years. Some school districts have negotiated treatment of the CCC as the same as national state teacher certification in their collective bargaining agreements. In addition, a growing number of states and local school districts have established salary supplements and/or are now providing stipends to holders of the CCC or other types of licensure. This practice has grown as a method of retention because of the shortages of speech–language pathologists across the country.

Although certification is important to establish credibility, licensing is required in many states to legally practice speech–language pathology. In many states, ASHA certification satisfies many or all of the state requirements for licensure.

ASHA also offers clinical specialty certification in the areas of child language and language disorders, fluency and fluency disorders, swallowing and swallowing disorders, and intraoperative monitoring. This certification provides holders an opportunity to earn a formalized credential recognizing advanced knowledge and skills in a specialized area of practice. Specialty certification boards work with the Council for Clinical Certification (CFCC) in Audiology and Speech–Language Pathology to establish requirements and oversee the programs. Speech–language pathologists in schools are not required to have such professional certification, but they may wish to pursue one of these advanced certifications if their area of practice is highly specialized, and after years of practice, when they can demonstrate advanced skills. (See "Clinical Specialty Certification" at www.asha.org/Certification/specialty/Clinical-Specialty-Certification/.)

TABLE 9.1. Certification and Licensing Requirements for Speech–Language Pathologists

Certification	Agency	Purpose	Academic preparation	Test	Practicum	Renewal	Required for school services
Certificate of Clinical Competence in Speech–Language Pathology (CCC-SLP)	American Speech–Language–Hearing Association (ASHA)	Recognize clinical competence	Graduate degree in the discipline	Praxis II®: Examination in speech–language pathology	A total of 250 hours clinical practicum, and 36 weeks of supervision on the job	Pay fee every year	No
Speech–language pathology license	Designated state agency	Protect the public from untrained practitioners	Determined by the state, many mirror the ASHA guidelines for the CCC	Praxis II®: Examination in speech–language pathology	One to 2 years of supervision on the job	Pay fee every year or every other year, plus obtain continuing education units (CEUs) per state law	Only in states with universal licensure
State education agency credentialing or teacher license	Designated state agency	Ensure training to work with children in an educational setting	Determined by the state; may align with ASHA guidelines and state license requirements	Praxis II®: Examination in speech–language pathology	Per state laws, may have beginning teacher programs for all new employees working with students	Pay fee every 3 to 5 years, depending on state; may require CEUs	Yes, in some states

State Licensing

A school district may not use the ASHA CCC as the sole licensing requirement for employment, but rather, the state department of education may have its own state certifications or licensure. Some school districts do require the CCC in addition to any state requirements. ASHA's Web site contains specific up-to-date information on state trends and requirements. (See www.asha.org/advocacy/state/State LicensureTrends/.) In some states, licensing and credentialing for school services are separate. In other states, licensing covers both education and health-care settings. The difference between these various licenses and certifications is important, especially as it pertains to billing for Medicaid. In years past, some speech–language pathologists resented needing to hold several licenses, especially if they were using their license to bill. However, holding several licenses and certifications is common in many professions, and speech–language pathology is no different. State licensure requirements are overseen by the agencies that are concerned with consumer protection, so they have a purpose that is different from that of education credentialing agencies. Fortunately, all state agencies work collaboratively and currently coordinate with ASHA for requirements. Continuing education requirements are in place in nearly all states.

Teacher Certification

Each state education agency (SEA) requires a credential that shows a speech–language pathologist has completed a course of study in a university communication sciences and disorders program with certain elements, courses, and field experiences approved by that state. These state authorizations may be called teacher permits, teaching certificates, teacher licenses, or clinical service credentials. In this way, the SEA has final approval of all speech–language pathologists who work with students in that state.

Speech–language pathologists must have some type of state teacher certification to work in a public school setting. Some states have reciprocity with other states (e.g., New England states have reciprocity with each other), but most states accredit only their own state universities and teaching staff. Speech–language pathologists must have a state teaching or clinical license to bill a third party, such as an insurance company or Medicaid, for a student's services in schools.

Ideally, school-based speech–language pathologists should possess all three credentials—ASHA's CCC, a state license, and a teacher certification—in states that have licensure; however, the legal requirement is to hold whatever state certification is needed for providing speech–language services in a particular state's public schools. The requirements for the three credentials do overlap, especially academic requirements, clinical clock hour requirements, and the required professional years of supervised practice. Simultaneously completing these national and state requirements right after university graduation is easier than trying to return to a university to complete one or more credentials later in one's career, because test scores often become outdated, logs of courses and hours can be misplaced or lost, and requirements change, which may mean returning to university or retaking the Praxis. Speech–language pathologists in certain states may become frustrated with the need to hold multiple certifications and licenses. This occurs in government-related systems that have overlapping oversight from various agencies. Maintaining all requisite certifications is a recommended professional practice and may become a point of defense if credentials are challenged in any sort of due process action (see Chapter 8). In addition, lapsing certification or licensure, even if an individual is taking a sabbatical from working in a particular work setting, may prove misguided when life circumstances change and the individual would like to have the option to return to work in that setting. So the rule of thumb is for speech–language pathologists to obtain all of the certifications and licenses in their state and maintain them through paying the fees and keeping up with continuing education requirements.

The current requirements for ASHA's CCC are available on the ASHA Web site (www.asha.org), as is an overview of teacher licensing requirements for each state and contact information for each SEA. Applications for a state teacher certificate must be requested from each SEA, and licensing applications must be requested from the state licensing panel or board, usually housed in a social services or health-care department. Although the requirements for certification and licensing might initially appear confusing, Table 9.1 should help school-based speech–language pathologists understand the details of certification and licensing.

Speech–language pathologists are considered related service providers under IDEA. Under IDEA 2004, related services personnel and paraprofessionals must have qualifications that are consistent with any state-approved or state-recognized certification, licensing, or registration (§ 612 [a][14][B][i]). Emergency, temporary, or provisional certifications are prohibited (§ 612 [a][14][B][ii]). It should be noted that the language for highest requirements in the state found in the IDEA Amendments of 1997 at § 612 (a)(15)(B)(ii) was removed from IDEA 2004. Speech–language pathologists must be vigilant in their states to monitor any attempt to reduce professional standards. ASHA will help state associations resist efforts to lower professional personnel standards. It is tempting for states, especially in times of shortages, to lower standards; however, maintaining high personnel qualification is critical for ensuring quality services for students.

An Ideal Timeline

Typically, candidates who intend to work in the public schools complete their bachelor's degree in communication sciences and disorders, become full-time graduate students, attain their master's degree, pass the national examination (i.e., Praxis II®), complete a clinical fellowship (CF) during their first year on the job, and meet ASHA's certification requirements by the end of their first year of work. This process may take longer for some candidates to accomplish than others. Some states do not require a master's degree in communication disorders for candidates to begin working in public schools; however, this is not endorsed by ASHA or recommended by professionals in the field.

Speech–language pathologists must realize how important it is to schedule these personal benchmarks carefully and completely, with guidance from mentors in the school district and a graduate school adviser. This scheduling may help speech–language pathologists avoid suddenly realizing that they cannot finish all the requirements in the first year and then losing the momentum needed to complete the academic preparation. Many candidates report that keeping the goal in sight can be hard, especially when others in the school community do not have to earn two more certifications after earning their teaching credentials. However, the CCC and the state license (in states requiring licensure) are critical steps in the preparation of a fully qualified professional. To work through a 3- to 5-year plan for completing these three certifications, speech–language pathologists will find it imperative to keep complete and accurate records of all courses, classes, clock hours, registered supervision plans, and test scores in a personal file for solid documentation. The candidate is always responsible for providing proof of meeting all requirements.

Securing a Position

The Job Market

ASHA reported that prospects are excellent for employment as a school-based speech–language pathologist in the near future and beyond because of mandated services under IDEA 2004, the increase in special education students, and the need for services by culturally competent practitioners for individuals, including children, who are from culturally and linguistically diverse backgrounds. The ASHA Web site reported, "The U.S. Census Report indicates that the number of special education students in need of services is disproportionate to the number of qualified Speech–Language Pathologists who can provide these services" (ASHA, n.d.-e). Shortages of special education teachers and specialists have been documented since the mid-1990s (Cross, 2016). This situation makes the job market competitive for speech–language pathologists. "According to the U.S. Department of Labor's Bureau of Labor Statistics' Occupational Handbook, 2013–2014 edition, speech–language pathology employment is expected to grow by 23% from 2010 to 2020—faster than the average for all occupations" (ASHA, n.d.-e).

The quality of the nation's speech–language pathologist workforce depends on having an adequate supply of qualified individuals. Should shortages occur, local districts may be forced to hire less qualified personnel or assign staff to positions for which they are unprepared.

ASHA has undertaken an active role in trying to create solutions to the shortage problem (see ASHA's Forum on Strategizing Solutions to Personnel Shortages in Speech–Language Pathology at www.asha.org/slp/slppersonnelforum/#_ga=1.2220752 92.509329459.1419034974), but the reality is that the shortage and social issues have created employment opportunities for speech–language pathologists. *U.S. News and World Report* identified speech–language pathologist as number 2 on the Best Social Service Jobs and number 30 on the Top 100 Best Jobs for 2014 ("Speech–Language Pathologist Overview," 2016). In the meantime, existing speech–language pathologists and those entering speech–language pathology university programs are much needed; therefore, their negotiating power is increased.

The Application

Obtaining a job in a school setting is a formal process. Schools typically have an application process for all prospective employees that can be obtained through the personnel or human resources department online at the school district's Web site or through a comprehensive employment Web site for the state. Before submitting an application to a local education agency (LEA), the applicant may wish to determine whether that agency has a speech–language pathologist opening. Such information may be found by calling the agency's personnel or human resources department, calling the special education department, searching for job postings on agency or statewide Web sites (e.g., ASHA, state speech–language–hearing associations, the Council for Exceptional Children, state departments of education, local school districts, regional service agencies, Web sites that specialize in posting employment opportunities), looking at job postings at a local university, or reviewing national or regional publications with classified advertisements.

Include a cover letter with all applications. In this letter, state what type of position is being sought, how your qualifications match the desired qualifications for the position (i.e., certification and licensure), and why you are interested in that particular agency. This letter should be short (no more than one page) but should allow readers to see qualifications that might interest them as an employer. Emphasize your interest in working with children. Identify any specialized training received while in graduate school, or any other unique experiences that show involvement with education or children. Do not underestimate the importance of the cover letter, as it is the first introduction the potential employer has to new candidates, and initial impressions can make the difference between being called for an interview and not being called. Remember that although there are shortages in the field, some districts are considered highly desirable, so there may be several applications. This is still a competitive process, and so candidates need to represent themselves well in their cover letter in order to capture the attention of their potential employers.

In addition to the cover letter, some applications include an essay question. Such questions will typically be broad in scope, for example, "Describe your belief system about education," "Describe some noteworthy experience you have had in the past 3 years," or "Who was the person who most influenced your decision to become a teacher?" Time and consideration should be taken in answering any essay question. Your response is a prime opportunity to communicate to the potential employer your interests, energy, and beliefs about education, special education, and speech–language pathology in the schools. The essay plays an important role in forming the first impression for those who are screening applications, so details such as organization, clarity of ideas, spelling, and legibility should not be overlooked.

Job applications will generally also require letters of recommendation. These letters should come from individuals who have knowledge of your clinical skills, meaning clinical supervisors or university professors. Letters should be from professionals in the field. Letters from ministers or family friends will not be able to provide the information that an employer needs regarding work skills pertaining to the job duties and requirements. If you have worked in a related field with children (e.g., as an instructional aide, as an in-home behavior interventionist), letters from these supervisors may be included. Generally, at least two or three professional recommendations are required as part of the application.

The Interview

Applications will be screened by one or more persons at the school district or agency prior to an invitation to interview. The interview process will vary from agency to agency, but candidates should expect to be interviewed by individuals who may not have expertise in speech and language. Candidates should expect a panel of two to five people to conduct the interview. In addition, there may be several different panels or meetings with various individuals. For example, the first-level interview might be with a building principal and staff members from a school site. Other special educators, including speech–language pathologists, may or may not be included. Usually someone from the district special education department, such as the director or program manager, will participate as a member of the first interview panel. Second- and third-level interviews may be part of the process and may include other professionals, administrators, parents, PTA members, or teacher organization representatives.

Questions will vary depending on who is conducting the interview. Be prepared to answer questions of a technical nature about speech and language, including questions regarding service delivery and student eligibility. Questions about student discipline and classroom management are likely to be included. It is also advisable to know something about the current educational issues in the local school or in the nation. Reading articles in recent issues of state speech–language–hearing association newsletters or ASHA publications and checking the agency's Web site are effective ways to prepare.

Personal presentation is very important in an interview. Practice responding to interview questions with familiar people a few days before the actual interview. Practice answering questions that are likely to be asked, such as "Tell us about yourself, your background, and your educational training." The culture of schools can be very "student friendly," and interviewers will also want to know if you can provide this level of concern. Educators seek a caring and kind speech–language pathologist who is interested in students first, wants to be a member of their school team, and has a solid knowledge base in the profession so as to be a good resource for them. These traits should be communicated in an interview. With current requirements for access to curriculum, it is also critical that a candidate can explain the role of the speech–language pathologist working with a curriculum.

When interviewing for a school position, especially for the first time, do not be surprised if there are questions that are unfamiliar. Do not try to make up answers. Feel free to say "I do not know" or "I am not familiar with that area." When in an interview, remember that someone in the room wrote the question and does know the answer, so fabricating an answer is usually not successful. Another good answer is usually "I don't know, but I am willing to learn." The most important advice is to relax and let your personality and experience be your guide. An example of possible interview questions can be found in Table 9.2. Use these questions as a starting point for practice.

There is usually a time in an interview when the candidate may ask questions. It is not advisable to ask questions about money or benefits at that time. That information, especially salary, can be obtained either through the agency's Web site or through the human resources department. It is considered appropriate to ask questions about working conditions, caseload size, continuing education opportunities, and budget.

Accepting the Position

When an offer of employment is made, make sure all questions about employment conditions are asked and answered fully. Now is the appropriate time to ask questions about the following:

TABLE 9.2. Possible Interview Questions for Speech-Language Pathologists

Please begin by telling us about your professional training and experience, including your job-related experiences and education.
Describe how a student qualifies to receive special education services. What are the specific criteria to determine whether a student is eligible to receive speech and language services?
A fourth-grade student has been referred for a language evaluation. How will you conduct the assessment? What tools and procedures will you use?
Describe your experience working with bilingual students. Discuss the issues related to students who come from a monolingual Spanish-speaking home but have received English-only instruction.
Review for us your experience with the following disorders. Discuss both assessment and intervention: • Fluency • Voice • Articulation and phonology
Describe your experiences with the following: • Alternative and augmentative communication • Assistive technology • Students with significant disabilities, including autism spectrum disorders • Speech-sound disorders • Literacy
Discuss the various types of service delivery models that you might use and how you would determine what is appropriate.

- Salary
- Payment schedule (10 months or 12 months)
- Work calendar
- Benefits (including health, dental, vision, and other insurance, including workers' compensation; also inquire about tax shelter opportunities that may be available to public employees)
- Retirement system
- Union membership (required or optional)
- Site assignments
- Clinical supervision, if needed

If a candidate is in the enviable position of having two or more viable offers, he or she may be able to negotiate. However, be cautious so as not to lose both offers. It is acceptable to be straightforward and tell the prospective employer that another offer is being considered, describe the pros on that side, and see what each district will offer. Some agencies offer stipends and incentives on their salary schedule to increase the pay for speech–language pathologists. In addition, some agencies may qualify for loan forgiveness, if this is applicable to the candidate. Loan forgiveness may apply when the school or district is in a high-poverty area. (See ASHA's Web site for information on loan forgiveness programs or the U.S. Department of Education's Web site on federal student loan forgiveness at https://studentaid.ed.gov/repay-loans/forgiveness-cancellation.)

Remember that unlike in the private sector, salary schedules in public institutions are negotiated as part of collective bargaining, so there may be little wiggle room for the district to negotiate pay. Salary schedules are typically posted on the district's Web site. An advisable practice is to review the schedule prior to applying. Salary schedules are generally set up based on years of experience and amount of education. Potential candidates can generally review the salary schedule and determine their potential placement. Stipends or salary supplements will also be listed on the salary schedule, as these too are negotiated items. There are many different aspects to consider when selecting a place to apply and to work. Salary and benefits are two such considerations. Location, personal history with the district, professional support, the district's reputation, and other factors may also affect why an individual would select a certain district or educational agency for employment. The place one chooses to work is a matter of both the agency selecting the candidate and the candidate selecting the place of employment. Doing as much research on the district as possible prior to applying is recommended to ensure that it is a desirable place to work. If certain factors, such as salary, are not attractive, then do not apply at that agency.

Another option for working in school-based settings that some speech–language pathologists may increasingly consider is the option of working for a contract company. Such companies may offer flexibility and benefits that may be enticing, especially to candidates who do not anticipate committing to a full career with a specific educational system. In some cases, the salary may be higher than it is in the school district. Another advantage of working for a contract company is that the company may provide moving costs or certain living expenses.

School districts look to contract companies when they are unable to fill open positions on their staff. There are pros and cons to working for a contract company that speech–language pathologists should consider. Salary and flexibility may be among the pros, as well as other benefits such as the payment of association dues and licensing fees. On the other hand, contract companies often do not offer sick days or retirement systems. Working directly for a school district also has its benefits. Security in terms of earning tenure in the school system, paying into a retirement system that has strong benefits after a full career, getting sick days, and earning seniority that comes with a broader say in assignments may be among some of the advantages of working directly for a school district. As a member of the school district staff, speech–language pathologists will also be involved with the reform efforts in that district and have influence in the role that special education takes. Most contract individuals will not be asked to sit on committees or to contribute in a decision-making manner to school issues. Contractors also may not be allowed to participate in continuing education events.

Organizational Structures

Schools in the United States are created under many different types of organizational structures. Schools themselves usually are part of a district, with names that may sound familiar, for example: Jefferson County Public Schools (Louisville, KY), Los Angeles Unified School District (Los Angeles, CA), and Sunnybrook School District (Lansing/Lynwood, IL). School districts vary by size, organizational structure, geography, historical events, and state fiscal procedures. The Los Angeles Unified School District encompasses a massive area, not only in terms of land but also in the more critical responsibility of educating nearly 900,000 students (nearly as many students as in the entire state of Wisconsin). The state of North Dakota has slightly over 104,000 students enrolled in its entire state's school system. And in Hawaii, the entire state encompasses only one school district, serving approximately 184,000 children.

The organizational structures that provide services to children with disabilities vary greatly from district to district and from state to state. Throughout this book, reference has been made to local, regional, and state services. *Local* usually refers to a school district, but not always. For example, in a rural or smaller suburban district, special education services may be provided on a regional basis. Regional systems are typically cooperatives of smaller school districts that join resources together to provide services to children with specialized needs. State systems typically support schools for students who are blind or deaf and who require highly specialized forms of instruction. States may also run diagnostic centers. The federal law frequently refers to the LEA to denote the organizational entity that has responsibility for the provision of services to students with exceptional needs.

Special education services may be provided through a variety of organizational structures. In some circumstances, the related services are provided by speech–language pathologists and other service providers employed by the school district. In other circumstances, a regional area system may be the employing agency for speech–language pathologists or other support personnel. In these situations, the related service providers are then assigned to schools or districts in the surrounding geographical area. When services are provided through a regional system, it may be that the school district is too small to support a full-time specialist staff, or there may be a belief that a higher level of expertise can be maintained by supporting specialist staff through a regionalized service area. Both district and regional systems will have administrative and program support personnel. Depending on the size of the agency and the administrative structure within the local school system, the speech–language pathologist may or may not have much contact with the administrative regional and support staff.

Funding

Education is considered a constitutional property right in the United States and so is funded through government resources. Funding for schools is complex and often political. Before trying to understand how funding occurs for special education, the prudent employee (and citizen) should have a basic understanding of how public education is funded in the United States. Education is compulsory for children through age 15, 16, 17, or 18 years, depending on the state. Each state constitution requires that a comprehensive educational program exist and be funded for either kindergarten or Grade 1 through Grade 12. Some states have state-operated preschool programs, and some states have 2-year postsecondary educational programs that are open to all high school graduates at little or no charge. Sometimes such systems articulate with a statewide university or technical college system. School funding is often subject to economic fluctuations, which is especially difficult for school district personnel trying to meet educational mandates for students in both general education and special education.

School Finance

The massive K–12 educational system is free to the citizens of all states, a concept found in few nations in the world. Revenue for school districts comes from a combination of local, state, and federal sources. Relatively small parcels of money come from the federal government, although people are often under the misunderstanding that the federal government funds special education. A larger amount of money comes from state governments, and the largest pool of money to support special education generally comes from local agencies.

Federal funds for education are quite limited and targeted to specific programs, with strict usage guidelines. State taxes for education are derived from revenue sources that are relatively constant but often variable in terms of consistency—income, property, and sales. These revenue sources are identified in the state constitution. Local funding is typically generated through levies on property values and sales tax charged in addition to state-mandated taxes.

The actual dollars realized from each different revenue source can vary dramatically across states. In some states, city or county taxes are used for education, contributing to great variations between affluent and low-income areas, urban and rural districts, and districts where property values are high versus low. Since the late 1970s, equity in state educational funding between school districts has been a controversial issue and the topic of many legal challenges.

Funding for Special Education

Since the inception of the Education for All Handicapped Children Act (EAHCA) of 1975, the funding of special education has been one of the more controversial aspects of the entire school funding picture. When EAHCA was enacted, federal funding for this program was originally promised by Congress at 40% of the excess cost of special education in each state. This level of funding has never been realized. Parents, professionals, and politicians have been advocating for full funding of special education for many years. Special education is an example of an unfunded mandate of the federal government, meaning that state and local entities are required to implement programs legislated by Congress for which they do not receive adequate federal funding.

In spirit, the concept of full funding has bipartisan support. In the reauthorization of IDEA 2004, Congress built in a formula designed to bring the allocation for special education to full funding within 10 years. In this formula, there are recommendations for the funding levels that need to be reached each year to achieve the full funding goal. Unfortunately, each year since the reauthorization, the finance committee has cut the recommended allocations. Although the recommended levels are stated in the law, IDEA funding continues to be discretionary and not mandatory; other priorities are put ahead of full funding for IDEA. When federal funding does not meet its intended level, state and local contributions need to be increased to cover the costs of special education. These funds come from the general fund, depleting funds available for other education programs and purposes and creating tension between general education and special education.

The term *full funding* may be misinterpreted. Since the federal component of special education is intended to fund 40% of the excess cost of special education, state and local districts would always be expected to fund the basic per-pupil funding that all students in a state receive and then also 60% of the costs beyond the per-pupil funding. The challenge for districts is that the cost of specialized programs, including teachers, smaller class sizes, and specialized equipment and materials, has risen dramatically in the past 40 years. So when the federal obligation is less than originally promised, the extra burden on states and local agencies can be in the millions of dollars, meaning that other programs and services in the district cannot be supported. This creates tension between special education and general education, as special education programs need to be provided regardless of the funding flow. Speech–language pathologists need to be sensitive to the complexities of budgets and the reasons why some fiscal decisions are made that may seem unreasonable to a practitioner at a site. Ultimately, school-based personnel must always remember that funding comes from the government and thus is not limitless.

Categorical Funding

Special education funding is considered categorical or restricted, meaning that the dollars in the special education fund are restricted to being spent on that category of services and related costs only. General education funding is considered unrestricted because those dollars can be spent on any program in the schools. The costs of special education programs represent approximately 19.1% of total spending on elementary and secondary education in the United States (New America Foundation, 2014a). The money allocated to fund special education typically falls short of the true cost of the programs. There is an expectation applied to most state special education funding formulas that the general education fund will contribute to the cost of special education programs. Rising costs and inequitable formulas for special education programs have created the need to increasingly draw on the general fund of most local education agencies. General educators, school board members, and parents may blame special education costs for the inability of their system to provide items for the students in general education. Advocacy in this area has involved lobbying and joint efforts on the part of interested organizations, including ASHA, to encourage Congress to live up to its obligations and fund IDEA at the promised level.

Funding systems are variable across states and are in flux. As mentioned, the recession beginning in 2007 saw school districts suffer with budget cuts, yet expectations to provide services remained. Recent efforts in school funding are examining models of funding that will not devastate school funding if there is an economic downturn. ASHA's School Finance Committee is a standing committee in ASHA that keeps diligent watch on these and other issues related to school funding and finance. Information is available on School Funding Advocacy on the ASHA Web site (see www .asha.org/Advocacy/schoolfundadv/default/).

Speech–language pathologists, and other special educators, need to understand how funding systems work for their state and local entity. Providers of special education services are frequently frustrated by the seeming lack of support or funding for the programs in which they work. Questions about why staff is not added or why supplies and materials or conference budgets are tight or nonexistent frequently plague service providers. In addition, pressures may be put on speech–language pathologists by parents and other educators to provide services or equipment when the resources to do so are not available. In these instances, speech–language pathologists may find themselves caught in the middle of the unfunded mandate quandary. Solving this quandary is clearly not the responsibility of speech–language pathologists, but understanding the issues may help them deal with the questions.

Growth in Identification: Costs and Funding Issues

Special education enrollment is reported to have grown at nearly twice the rate of general education between 1980 and 2005. Historically, it was estimated that approximately 10% of the student population would be students with disabilities under IDEA, when they currently represent approximately 13% of the total population of students. There are many reasons for this, including

- greater identification of students with disabilities from birth to age 5 years, who then participate in early intervention and preschool programs; and
- inclusion of "developmentally delayed" individuals ages 3 to 9 years.

In addition to increasing enrollment, special education expenditures have increased at a faster rate than have general education expenditures, stressing local dollars. Service costs and higher cost for students with high-need disabilities are responsible for this increased spending (New America Foundation, 2014a).

Changes in Funding Systems

Federal funding for special education comes to states in a number of different types of grants. These are allocation grants, not competitive grants, meaning that the states automatically receive the funds. These grants are distributed to states, which then distribute the funds to LEAs. The grant funds are to cover various costs, such as personnel development, direct and support services to children in various age categories, administrative costs, and other related activities.

IDEA 2004 funding builds on the intentions set in the IDEA Amendments of 1997 to give greater flexibility in the use of special education funds and also to blend funds with other categorical programs, specifically Title I and other programs under ESEA. These funding changes mean that school-wide plans may be developed that assign speech–language pathologists as a part of prevention or intervention programs. Speech–language pathologists may include student peers without disabilities in groups when working in class, and joint services may be provided to students who qualify for several programs. Speech–language pathologists in schools must know and understand local restrictions and allowances because each state and LEA will interpret these new regulations in slightly different ways.

Early Intervening Services

In an effort to encourage flexibility and also to move away from the "wait to fail" model of special education identification, IDEA 2004 includes a new funding mechanism for the use of up to 15% of an LEA's allocation to develop and implement early intervening services. This provision encourages coordination with other funding structures (i.e., ESEA, Title I) to provide these services (34 C.F.R. § 300.226 [e]) but is not intended to deny or delay the provision of FAPE or an evaluation for a student who is suspected of having a disability (34 C.F.R. § 300.226 [c]). These funds are intended to be directed at students who are not currently identified under IDEA but who are "in need of additional academic and behavioral supports to succeed in the general education environment" (34 C.F.R. § 300.226). Although these services can be directed at all students in kindergarten through Grade 12, the C.F.R. calls for specific emphasis to be placed on students in kindergarten through Grade 3. For school districts where significant disproportionality has been identified (i.e., the overrepresentation of minority students in special education), early intervening services must be reserved and used to the maximum extent possible.

The activities allowed to implement coordinated early intervening services (34 C.F.R. § 300.226 [b]) include the following:

(1)   Professional development (which may be provided by entities other than LEAs) for teachers and other school staff to enable them to deliver scientifically-based academic instruction and behavioral interventions, including scientifically-based literacy instruction and, when appropriate, instruction on the use of adaptive and instructional software.

(2)   Providing educational and behavioral evaluations, services, and supports, including scientifically based literacy instruction.

The provisions for early intervening services (EIS) are where the development and use of some response to intervention (RTI) programs may be realized. This component of the law then allows speech–language pathologists and other special educators to support and work directly with students who may be struggling in general education without waiting until the students are identified through a formal assessment as meeting criteria under special education law. The language of the law emphasizes the mandate that prior to any identification for special education, students need to be provided with scientifically based instruction.

States and local districts have established guidelines for the implementation of these provisions, as there are reporting requirements under the law (34 C.F.R. § 300.226 [d]), in addition to the necessity to ensure that misuse of the provision does not occur.

EIS and the use of RTI programs are examples of the system response to implementing program and practice changes that should not only result in more immediate assistance for struggling learners but also result in financial savings. As has been illustrated, special education enrollment has climbed, significantly straining and affecting the overall system. The use of funding and resources of special education to provide interventions prior to identification is a blend of current research, policy, and fiscal solutions.

Medicaid

One way that many school districts increase available revenue to support special education programs is through Medicaid reimbursement. This program is authorized under the administration of the Centers for Medicare and Medicaid Services. The Medicaid program authorizes payment for speech–language pathology services provided in schools under IDEA Part B when the following criteria are met:

- Services are provided to Medicaid-eligible children.
- Services are medically necessary.
- Services are delivered and claimed in accordance with all other federal and state guidelines.
- Services are included in the state plan.

Under the Early and Periodic Screening, Diagnosis, and Treatment (EPSDT) program, a child health component of Medicaid, speech–language pathology and audiology services are covered for the following:

1. Identification of children with speech or language impairments
2. Diagnosis and appraisal of specific speech or language impairments
3. Referral for medical or other professional attention necessary for rehabilitation of speech or language impairment
4. Provisions of speech and language services
5. Counseling and guidance of parents, children, and teachers
6. Augmentative devices, hearing aids, and services

ASHA provides extensive information that gives guidance to school-based professionals who bill Medicaid. These resources are available to members on the ASHA Web site and include general information about the Medicaid program, both a position statement and a technical report on the "under the direction of" rule, and other information (see "Additional Resources" at the end of this chapter).

Under this program, the revenue generated through the cost of medical assistance is intended to go back to the programs that provided these services. Decisions about how this happens at the local level are made by a collaborative, as required under the program. Speech–language pathologists who participate in billing for Medicaid services should inquire about participating on the collaborative or at least ensure that there is representation of the professional group. Although some speech–language pathologists may feel that Medicaid billing is cumbersome, the funds realized would otherwise not be available to the program. Congress put this program in place, and it is important for most systems to realize the revenue available under the program.

Speech-Language Pathologists' Roles and Responsibilities

The position statement (ASHA, 2010b) "Roles and Responsibilities of Speech–Language Pathologists in Schools" can be found at www.asha.org/policy/PI2010-00317/. This statement outlines the critical roles and range of responsibilities that school-based personnel assume. These roles are all directed toward improving student outcomes. The statement asserted that *speech–language pathologists "have integral roles in education and are essential members of school faculties"* (ASHA, 2010b) and do the following:

- Work across all levels
- Serve a range of disorders
- Ensure educational relevance
- Provide unique contributions to curricula
- Highlight language and literacy
- Provide culturally competent services

The following are included in speech–language pathologists' range of responsibilities:

- Prevention
- Assessment
- Intervention
- Program design
- Data collection and analysis
- Compliance

The statement continued to define collaborative partnerships and leadership that fall within these roles and responsibilities. The authors strongly recommend that readers access this position statement, read and discuss it, and compare it to their own work setting.

Some states have guidelines that are the state department officials' interpretations of federal laws within the funding and political structure of their state and consequently are more flexible and subject to more frequent changes than federal regulations. ASHA's guidance is from a national professional organization and is not binding in any state. Local school districts, consortiums, and regional areas can also assemble such lists to guide their speech–language pathologists in a particular area. Many times, school-based speech–language pathologists and their state professional organizations will help write these lists so that they accurately reflect the professional aspects of the position that may not be known to education officers who are assigned these tasks (see "State Consultants" later in this chapter).

Lists of roles and responsibilities may cast a longer shadow in school districts than they do in health care or private practice environments because of employee unions. The conditions of work, the demands made on management on behalf of an employee, and, most importantly, the relative fairness of one employee's job responsibilities compared to another's are critical issues. Therefore, lists of assigned primary duties are important to know and follow in public education. Additional roles and duties, and who assigns them to the speech–language pathologist, are equally important.

Every work environment will place additional responsibilities on speech–language pathologists. These will vary according to an interesting set of criteria inherent in the individual school or school district and determined by school characteristics, such as the size, grade levels, ages of students, location (rural, suburban, or urban), degree of security needed, discipline codes, student transportation, teacher and staff relationships, community expectations, personal interests, and administrator's style. Speech–language pathologists have often taken on additional roles that are voluntarily, based on their personal interests (see Table 9.3), because the previous speech–language pathologist did them, because the school was shorthanded, or because everyone took on extra duties to cover the territory. It is easy to see how involved speech–language pathologists can get in their schools.

Although taking on extra activities may not appeal to every speech–language pathologist, the authors engaged in one or more events each year and found that doing so enhanced their speech and language service delivery in unexpected ways. Additional school roles can increase the visibility of speech–language pathologists school-wide, offer opportunities to observe students communicating with their peers in a generalizing environment, build staff relationships, attract administrator support, and integrate speech–language pathologists into more aspects of the school and community.

Speech–Language Pathology Assistants and Aides in Schools

Extending Service With Paraprofessionals

Professionals in many fields work with paraprofessionals who support professionals and enable them to accomplish more. Physicians work with physician assistants, attorneys

TABLE 9.3. Additional Roles and Responsibilities of School-Based Speech–Language Pathologists

• Recess duty	• Bulletin board decoration	• Club adviser
• Play director	• Dance chaperone	• Magazine sales coordinator
• Athletics coach	• Student government	
• Social committee chair	• Head Start read-aloud	• Field trip assistant
• Preschool monitor	• School accountability team	• Parent education programs
• Parent-teacher organization	• Triathlon coach	• School discipline team
• Curriculum committees	• School Web site	• School newspaper
• School yearbook	• Candy sales	• Assessment team
• Assistive technology	• Bilingual assessor	• School store
• School post office	• Internet pen pals	• After-school care
• Homework club	• Department chair	• Literacy lab
• Grant writer	• School improvement committee	• Assessment committee coordinator
• Assistant principal	• Science fair mentor	• Administrator's designee
• Principal's designee	• Morning duty	
• Bus duty		

work with paralegals, physical therapists work with physical therapy assistants, and occupational therapists assign duties to certified occupational therapy assistants. Speech–language pathologists can extend their services through the use of speech–language pathology assistants (SLPAs) and aides.

Support personnel in school speech–language programs may be called SLPAs, aides, assistants, technicians, paraprofessionals, and other related job titles. Some positions require entry-level skills; others seek applicants with advanced training, such as a postsecondary degree or a certificate to show educational accomplishments. More-skilled support personnel take a greater responsibility for the instructional program and enable speech–language pathologists to be more effective and assume some or many of the tasks necessary to implement a single-school or multisite program. Because of their training, SLPAs are able to provide therapy and monitor student progress, under the supervision of a speech–language pathologist.

Although, historically, untrained support personnel provided a valuable addition to speech and language programs, their contribution was constrained by their training and experience and the limitations placed on them by regulations of the state or district. Today, however, SLPAs and aides are regulated by the state in which they work.

ASHA's Guidelines for SLPAs and Aides

In 2013, ASHA approved a Scope of Practice document for SLPAs (ASHA, 2013b). In 2014, an Issue in Ethics for SLPAs statement was approved (ASHA, n.d.-n). These documents and ASHA Web site information on SLPAs' new service delivery models in health care and education demanded that support personnel be an integral part of the many new levels of service proposed to both reduce costs and compensate for the shortage of professionals. Paraprofessional support is vital to the provision of special education services in schools, including speech–language services.

Instructional aides, also known as speech aides, are support staff who have been trained by school-based speech–language pathologists to assist with programs. Generally, these individuals do not have training in specific areas, such as special education or speech–language pathology. Aides are able to assist with contacting parents, locating and collecting identified students, developing materials, repairing equipment, and preparing a wide range of clerical work necessary for a school-based program. Aides cannot work with students unless they are supervised, but they can be very helpful to busy speech–language pathologists. Aides may work in more than one general education or special education program and extend the activities of the speech–language pathologist to more corners of the school. In some cases, speech–language pathologists may train classroom aides to support students with their communication needs.

SLPAs, on the other hand, are persons with a minimum of an associate's degree or equivalent course of study in speech–language pathology. They work with students under the supervision of speech–language pathologists. They take course work at community colleges or universities in child development and speech–language pathology and have the recommended number of hours of field experience with a variety of communication disorders. Although a bachelor of arts or science degree in communication disorders could be used as the course work, the person would still need to take the practicum or field experience to be registered, or licensed in some states, as an assistant.

Aides and assistants can be used in school speech, language, and hearing programs if they are properly trained and appropriately supervised by a certified speech–language pathologist. Both the speech–language pathologist and assistant must follow their state licensing laws if they work in a state with licensure requirements.

SLPAs and aides can make a significant difference in how services are offered in many schools. Speech–language pathologists need to know how to design quality programs that include these assistants and aides in order to extend services to students on the caseload.

The Role of States in Regulating SLPAs

State licensing laws take precedence over ASHA guidance for the use of SLPAs. The ASHA (2013b) "Speech–Language Pathology Assistant Scope of Practice" outlined good clinical practice, responsible supervision, concern for students, and ethical conduct. Generally, ASHA guidance is considered when state laws are established.

There is wide variation in how states regulate aides and assistants in speech–language pathology. Speech–language pathologists in schools have the responsibility of knowing their state licensing regulations and ASHA's guidelines for support personnel to ensure that students receive the most effective services from qualified personnel. Most states do have supervision requirements. The *Code of Federal Regulations* requires paraprofessionals in special education programs to be trained and supervised (34 C.F.R. § 300.156 [2][iii]). This includes aides or assistants who are assigned to school districts' speech and language programs (Moore-Brown, 2001).

SLPAs' Responsibilities and Limitations

The list of responsibilities of an SLPA are found within the ASHA Scope of Practice for SLPAs (2013b). State laws may differ slightly from these guidelines in regard to the roles of SLPAs. How SLPAs are used will differ on a local or building level as well. SLPAs will be in contact with aides in the special education program who have vastly different duties. Some administrators may require greater uniformity at their schools and require that all support staff carry additional duties. SLPAs may be assigned by the principal to contribute to some of the overall activities of the school, such as the following:

* Bus or recess duty
* Field trip assignments
* Office assignments
* Health monitoring
* Fire drill assignments
* School fund-raising campaigns
* Homework correction

The primary function of SLPAs should be serving students. If schools assign SLPAs to duties that disrupt services to students on the caseload, speech–language pathologists may need to advocate for a change with the supervisor. Each SLPA's role must be managed by the supervising speech–language pathologist, with appropriate attention to other educators and administrators. The value of trained SLPAs, of course, is their knowledge of communication disorders, sensitivity to child development, and availability to continue therapy when speech–language pathologists must complete evaluations or visit another site or home. The SLPA can also maximize the use of the augmentative communication system during instruction. If SLPAs speak another language besides English or have a culture that is different from that of speech–language pathologists, they can be tremendous assets to programs. Many SLPAs represent the cultural and linguistic diversity of their communities and can be powerful extensions of the speech and language program in the community.

Both high-school and elementary speech and language programs with SLPAs can provide highly effective services, including helping students with moderate to severe disabilities who require close monitoring in the classroom.

Speech–language pathologists who use SLPAs report that it is "energizing," "more interactive during the day," "easier to reach more students," and "refreshing" and that the speech–language pathologist's role "extends into many more classrooms and increases my visibility throughout the school" (Montgomery, 2000).

School-based speech–language pathologists may need to educate their school districts, directors of special education, colleagues, and other administrators about the benefits of having SLPAs. These individuals may be unaware of the contribution SLPAs can make, as well as the way they are trained, hired, and compensated for their work in the comprehensive speech–language program. Speech–language pathologists may need to provide information on how SLPAs enhance the therapy program to parents who may be unaware of the training and skills of supervised SLPAs and may not recognize how beneficial such services can be. Speech–language pathologists need to constantly examine what all the students in a school need, how staff are attempting to meet those needs, and the possible advantages of having one or more SLPAs to improve overall productivity and educational outcomes.

The Roles and Responsibilities of Educational Audiologists

Educational audiologists serve a variety of functions within the school setting beyond the diagnosis and management of hearing loss. These professionals work as members of a team that designs an educationally appropriate program for students with hearing loss. IDEA 2004 mandates that services related to hearing conservation and hearing loss be provided in public schools.

Because educational audiologists are working as members of the multidisciplinary team for individual children and as consultants to the overall school system, their roles extend beyond that of a consulting audiologist or one who may be seeing a child through a hospital program or physician's office. While audiology services include clinical diagnostics, the Educational Audiology Association's (EAA, 2009) position statement also contended that these services include planning and delivery of (re)habilitation services and counseling. Comprehensive audiology services in schools include the following: prevention, identification, assessment, (re)habilitation, providing follow-up and monitoring, equipment and materials, administrative support, evaluation, and research.

Recommended Professional Practices for Education Audiology

The following are recommended practices for education audiology (EAA, 2009):

1. Identification of children with hearing loss, including (a) collaboration with state and local agencies, (b) development and oversight of identification programs, (c) utilization of objective screening tools, (d) assistance in training and support of individuals who conduct hearing assessment, and (e) documentation of program effectiveness
2. Determination of the range, nature, and degree of hearing loss, including referral for medical or other professional attention for the habilitation of hearing
3. Provision of habilitative activities, such as language habilitation, auditory training, speech reading (lipreading), hearing evaluation, and speech conservation, including (a) development and implementation of evidence-based guidelines for habilitation services, (b) provision of functional assessment of students and preparation of necessary documentation for qualification, (c) collaboration in development and development of Individualized Education Programs (IEPs) and Individualized Family Service Plans, (d) application of research-based protocols, and (e) provision of training of personnel and parents

4. Creation and administration of programs for prevention of hearing loss, including (a) provision of comprehensive curriculum, (b) collaboration with other school professionals, and (c) provision of resources and materials for personnel and parents

5. Counseling and guidance of children, parents, and teachers regarding hearing loss, including (a) facilitation of supportive school-based learning and social environment, (b) provision of informational and effective counseling for personnel and parents, (c) collaboration with and referral to additional school and community resources, and (d) assistance with transition and support

6. Determination and implementation of children's group and individual amplification needs, including (a) selecting and fitting an appropriate aid and evaluating the effectiveness of amplification, (b) collaborating with school personnel and manufacturers in this process, and (c) serving as a resource for methods of meeting standards of the American National Standards Institute

EAA (2002) also outlined roles and responsibilities for educational audiologists in the early detection and intervention of hearing loss. The position statement made the following assertion:

> Audiologists who are employed in school settings have an opportunity as well as the responsibility to promote the early detection and intervention of hearing loss. While the definition of audiology, according to the Individuals With Disabilities Act, includes identification of children with hearing loss, the responsibility of population-based screening activities are generally considered health initiatives rather than special education responsibilities.

The roles and responsibilities of the educational audiologist in this area are identified as follows:

1. Identification of children with hearing loss
2. Determination of the range, nature, and degree of hearing loss and communication functions
3. Referral for medical and other services necessary for the habilitation or rehabilitation of children with hearing loss
4. Provision of auditory training, speech reading training, listening device orientation and training, and other services
5. Provision of services for prevention of hearing loss
6. Determination of the need for individual amplification, inclusion selecting, fitting and dispensing appropriate listening and vibrotactile devices, and evaluating the effectiveness of those devices
7. Counseling and guidance of children, parents, and teachers regarding hearing loss

Educational audiologists are uniquely skilled to assist with several current areas of practice, which have affected how and to whom schools provide service because of technological advancements. One area is the treatment and management of children who are identified through universal newborn hearing screening, plus the management of children and students who have been implanted with cochlear devices. The mapping of these devices, as well as the auditory training that is necessary, is highly specialized treatment involving both speech–language pathologists and audiologists (EAA, 2009).

Another more recent area of practice receiving increased attention is the area of hearing conservation. ASHA's 2006 campaign "Listen to Your Buds" (see www.asha .org/buds/) is an example of consumer awareness efforts about how normal hearing can be damaged by listening to personal amplification systems, such as iPods, too loudly. Because of the noise inherent in schools due to classroom environments, bands, and the activities of students, the educational audiologist is a wonderful resource for health conservation initiatives. The EAA (2014) noted that

> consequences of NIHL [noise-induced hearing loss] in children include communication difficulties, lower academic performance, reduced productivity, social isolation, depression, and tinnitus (Dobie, 1995, as cited in Folmer, Griest, & Martin, 2002). *School-age children and young adults do not appreciate the long-term impact of noise-induced hearing loss and may find that they are denied entry into a chosen occupation, e.g., military service, law enforcement, flight school.* Therefore, the purpose of this document is to provide the resources needed to develop and implement a hearing conservation educational program for school-aged children, with the goal that these educational efforts can eventually help to reduce the prevalence of NIHL. The audiologist working in the school can facilitate the success of these programs.

Speech–language pathologists and audiologists have many frontiers for collaboration that did not exist just a few years ago. Current practice in schools finds students requiring management of cochlear implants, students who may be in need of testing for central auditory processing disorder (CAPD), students who have noise-induced hearing loss or head trauma from a concussion that causes hearing loss, students with hearing loss due to congenital anomalies or other medical conditions, and students with other hearing issues that have educational impact. These issues require both collaboration and expertise. Speech–language pathologists will be called on to take the lead on case management for these types of cases. Collaboration with the educational audiologist will be critical in designing intervention plans and educational programs that are meaningful and beneficial for students based on their unique learning needs.

Ethics

Ethical behavior is expected of all professionals. Speech–language pathologists in public schools will find themselves in situations that call on their ethical code of conduct. Any speech–language pathologist who is an ASHA member with a CCC or who is in a clinical fellowship (CF) is bound to abide by ASHA's (2010c) "Code of Ethics." State speech–

language and hearing associations also typically have a code of ethics that members are expected to uphold. Although membership in professional associations is recommended, the code of ethics should serve as a guideline for any individual who practices as a speech–language pathologist, regardless of membership in these organizations. Under the code of ethics, speech–language pathologists have a reporting responsibility if they are aware of unethical behavior on the part of a fellow professional. ASHA's Board of Ethics responds to violations that are reported against ASHA certificate holders.

Americans generally hold honesty and integrity as important values and do not anticipate situations that would compromise such values. In the everyday work world, unfortunately, situations may arise that create uncertainty regarding appropriate behavior. In more extreme situations, a speech–language pathologist may encounter people who do not behave ethically and who put the speech–language pathologist in a compromising position. In all cases, speech–language pathologists must follow federal and state regulations and laws. Consider Cooper's example given in the ASHA Ethics Roundtable (Moore-Brown, 1998) titled "When Supervisor and Supervisee Disagree" (ASHA, n.d.-g). In this case study, the speech–language pathologist made recommendations for an intervention plan in her report, and the supervisor changed the recommendations. In dealing with this type of situation, speech–language pathologists may find themselves in an ethical conflict between doing the right thing for the student and possibly compromising their employment position if questioning the supervisor presents a threat to employment.

Other situations that may arise in public schools include the following:

- A student needs a type of intervention that the speech–language pathologist does not feel competent to provide.
- A teacher or parent demands services when a student is not in need of such service.
- The speech–language pathologist believes that a student should be referred to a private speech–language pathologist for specialized treatment or evaluation services, but the school district will not pay for the referral.
- The speech–language pathologist believes that a student requires more intervention time than is available in the schedule.

If speech–language pathologists are challenged in this way, it is wise for them to seek advice from a mentor, such as another colleague or an administrator (e.g., principal, program specialist, director). Be certain that whoever is selected will keep the issue confidential. Maintaining professionalism and confidentiality in communications regarding an ethical situation are equally important. Speech–language pathologists can also contact the state department of education or regional education agency for assistance. The ASHA Web site (www.asha.org/practice/ethics/) maintains educational resources on this issue.

State and national speech–language–hearing associations are good places to turn when situations arise that provide ethical challenges. These organizations may provide guidance to those in the field regarding a variety of professional or ethical challenges, such as the following:

- Caseload size and management
- What to do when a supervisor directs an evaluation be conducted when the speech–language pathologist has screened and indicated no evaluation is necessary
- What to do when a parent demands to be present during an evaluation
- Use of new therapy techniques that are controversial

One legal and ethical challenge that often faces speech–language pathologists in schools is the issue of providing services to children outside of the school setting in a private practice situation. If a speech–language pathologist is serving a student in the school setting, it would be considered a conflict of interest to provide that same student outside services that address his or her IEP goals. The reason for this is that IDEA 2004 calls for programs and services to be provided to children through the IEP in order to provide FAPE. The parent would have recourse, through due process, to argue that the services provided outside the school should be provided or paid for by the school district. These are sticky situations, so it is recommended that speech–language pathologists avoid private practice with students who are being served in their employing school system under an IEP.

Another scenario that might present itself is a request for the speech–language pathologist to serve the student during the summer or when the student is off track in a year-round setting. Regulations pertaining to the provision of extended-year programming do not allow school districts to categorically exclude certain students from services during break periods. Therefore, while speech–language pathologists previously may have felt comfortable serving students on a fee-for-service basis during the summer or over school breaks, the new regulations make it clear that some children may be eligible for extended school year programs if the service is required for the child to receive FAPE (34 C.F.R. § 300.106). It is recommended that speech–language pathologists be very cautious about serving students in a private practice setting if they are also providing services to these students during the school year. Some school-based speech–language pathologists avoid any potential conflict by doing summer work in hospitals, skilled nursing facilities, or private practice offices that serve geriatric patients.

Ethics and ethical practice are of critical importance in the current era. Licensing requirements in some states may have mandates for some continuing education in the area of ethics. Violations of ethics, including accusations of ethical violations, can be devastating personally and professionally. In addition, licensed practitioners and those holding the ASHA CCC have a responsibility to report ethical violations to the ASHA Board of Ethics. Surprising or not, some actions could potentially be considered an ethical violation but are not necessarily illegal. Practitioners who have questions about ethical issues should seek guidance from ASHA or a fellow ASHA member who can help to guide their actions, if an action is required. Also remember that as new practice areas are established, the ethical parameters related to these emerging areas may be murky at first and need consideration. Contacting someone for guidance is always a prudent way to approach matters in question.

Professional Organizations

Professional organizations provide a needed link to current developments in the field, legislative information, and networking with others. Speech–language pathologists who work in schools have many professional organizations they can join. Speech–language pathologists typically want to affiliate with organizations that will keep them in contact with at least three aspects of their employment: (a) the discipline of speech–language pathology nationally, (b) their discipline within the state, and (c) the broader field of schools and education. In many cases, speech–language pathologists will also wish to become members of an organization for a specialty area within speech–language pathology, such as fluency, autism spectrum disorders (ASDs), or family counseling. Although there are some costs involved in maintaining one's membership dues and in attending conferences, professionals should view membership in more than one organization as a necessity, not a luxury. The following suggestions are designed to help speech–language pathologists decide which are the most appropriate organizations to join.

The National Organization:
The American Speech–Language–Hearing Association

ASHA is the primary professional, scientific, and credentialing association for the professions of speech–language pathology and audiology (www.asha.org). Speech–language pathology and audiology are known to be two professions but one discipline. ASHA represents both professions and one discipline through many avenues. ASHA is held in high regard in the scientific and service communities of education and health care and related or allied fields. According to Haynes and Johnson (2008), professional credibility is established through the following:

- Licensure and certification
- A professional association that facilitates research
- A profession that produces its own independent research
- Professional peer-reviewed journals that publish research
- Professional meetings to present research
- A code of ethics that includes research ethics
- Accreditation of training programs that expose students to research
- Continuing education requirements and keeping up with research

Professions that establish their own scientific base prevent others from directing or questioning their professional actions. Understanding the importance of all of these parameters helps speech–language pathologists understand why ASHA certification and membership are important and how they hold each member out to the professional community as an individual with connection to this professional community. Because certification and membership are separate entities in ASHA, speech–language pathologists who have a CCC need to request membership if they wish to join the organization. Membership in ASHA should be viewed as a responsibility and a privilege of school-based speech–language pathologists. Working in a school district with many other ASHA members is a distinct advantage and increases speech–language pathologists' professionalism. A school district with speech–language pathologists on staff who hold ASHA memberships will attract new professionals to complete their clinical fellowship (CF) there to take full advantage of the valuable mentoring opportunities. Many other professionals who work in school settings do not have the opportunity to hone their new skills in a nurturing CF environment their first year on the job. Related fields have adopted this model through externships for special education teachers and through state-sponsored mentor-teacher positions to enable more skilled educators to help new employees during induction.

Membership in ASHA provides access to journals, newsletters, conventions, and other continuing education offerings; special interest groups; important lobbying and political action committees; position papers and technical resources for service delivery; the latest information on a clinical population or new assessment tools; and a code of ethics to guide one's practice and decision making. The network of over 186,000 members and affiliates in speech–language pathology and audiology is a tremendous resource. The interests of each state are represented in the governing body of ASHA and in the work of national committees and task forces that influence school-based practice. Attracting school-based speech–language pathologists to ASHA committees is very important to the viability of the national organization, but it is even more important to the practice of speech–language pathology in public schools. National regulatory agencies, particularly the Office of Special Education and Rehabilitative Services (OSERS), can interact directly with ASHA on key issues. This type of access to key policy makers is nearly impossible for school district employees to get on their own. ASHA also provides its members such benefits as low-cost professional liability insurance, continuing education options to maintain a license or increase one's skills, and critical resources on professional practice.

Special interest groups (SIGs) are an important part of the organizational structure of ASHA. Divisions allow for an in-depth professional connection around a particular aspect of the profession. ASHA has the following SIGs:

1. Language Learning and Education
2. Neurophysiology and Neurogenic Speech and Language Disorders
3. Voice and Voice Disorders
4. Fluency and Fluency Disorders
5. Speech Science and Orofacial Disorders
6. Hearing and Hearing Disorders: Research and Diagnostics

7. Aural Rehabilitation and Its Instrumentation
8. Hearing Conservation and Occupational Audiology
9. Hearing and Hearing Disorders in Childhood
10. Issues in Higher Education
11. Administration and Supervision
12. Augmentative and Alternative Communication
13. Swallowing and Swallowing Disorders (Dysphagia)
14. Cultural and Linguistic Diversity
15. Gerontology
16. School-Based Issues
17. Global Issues in Communication Sciences and Related Disorders
18. Telepractice

SIG 16 was established in December 1999 as the division dedicated to school issues and service delivery. SIG 1 also addresses the language and learning aspects of students in educational settings. School-based speech–language pathologists are likely to find that belonging to one or more divisions will provide them with a strong base of information about topics specific to their needs. SIG 11's focus is administration and supervision, which is useful for school-based members who are in administrative or quasi-administrative roles. SIG 14's focus on issues related to serving individuals from culturally and linguistically diverse backgrounds can provide specialized resources for school-based personnel. Each SIG has a newsletter and a LISTSERV that provides both scholarly and practical information for practitioners in that area. SIGs also sponsor or cosponsor conferences and workshops for continuing education credits that are responsive to member needs.

ASHA's School Services division is dedicated to assisting school-based personnel. Because 55% of ASHA's membership is school based, the association is intimately familiar with issues in the schools and strives to provide resources and support for school-based professionals. Although holding a CCC is not required in many states, school-based ASHA members find the membership benefits valuable in their daily work, including legislative, professional, and practice information and networking. To establish a solid connection between ASHA and state issues, State Education Advocacy Leaders (SEALs) are appointed by state speech–language–hearing associations to work directly with ASHA on their specific state issues.

State Speech–Language–Hearing Associations

Another discipline-specific organization of interest to speech–language pathologists in schools is the state speech–language–hearing association. The District of Columbia and all states have such an organization, plus there is an organization for those who work overseas, mainly in American schools and Department of Defense Schools (DODS) for dependents in the U.S. Armed Forces. All state speech–language–hearing associations have Web sites that can be located through an Internet search, or they can be found through social media.

State associations are independent entities, not chapters of the national association. They address their members' state concerns, represent them before legislative bodies, create continuing education opportunities, and determine their own membership criteria. Nearly all state organizations have a student membership at a reduced membership rate. Many also have membership categories for SLPAs. A state organization is also discipline specific but carries much more weight than ASHA does with state governance, funding sources, higher education agencies, and state licensing bureaus. In fact, many times a state organization is the only entity that can address inequities for speech–language pathologists in a school system at the state level, because public schools are state-funded enterprises. State associations vary in size from approximately 100 to 5,000 members and have a loose relationship with ASHA as "recognized associations." The state organizations can band together at times to push for federal changes, led by the Council of State Association Presidents (CSAP).

Membership in a state association greatly helps school-based speech–language pathologists with licensing requirements, continuing education offerings, state news, and connections with a network of professionals who work under the same state regulations. Some state organizations work very closely with their state departments of education, interpreting and influencing state policy. Although membership in a state speech and hearing association is certainly not required to work in schools, this is the organization that will be advocating for state issues that will affect education, health care, and local decisions about funding and other related issues. Being part of this process is important to speech–language pathologists and their school districts. Participating in SIGs and committee work in state associations can enhance speech–language pathologists' effectiveness. Having held state association presidencies, both authors are convinced that membership in one's state association is critical for speech–language pathologists and for the profession.

Associations of Related Interests

Another association type is one reflecting general education, special education, or both. Some speech–language pathologists find that they can appreciate and be appreciated by their general education colleagues if they feel a connection with the greater education environment. Organizations that are popular choices for speech–language pathologists may be ones that either combine educational approaches or give another perspective on public schools. One of the authors of this book found that joining the National Association for the Education of Young Children (NAEYC) was like looking up from the microscope and seeing a whole laboratory for first time. The central focus of the Council for Exceptional Children (CEC) is special education in the schools. CEC, like ASHA, has divisions for special interests. The Division for Communicative Disabilities and Deafness (DCDD) provides a common network for those working with children with these issues. The International Literacy Association and the Association for Supervision and Curriculum Development (ASCD) provide great resources at a time when understanding general education curriculum and instruction is necessary. These organizations are national; however, states and regions have similar organizations on smaller scales that focus on state issues. Again, these groups have great value for speech–language pathologists because education is a state issue, and the decisions about education are made by local legislatures and school boards who listen to their constituents, not to a group that represents other states. Bigger is not necessarily better when it comes to influencing opinion makers about their personal ideas of quality.

It is important to recognize the key organizations for other school professionals even if you cannot or do not join them. A few national organizations focused on the broader view of general or special education include the National Association of Secondary School Principals (NASSP), National Association of Elementary School Principals (NAESP), and National Association of School Psychologists (NASP).

As noted earlier, some speech–language pathologists find it advantageous to join an organization that specializes in a particular disorder, approach, philosophy, or subgroup. Although special interest groups in both ASHA and state associations may have similar subgroups, these are still managed by the parent organization and have the same basic orientation and resources.

Professional organizations play an important part in the school-based speech–language pathologist becoming someone who knows the discipline within the larger context of education, plus one or two specialty areas in great depth. Membership in more than one organization allows speech–language pathologists to hone skills in one activity and use them with another, related group. The new energy that professional organizations add to the practice of speech–language pathology in schools is a great reason to join them.

Teacher Unions

Having a professional career as a speech–language pathologist in the schools means working in a specialized environment. The speech–language pathologist is an employee of the school district but is not a teacher in terms of classroom instruction. The speech–language pathologist is a related service provider who determines which students will receive speech–language services and to what extent, but typically is not an administrator. These positions exist to provide supports to students who require specialized assistance to enable them to be successful in the classroom and curriculum.

In some states, speech–language pathologists are viewed as teachers for purposes of credentialing, union membership, and salary placement. In other states, they have all of these teacher rights but are considered nonteaching employees when they apply for related credentials or mentor-teacher pay. Within states, some districts will place their speech–language pathologists on the management or support services track (i.e., nonunion) to receive additional pay but not management responsibilities.

Unions are prevalent for educators in some states and nonexistent in others. Teacher union employee groups are organized for the purpose of collective bargaining and work-related representation issues. Unions seek to cover fragmentation groups, such as nonmanagement employees, but may not always do so. Unions may have local chapters, and most are aligned nationally with either the National Education Association (NEA) or the American Federation of Teachers (AFT).

When a speech–language pathologist is hired by a school district, county agency, or regional special education unit, the local leader of the teachers' bargaining unit usually contacts the new employee to provide information on the union. If the union is a closed shop, all teaching employees—which may or may not include speech–language pathologists—must pay dues to that union. If it is an open shop, the speech–language pathologist may choose whether to join the union that bargains on behalf of the members but can select only the currently situated union. The determination of closed shop versus open shop may be done at the state level or at the local district level, depending on the state. Advantages of union membership are hotly debated, though the issue of joining is often moot for speech–language pathologists if the employing district is a closed shop union. However, they are generally well represented by unions if they bring their issues to the attention of the union's leadership. Speech–language pathologists may find, however, that they will need to educate the union leadership on the specifics of issues such as workload, salary stipends, or other issues if these are unfamiliar to the union.

At times, speech–language pathologists will bring concerns about employment conditions to the attention of ASHA or a state association and seek intervention from the professional association. When these issues are not professional issues but rather bargaining issues that must be worked out between the parties in the employment contract (i.e., the school district and its employees), then the professional association may not be able to directly assist but can provide advice. Often one district will assist colleagues in a neighboring district with contract wording or work conditions that have been successfully resolved.

Liability and Insurance

General educators and special educators may find they work within a highly litigious environment at times. Although most professionals do not expect to be involved in litigation or to have their ethics or professional behavior questioned, this does happen. Occasionally, spurious accusations are made, or, unfortunately, unprofessional conduct occurs. The vast majority of the time, if professionals conduct themselves in a professional manner, their work behavior will not be challenged. The realities of a modern society dictate, however, that speech–language pathologists in public schools be informed and take adequate precautions regarding their own professional liability. Throughout this book, the importance of documentation and using research-based practice patterns has been emphasized. These habits will serve speech–language pathologists well should they become involved in litigation. In addition, speech–language pathologists should take the steps that professionals in related fields take and carry professional liability insurance.

School-based practitioners are often concerned when they hear about due process cases, thinking that parents may sue them. In due process cases, the litigation is against the school district, not against a person who is an agent of the district. In these matters, personal liability is rarely a concern. In other matters, the only time personal liability would be in jeopardy is in instances where someone refused to provide services or committed an action that was an intentional violation of a child's civil rights. Regardless, we live in a litigious society, so carrying professional liability insurance is considered prudent and recommended by the authors.

Professional liability and related insurance has several applications in the public school setting. There are basically three aspects to the liability issue:

- Liability for one's professional conduct in assessment and treatment of students with communication disabilities
- Liability for working as an educator of children to carry out the school district's curriculum, policies, procedures, and expectancies
- Liability as a citizen to abide by the civil laws and regulations of the city, state, and country (including laws that protect against discrimination toward persons with disabilities)

In the first case, to protect oneself from a claim regarding the conduct of professional practice, the speech–language pathologist needs to purchase professional liability insurance through an ASHA-approved agency or a similar service. Union membership sometimes provides this coverage. In the second case, the school district's insurance will cover an employee who is accused of negligence or incompetence if the person has operated under the district's policies and guidelines. In the third case, the person is liable for his or her own conduct as a law-abiding citizen.

It should be noted that being accused and being liable might be two different things. In certain circumstances, the liability coverage of the school district may not be able to cover legal representation, even if the accusations are unfounded. Such is the case when criminal accusations are involved. This is one of the reasons why it is prudent to carry liability insurance. Again, no one can prevent a lawsuit from being filed, but being able to have adequate defense is very important in all situations.

After investigation, if the speech–language pathologist is found responsible for inappropriate action, reprimands can take many forms. One's certification and/or state license could be forfeited if the speech–language pathologist is found guilty of a violation of professional practice. One's job, credentials, or both could be forfeited for not properly carrying out district procedures; and one could face civil action for a violation of civil rights laws.

Because school district policies are understandably silent on many aspects of a communication intervention program and permit speech–language pathologists to make their own judgments for assessment and intervention, the wise professional should carry professional liability insurance in addition to the coverage the school district provides. The scope of practice of the speech–language pathologist is an ever-changing landscape. Speech–language pathologists who are covered by liability insurance can be reassured that they are protected when engaging in appropriate practice in the event that their practices are challenged. In general, if the speech–language pathologist is acting within his or her scope of practice, the school district will defend the action. If, however, negligence or intentional wrongdoing is found, other consequences may apply as indicated previously.

Teacher associations and unions are also very helpful with insurance arrangements or immediate assistance if allegations of wrongdoing are brought against one of their members. Assistance with insurance and liability issues may also be available from school-based colleagues, ASHA, state associations, unions, and insurance brokers. All professions have well-structured insurance plans to protect clients against workplace hazards, such as false claims against the insured, unsubstantiated terminations, costly defense actions, and unfair treatment.

Whom to Ask When You Have a Question on the Job

No matter how long someone works in the schools, he or she will frequently have questions about situations that are new and novel. The first rule of working in public schools is "Don't be afraid to ask for help!" Where to go for that help may vary depending on the nature of the question. One thing to remember is that public school staff members are generally thoughtful and helpful, because this is the nature of people drawn to working with children. As a new person, though, seek advice from someone who has the knowledge to answer your question and has the experience to help you learn the expected methods of working within your school culture.

Support Networks

Speech–language pathologists need to develop several networks to acquire the types of information they need. Table 9.4 provides helpful information on who may be able to provide specific information for speech–language pathologists working in public schools.

There are other important people who can be a resource to both beginning and veteran speech–language pathologists. Such people might include the following:

- Other speech–language pathologists and audiologists in schools
- Speech–language pathologists and audiologists in health care
- District or regional resource support staff for technology, staff development, categorical programs (e.g., Title I, bilingual education, American Indian education, school-to-work), child welfare and attendance, and research and evaluation
- Directors of curriculum and instruction
- Assistant superintendents
- Business managers
- Superintendents (depending on the issue and size of the district)
- Parent groups
- Advisory groups

TABLE 9.4. People and Places for Finding Assistance

Person	Nature of information	Type of question or request
Site level		
Secretary	Supplies, equipment, meetings, schedules, absences	• Where do I get pencils and other supplies? • Can I use the copier at the school site? • Where do I report my absences? • To whom do I report regarding changes in my schedule? • Where do I get a key for my room?
Custodian	Furniture, cleaning, supplies	• How often is my room cleaned? • Could I get another chair for this room?
Principal	Schedules, meetings, resources, books and materials, funds, families, curriculum trends	• Where is my room? • Where can I obtain curriculum material? • Who will chair the Individualized Education Program (IEP) meetings? • When do you want those meetings scheduled? • What school-wide and district meetings should I attend? • What are the special programs that I should know about?
Special education teacher	Policies and procedures for special education, service delivery models used at the site, student data, strategies for instruction	• Which students receive duplicated services? • How can we work together to provide services?
General education teacher	General education curriculum, instructional support team (IST) practices, student performance information, current instructional methodology	• How is a particular student doing in class? • What modifications or accommodations are being used? • What is the program or curricular emphasis in the classroom?
District or region level		
Secretary (special education)	Student database, forms, ordering and budget	• Who sets up the IEP meetings? • What is the process for turning in paperwork? • What data am I required to keep? • How do I order supplies?
Psychologist	Behavior and social issues, testing, program issues, eligibility questions	• Are there characteristics being demonstrated that might be considered emotional disturbance? • What is the student's performance on processing tests? • What programmatic considerations should we be making? • What if the student does not qualify?
Program specialist or manager	Assistance with student issues, referral to more restrictive environments, assistance with referrals to outside agencies, assistance with issues involving advocates or attorneys	• What is my assignment? • What is my budget? • Can I discuss suggestions for program changes with you? • Who is conducting my performance evaluation?
Program administrator (coordinator, director)	Allocations of funds and resources, assignments, assistance with student issues, due process issues, hiring, supervision, program coordination	• What is my assignment? • What is my budget? • Can I discuss suggestions for program changes with you? • Who is conducting my performance evaluation?
Regional administrator	Legal assistance, allocations of funds, assignments (in some organizations)	The same as those for the program administrator, depending on the organizational structure.

When seeking information, speech–language pathologists should know the culture of the district and understand the hierarchy for gaining information or obtaining resources. Although most people will be relatively friendly, some school districts are very sensitive about the ways that employees go about getting what they need. Although a new person should feel comfortable asking questions, he or she should be sensitive in terms of from whom and where the information is sought. Sometimes employees will be told they "do not need to know about that." In such a circumstance, speech–language pathologists should simply ask who handles the matter and find out how to work with that person.

Existing structures for problem solving will also likely be in place. Examples include department, job-alike (i.e., people with the same job titles), regional, or school site meetings. Another example of problem-solving systems is to hold lunch meetings to discuss cases, which the authors have found to be a most successful learning and team-building experience. If such a system does not exist where you work, you might set it up!

Speech–language pathologists should also go to their state and national associations for guidance on specific issues. Such organizations often have policy and practice statements that may be useful in making decisions or communicating a position to administrators, parents, or teachers. The following helpful ASHA practice management resources are available on the ASHA Web site (www.asha.org/practice/):

- *Scope of practice statements:* A list of professional activities that define the range of services offered within the professions of speech–language pathology
- *Practice portal:* A one-stop access point to resources to guide evidence-based decision making on clinical and professional issues
- *Position statements:* Statements that specify ASHA's policy and stance on a matter that is important not only to the membership but also to other outside agencies or groups
- *Practice guidelines:* A recommended set of procedures for a specific area of practice, based on research findings and current practice, that details the knowledge, skills, and/or competencies needed to effectively perform the procedures

The following box provides activities for aspiring speech–language pathologists to begin engaging in professional activities common to the work world of school-based speech–language pathologists.

Activities for Aspiring Speech-Language Pathologists

Invite an officer of your state association to class, or interview him or her on your own. Prepare questions about the role that your association plays in legislation, recruitment, and retention of school-based speech-language pathologists. Inquire whether there is a committee or a board position to represent school issues. Inquire about whether there is a student chapter or reduced student membership fee and how you can get involved.

Plan to attend the next state or national conference for speech–language and hearing professionals held in your geographic area, or plan to travel to one. Register in advance, and review an online copy of the program and note how many topics are on school-based issues. Plan to attend those sessions, especially any committee meetings or task force meetings that are open to you. Ask questions, and get to know the professionals involved in these issues in your state.

If you are a student, join or become more active in your campus National Student Speech Language Hearing Association (NSSLHA) chapter. Bring issues from this class or this book for discussion at the next meeting. Record the responses, and keep track of the certifications, regulations, and procedures in your state for the topics discussed in this chapter.

Create a personal portfolio of your continuing education and professional development activities thus far. Begin to collect documentation of conference and course attendance that is necessary to maintain your state and national certifications. Record activities that have developed your professional skills even if they are not immediately needed for minimum requirements. List professional organizations, volunteer activities with children, leadership tasks in your school, and extracurricular activities that demonstrate your knowledge and commitment to public education.

Local and Regional Supervisors

Speech–language pathologists in public schools work with a variety of individuals who serve in different supervisory positions. The person who writes the speech–language pathologist's performance evaluations may or may not have a background in speech–language pathology or even special education. However, speech–language pathologists, as much as any other professional in the system, may be promoted into general or special education administration.

Building-level staff, including speech–language pathologists, are likely to report to a principal. In some systems, the supervisor is from the special education department and may have a background from either general education or special education. There is not one particular career track for general education or special education administrators.

Many special education systems have a middle management person called a program specialist, program supervisor, or program manager. These individuals may or may not be administrators, but they have significant involvement in program development, program placement decisions, and professional development. Some also are involved in employment decisions, such as making recommendations for hiring and termination. Job performance evaluations are typically conducted by individuals who are administrators, which is why a principal often performs that function for the specialist staff. ASHA's (2014b) instrument the Performance Assessment of Contributions and Effectiveness (PACE) provides an evaluation tool for speech–language pathologists in

schools that is designed specifically to capture the roles, duties, and responsibilities of the school-based speech–language pathologist. This instrument was developed in accordance with the trend toward value-added evaluations in schools. (See the ASHA Web site on PACE at www.asha.org/Advocacy/state/Performance-Assessment-of-Contributions-and-Effectiveness/.)

Depending on the size of the district, the special education department may also have a director or coordinator who oversees the entire operation of special education in the district. This person may also have job responsibilities other than special education, such as other pupil services functions (e.g., health, psychological, counseling, student discipline, home study). The speech–language pathologist may or may not interact on a regular basis with the district-level special education administrator. If the district is large, program support staff will provide guidance. A large district or consortium of smaller districts may even have one individual who oversees only the speech–language and audiology programs. In a midsize or smaller school district, the speech–language pathologist may have regular contact with the district-level administrator.

Speech–language pathologists who have moved into supervisory and administrative roles in public schools have access to groups such as ASHA's SIG 11, Administration and Supervision, and the Council for Administrators and Supervisors of Speech, Language, and Hearing Programs (CASSLHP) to provide support and collegial interaction. Supervisors who are speech–language pathologists may need input regarding program goals, the speech–language pathologist's role, and the work of the field. When you share information with a supervisor, you will usually find it helpful to recognize that person's perspective and what is important to him or her. Speech–language pathologists will find that discussing how their expertise can promote improved reading ability and academic skills is of great interest to a principal. Principals typically place high regard on the skills and training of the speech–language pathologist who works with the students on their campus. If the principal is not knowledgeable about how the skills of the speech–language pathologist can support academic success for the students on the campus, it is those professionals' responsibility to provide such information to the principal. Once the principal learns the extent of the skills and abilities of the speech–language pathologist, a great partnership can occur that will be rewarding for all parties.

State Consultants

In the early days of special education, most state education agencies (SEAs) had consultant positions for all specialty areas (e.g., visual impairments, deaf and hard of hearing, preschool, speech–language). By the end of the 1990s, several states still had consultants with a speech–language background, but these individuals had job responsibilities that extended far beyond the field of speech–language. Such responsibilities included working with the complaints and monitoring division of the SEA, working with school reform issues, and working with Medicaid billing. Despite these other job responsibilities, today's SEA consultants connect with speech–language pathologists in the field in a variety of ways. They also connect with each other through an ASHA-related organization called the State Education Agencies Communication Disabilities Council (SEACDC). Twenty-five states have representatives to the SEACDC group. To see if your state has a representative, visit www.seacdc.org.

The responsibilities of SEACDC members include the following:

- To advise and consult with appropriate federal agencies, state agencies, and other public and private organizations and committees on philosophies, principles, practices, and needs in all areas relating to services for individuals who have language, speech, or hearing disabilities
- To formulate and recommend policies and procedures in the field of language, speech, and hearing and to disseminate them to appropriate agencies and organizations
- To establish liaisons with other organizations and associations whose primary purpose shall be to promote the provision of appropriate speech, language, and hearing services to children from birth through high school graduation or age 21 years (www.seacdc.org)

Speech–language pathologists in public schools are encouraged to contact their SEA and find out who is the consultant responsible for speech–language and hearing programs. This person can be one more valuable resource for answers and ideas (Flynn, Ireland, & Hall-Mills, 2011).

Continuing Education

School-based speech–language pathologists have a professional responsibility to maintain and update their clinical skills to meet the needs of myriad developmental levels and the ever-expanding range of disabilities presented by students. When assignments change, speech–language pathologists often need new skills or need to update previously learned skills. This might be particularly true when speech–language pathologists encounter students in secondary school for the first time or students with specialized needs, such as those with autism spectrum disorder (ASD), with cerebral palsy, needing augmentative and alternative communication or assistive technology, or perhaps with a cochlear implant. In most schools, the speech–language pathologist is the only professional who can assess and implement a plan for these students' communication needs. Much of one's graduate program in communication sciences and disorders is devoted to recognizing and serving students with these disorders, as well as identifying sources of information that the speech–language pathologist can access later to stay current with the field. Part of the allure of this profession is the steady stream of new developments in so many areas and continued expansion into new areas. School-based speech–language pathologists also play increasingly important and expanding roles in reading instruction and classroom-based services, so continuing education in these areas is essential.

Continuing education is the vehicle to assure parents and other team members that qualified providers with state or national licensure and certification remain knowledgeable and qualified. In some states, a specific number of continuing education units (CEUs) must be reported for renewing credentials, whereas others rely on professional integrity, allowing professionals to be responsible for keeping track of their attendance at professional development workshops, seminars, and courses.

ASHA policy requires 30 certification maintenance hours (CMHs) over a 3-year period. These hours can be accumulated through a variety of continuing education opportunities, including ASHA or other professional development events that offer CEUs for speech–language pathologists. Although it is not required, one simple way to keep track of CEUs earned is to join the ASHA Continuing Education Registry (see www.asha.org/certification/maintain-ccc/). This service will automatically record and maintain hours earned, so that when necessary, the member can contact ASHA and receive a printout of approved CEUs earned. Information regarding ASHA requirements, as well as state and credential requirements, is typically included on the Web sites for the licensing or credentialing agency or organization, as well as in renewal mailings. Individuals are encouraged to always maintain a professional portfolio in order to verify and document trainings attended.

State organizations for speech–language pathologists are excellent sources of continuing education through their conferences, workshops, webinars, and professional study groups. ASHA offers the broadest array of continuing education formats, including the national convention, special topic conferences, workshops, seminars, audiotapes, video conferences, webinars, journal and newsletter read-and-test situations, study groups, special interest group (SIG) perspectives, and refereed scholarly journals. Universities offer classes and courses, but enrolling may be difficult if one is not pursuing a degree. University courses can be more expensive and time-consuming than training offered by professional organizations and may not have the advanced level of information the experienced professional is seeking. Continuing education offerings by school districts, state education agencies, and extended adult education programs are often free or low cost. These offerings can provide valuable information on general education curriculum and instruction, which may be very useful because of the new IDEA 2004 requirement to work with the curriculum. These courses may also suffice for school district salary schedule advancement (a local union or school district decision in most areas), but they may not be acceptable for state licensure or mandatory CMHs for ASHA. School districts will often pay for these trainings, but not always, or there may be some budget restrictions. When this is the case, the speech–language pathologist may find it necessary or wise to pay for the session to advance his or her education.

The certificate-granting body must approve CEUs for them to be counted as professional growth hours. This circumstance could require the speech–language pathologist to take multiple classes to accommodate what several boards, panels, and certification agencies require. Some states have developed arrangements that assist in coordinating these requirements. The speech–language pathologist should keep in mind that school districts, university curriculum and instruction departments, and SEAs are the only agencies likely to offer courses that help speech–language pathologists understand general education curriculum and instruction, a requirement of IDEA 2004. Keeping informed about the state and district curriculum frameworks and standards is the responsibility of speech–language pathologists in schools and can be met with teacher education CEUs. Participating and learning alongside teachers also gives speech–language pathologists insight into the expectations for teachers and helps to create partnerships.

Important advice regarding continuing education is as follows:

- Accrue CEUs toward certification maintenance on a regular basis.
- Choose professional development training options carefully.
- Learn the state requirements for maintaining credentials.
- Learn the state requirements for maintenance of speech–language pathology licensure.
- Know what is needed to extend clinical skills in schools.
- Learn which additions to your professional portfolio are needed for staying viable in the job market.
- Learn which additions to your professional portfolio are needed to help with defending your skills and training in a due process action if necessary.
- Look for continuing education providers who have received endorsement by all the certifying agencies to which speech–language pathologists must report to keep it affordable.
- Remember, all continuing education brings added value to your knowledge and skills, although some is more immediately evident than others.

IDEA 2004 stipulates that if the speech–language pathologist or any other member of the student's educational team needs specific training to be effective with that student, the training can be written into the student's IEP (34 C.F.R. § 300.320 [a][4]). This is referred to as "supplementary aids and services, program modifications, or supports for school personnel." If a team member needs specific training to help the child with a communication disorder (e.g., sign language, applied behavior analysis [ABA] training, augmentative and alternative communication), this training can be listed as a supplementary support for school personnel in the IEP. This could provide specific training for the speech–language pathologist or might enable a paraprofessional or another team member to learn a supporting skill for the classroom. The LEA representative is present on the IEP to authorize this type of commitment of LEA resources. Another type of training that may occur and should be written into the IEP is the training that the speech–language pathologist may need to provide to teachers, paraprofessionals, or parents.

Continuing education can take many forms, but it is always an important component of the school-based professional's role. Even if continuing education is not mandated, it is a professional responsibility, as is keeping track of one's continuing education growth activities each year.

Additional Resources

The following are ASHA resources on Medicaid:

- Medicaid (www.asha.org/public/coverage/Medicaid/#_ga=1.226082206.509329459.1419034974)
- Medicaid Toolkit: Credentialing (www.asha.org/Practice/reimbursement/medicaid/Medicaid-Toolkit-Credentialing/#_ga=1.262460040.509329459.1419034974)_
- Medicaid Toolkit: Documentation for Medicaid (www.asha.org/Practice/reimbursement/medicaid/Medicaid-Toolkit-Documentation/#_ga=1.18126653.509329459.1419034974)
- Medicaid Toolkit: Medicaid State Plans (www.asha.org/Practice/reimbursement/medicaid/Medicaid-Toolkit-State-Plans/#_ga=1.224705182.509329459.1419034974)
- Medicaid Reimbursement in Schools, including links to the following documents (www.asha.org/SLP/schools/prof-consult/medicaid/#_ga=1.19501756.509329459.1419034974):
  - Medicaid Guidance for Speech–Language Pathology Services: Addressing the "Under the Direction of" Rule: Guidelines 2005
  - Medicaid Guidance for Speech–Language Pathology Services: Addressing the "Under the Direction of" Rule: Knowledge and Skills 2005
  - Medicaid Guidance for Speech–Language Pathology Services: Addressing the "Under the Direction of" Rule: Technical Report 2004
  - Medicaid Guidance for Speech–Language Pathology Services: Addressing the "Under the Direction of" Rule: Position Statement 2004
- School-Based Medicaid Services (www.asha.org/practice/reimbursement/medicaid/SchoolBasedServicesAUD/#_ga=1.221032732.509329459.1419034974)
- Medicaid Payment for School-Based Services (www.asha.org/Practice/reimbursement/medicaid/school-based_services/#_ga=1.32037306.509329459.1419034974)

Explanation of the State Education Advocacy Leaders (SEALs) program and the names of the SEALs for each state can be found on the ASHA Web site (www.asha.org/advocacy/state/seals/).

Information about the Council of State Speech–Language–Hearing Association Presidents is available on its Web site (www.csap.org).

ASHA has mandatory continuing education requirements for all holders of the Certificate of Clinical Competence to maintain their certification (www.asha.org/certification/maintain-ccc/).

The Enhanced Future for School-Based Speech–Language Pathologists

In This Chapter

This chapter considers the influences shaping the future work world of speech–language pathologists. Trends and forces affecting the future are presented and discussed in terms of their impact on speech–language services in the educational setting. The trends and impact on service are part of broader influences that affect society, the professions of speech–language pathology and audiology, and all aspects of the educational system. The 21st-century skills that students need are revisited as evidence of the challenge for the educational system. Trends in classroom instruction, support services, and speech and language services are all reactions to the need to prepare today's students with disabilities to enter into the work world with these advanced skills and be able to successfully compete. Four areas influencing the change are access to the curriculum, professional shortages, legislative mandates, and research to practice. The chapter concludes with predictions of expanded scope of practice and professionalism of speech–language pathologists and audiologists in schools.

Chapter Questions

1. Consider the traditional practice models and beliefs and the new practices models and beliefs, and discuss which practices you have observed in your own school or a school where you have been involved. Also discuss what the responses of the speech–language pathologists and audiologists working in the school have been to these transitions.
2. Examine the 10 issues identified by the Council for Exceptional Children as those that most seriously affect its membership of special education teachers. How do these issues affect speech–language pathologists in schools?
3. Review the 21st-century skills needed by students, and discuss how your school, or a school you know, is involved in developing these skills in students. How do these programs affect students on the speech and language caseload?

4. Match the trends in classroom instruction, support services, and speech and language services to recommended practices for intervention discussed in Chapters 5, 6, and 7.
5. Discuss why change moves slowly in schools and what strategies are recommended to deal with change. Give an example.
6. How will persistent vacancies of speech-language pathologists affect the field in the next 5 years?
7. Conduct an Internet search on three of the predicted trends for expanded practice and professionalism. How do you see these trends affecting your own personal career?

Foundations for Envisioning the Future

Educational systems throughout the United States have experienced unprecedented change throughout the first two decades of the 21st century. The impact of the requirements of the Elementary and Secondary Education Act (ESEA) and the Individuals With Disabilities Education Improvement Act of 2004 (IDEA 2004) has been greater than simply adding new forms or procedures to schools and educational agencies. A backward glance at the system changes undertaken since the passage of these laws gives perspective to the profound changes that education is experiencing. Although this reflection may seem unnecessary to those new to the professions, we believe that this historical grounding is important, as we launched sea changes in schools that are still evolving. Speech–language pathologists who work in schools have experienced changes in policy, procedures, roles, responsibilities, and practice. Looking backward gives a perspective of how far we have come. Looking forward gives insight into how far we want to go.

The work of speech–language pathologists in the educational system provides essential communication links to students whose needs range from the struggling reader with literacy challenges to a student with a high-tech augmentative communication device designed to compensate for his or her lack of usable speech. The expertise needed by these professionals will directly determine how successful the student will be in his or her educational experience. Over the course of the history of special education, the roles of education professionals and specialists have evolved and changed along with political, legislative, social, and research influences. As we look to the future, the challenges facing the education system are significant. But within these challenges are opportunities for developing new methods of facing old problems and overcoming barriers that have been systemic and, unfortunately, sometimes even harmful to children.

Although new programs and mandates can sometimes feel personal, as individuals are asked to change how they do their jobs, educational reforms must always be considered within the broader context. One old adage that serves well in this context is to "think globally but act locally."

Beliefs and Actions: Thinking About Teaching and Learning

Special education services are extensions of the general education program. Too often in daily practice, the intentions of special education are forgotten: Special education is provided to help students benefit from their general education instruction; related services, such as speech–language services, are provided to help students benefit from their special education. Examining the daily and big-picture issues of the educational system is necessary for speech–language pathologists to know how to approach their work in the public schools. This includes understanding the belief systems on which legislative policy, research, and practice are built. Special education and general education programs are not separate; they are interconnected, especially now. What happens in one program directly influences and affects the other. Table 10.1 illustrates the beliefs and actions under an old model and those in the new model being advocated.

It is because of the evolution of new model beliefs and actions that some of the practices of the past are being eliminated, such as dual funding systems, the discrepancy model, and the one-way trajectory of special education referral and assessment. Special education services and personnel practices are changing to reflect updated thinking in the field. Once a belief system changes, old practices do not fit anymore. An example of how such change occurs can most dramatically be seen in the growth of Multi-Tiered System of Supports (MTSS) models throughout the country (see Chapter 3).

Future Forces Affecting Education

One of the most humbling aspects of working in schools is the realization of how our work affects students' futures. The question "Where will this student be when he or she is my age?" is always provocative. Considering "What type of work will this student be doing when he or she is 20, 30, 40, and 50?" might lead us to realize that the type of job the student might have might not even exist now. Think of all of the jobs that exist currently that did not exist even 2 years prior. It is this reality—the reality of a rapidly changing world—that is influencing changes in delivery models and expectations for students and educators. It is this reality that mandates our need to move from an Industrial Age of education to create learning systems that will better prepare students for their future in a world that does not currently exist. The Common Core State Standards (see Chapters 3, 4, 5) have attempted to lay a foundation for teaching and learning so that students can compete in a global economy and, indeed, thrive in that world. Even while old models of teaching and learning are evident in schools across the United States, economies, institutions, and societal structures are evolving, which will affect education (KnowledgeWorks, 2015). Why is such a discussion important to the work of speech–language pathologists? If you think about how health-care redesign is happening, then consider these forces in education.

The evolution from an educational system built on the current paradigm from the Industrial Age worldview to a learner-centered paradigm based in a Networked Age

TABLE 10.1. Comparisons of Old Models and New Models in Special Education Services

Old model beliefs	Old model actions
• Students are somehow different internally and instructionally. • Students with disabilities are not capable of learning higher level concepts. • Programs for students with disabilities should be separate from general education.	• Assessment searched for within-learner deficits. • Tasks in intervention worked on processes rather than content. • Provided students with watered-down curricula that does not include challenging content. • Did not expect students to succeed academically, socially, or vocationally, so there was no need to provide those opportunities (low expectations). • There were separate funding systems. • There was separate service delivery (e.g., pull-out, separate classes).
New model beliefs	**New model actions**
• All students need good solid core instruction; students who are struggling need more. • All students should master standards and grade-level curricula. • Have high expectations for all learners, including students with disabilities, English Learners, and those from minority and low-socioeconomic backgrounds.	• Assessment guides how the environment should be changed to support the learner (i.e., materials, delivery of service, instructional supports, intensity of instruction). • Tasks in intervention work on learning the material of the classroom. • Special education services should be designed to support students within the general education classroom where the core instruction occurs. • Funding should be blended to support student needs; up to 15% of IDEA funds can and should be spent on prereferral activities.

worldview calls for a learning system that will significantly change the way education occurs, focusing on personalized learning through technology and project-based learning. The previously discussed skills of communication and collaboration are essential to this learning system. In some ways, this personalization should seem familiar to speech–language pathologists and others who have supported students through Individualized Education Programs (IEPs) for several decades. As has been discussed throughout this text, the separation of general education and special education is an old-model way of operating. What if the overall system of education was transformed to be learnercentric? In fact, some aspects of this type of teaching and learning are already present in our schools. (See "A Transformational Vision of Education in the U.S." at http://education-reimagined.org/wp-contentuploads/2015/10/A-Transformational-Vision-for-Education- in-the-US-2015-09.pdf.)

Understanding that the pace of change is unrelenting, KnowledgeWorks's (2015) "Forecast 4.0" suggested a future that will be built on an *expanding ecosystem of learning*, *personalized learning*, and *new relationships with organizations*. Artificial intelligence, robotics, digital instruction, and neuroscience will be some of the influences on the future educational system.

ASHA's "Strategic Pathway to Excellence" (ASHA, n.d.-k) is built on an adapted model of Run, Grow, and Transform. ASHA includes initiatives that focus on accomplishing the Association's Strategic Objectives and embody revolutionary change within the profession or professions within the Transform level (www.asha.org/uploadedFiles/ASHA-Strategic-Pathway-to-Excellence.pdf). Examining the strategic objectives of ASHA provides a glimpse into where our professional association and its board of directors believe our professions are heading in the future. These objectives include the following:

- *Objective 1:* Expand data available for quality improvement and demonstration of value
- *Objective 2:* Advance interprofessional education and interprofessional collaborative practice (IPE/IPP)
- *Objective 3:* Enhance the generation, publication, knowledge translation, and implementation of clinical research
- *Objective 4:* Enhance service delivery across the continuum of care to increase value and access to services
- *Objective 5:* Increase the influence and demonstrated value of audiology and speech–language pathology services
- *Objective 6:* Increase the diversity of the membership
- *Objective 7:* Enhance international engagement
- *Objective 8:* Increase members' cultural competence

By examining the strategic goals of the association, speech–language pathologists can anticipate professional trends that will evolve within the transformational trends influencing educational learning systems.

Focus From the Curriculum Side

The focus on accountability and student outcomes has affected teaching and learning in both general education and special education. The implementation of the Common Core State Standards has led to widespread professional development so that teachers learn new methods of instruction. How teachers present information and how they assess and measure student learning are the center of professional development and discussions in professional learning community (PLC) meetings in every school in our nation. Schools also focus on all learners, with a great diversity of learning needs and challenges. As such, curriculum and instruction focuses on instructional approaches that accommodate all of these learners.

The Association for Supervision and Curriculum Development (ASCD) continues to be a leader in advancing effective practices for teaching and learning. The ASCD's work has been consistent with the national directions discussed: a focus on all learners, instruction for English Learners, and instruction related to the Common Core State Standards. Additional topics that are seen in ASCD publications and conferences include topics that focus on equity, differentiated instruction, academic vocabulary, mobile learning, and teaching and learning in the 21st century. ASCD's publications reflect a focus on the importance of teaching academic language and using differentiated instruction and universal design, as well as curriculum and thinking maps, instructional creativity, and interprofessional education, to address the needs of all students, particularly English Learners and other struggling learners. These initiatives, coming from the leaders in general education curriculum, are significant for those who work with students with disabilities and other struggling learners. These efforts reflect the melding of the interests of general and special education. The purpose of special education and related services, specifically the writing of goals based on the Common Core State Standards, will continue to evolve. The new era of accountability also, finally, includes standards for students who require alternate achievement standards. Expectations of inclusive education will include academic expectations for our most challenged learners. The conversations surrounding common core are not limited to students in general education but also include students with significant disabilities. The PLCs in schools and professional development that occur around these topics should be attended by speech–language pathologists, who can bring their lens on language and knowledge of language and learning to the rich discussions at such meetings. In addition, these venues allow for others to learn about the speech–language pathologist's expertise and how collaboration will be beneficial for improved student outcomes.

Advancement in the achievement of students with disabilities calls for a revamping of our organizational structures to affect curriculum and instruction and educational access. Calls for a "unified and coherent system of education" (Statewide Special Education Task Force, 2015; Thurlow, 2015) decry separating educational systems and advancing "a culture of collaboration and coordination" (Thurlow, 2015). The issues that are being discussed in the professional literature of curriculum and reading are important to review for several reasons. Not only can speech–language pathologists and other special educators learn from the advances in various disciplines, but this knowledge can also provide a common ground for all professionals as they search for effective interventions for students who struggle in these areas. This could have implications for the types of interventions used with students but could also affect whether students are ultimately referred for a special education assessment.

From the Special Education Side

Throughout this text, issues affecting special education, speech–language pathologists, and education in general have been discussed. Both in health care and in education, dramatic changes to systems of service delivery and funding are occurring. Accordingly, providing services to students with disabilities is an ever-evolving area of focus and practice. Chapter 1 discussed waves of reform. We continue to feel these waves in constant motion, as the issues that needed to be addressed still face us, including issues of inclusion, funding, discrimination, and evidence-based practices. What must be different in the era of common core and Digital Age technology is practice and delivery of services in an evidenced-based and inclusive environment. The tensions between general education and special education are real, as struggles for resources and instructional time face teachers and administrators. Struggles between the need for specialization and the need to ensure full access are practice area challenges that often tax the professionals who are trying to meet students' needs in the manner in which they have been trained. Accountability, serving the whole child (including families), paperwork, procedures, and evidence-based practices are but a few of the issues that special education shares with general education. In addition, big system issues of inclusiveness, positive behavioral supports, and funding are now joined by concerns related to mental health and serving the needs of an increasingly diverse student population. The education system has often turned to special education to solve these issues, but now we know that serving as "one coherent system" (Statewide Special Education Task Force, 2015) is likely the only way to address broad system needs.

All of these issues lay the foundation from which speech–language pathologists can view the future. We must not believe that we can operate independently or in a separate silo or room. We must link our thoughts and actions with colleagues in both general education and special education. By "thinking globally but acting locally," speech–language pathologists will be well positioned to consider additional information about services.

Educational Services in the 21st Century

In 21st-century schools, job duties are overlapping and synergistic with other colleagues, including psychologists, other therapists, classroom teachers, and even administrators. Collaboration, consulting, and networking are critical skills to have and develop as we work with other professionals. Training programs for speech–language pathologists and related services providers, including medical professionals, are being trained in models of interprofessional education and interprofessional collaborative practice (IPE/IPP). Funding models in health care are reflecting patient outcomes supported by an interprofessional team. Although education change is not driven by funding changes, the new focus on results driven accountability (see Chapter 2) means creating access to the general education curriculum, changing the methods that are used in delivering educational services. Former silo models of service delivery must be abandoned to bring all resources to bear in supporting student learning. In schools, speech–language pathologists will find their "value-added" role by supporting students in the curriculum. Speech–language pathologists and other special educators will increasingly be spending their time working in prevention activities with nonidentified students and in general education classrooms with identified students.

In the integrated world of educational services, frameworks of multitiered systems of supports will find speech–language pathologists and other specialists more involved with prereferral data collection and planning. This will affect how and when to conduct psychoeducational and/or speech and language assessments. The referral process will take on a whole new purpose. Defined questions regarding specific assessment issues will drive the data collection. In a world of classrooms operating with universal design for learning (UDL), student learning will need to be evaluated, questioning both the skill level of the student and the optimal learning environment needed for student learning. Assessment will need to reflect an academic focus in order to reflect the economic purpose of school. Assessment will be more dynamic and will need to reflect students' performance on standards, which is the currency of schools.

Twenty-First Century Skills

The 21st-century skills needed by students to thrive in a digital economy were identified in Chapter 1 as (a) Digital Age literacy, (b) inventive thinking, (c) effective communication, and (d) high productivity (North Central Regional Educational Laboratory and the Metiri Group, 2003).

If we take a look at this set of skills, we will agree that they represent what is necessary for future workers to be successful. Take a moment, however, and compare these skills to the old model beliefs discussed earlier in this chapter, where students with disabilities were removed from learning advanced skills because of how the service delivery models were operationalized. If educators are to ensure that students with disabilities and other struggling and at-risk learners are to develop Digital Age literacy, inventive thinking, effective communication, and high-productivity skills, then every opportunity must be afforded them, including the development of an educational system that has high expectations for these learners and ensures opportunities to develop these skills. For some challenged learners, their path to skill development may take new and different forms of experiences. That is the new job of special education. These skills should be discussed as part of transition planning for students aged 16 years and older, but work on the development of these skills should begin in elementary school.

Trends in Students Previously Unseen or Unserved

As the Every Student Succeeds Act (ESSA) and IDEA 2004 called for educators to improve student achievement for all students, each discipline reacts accordingly and will "meet in the middle" in its work. As we consider this, think about the examples of new student populations that speech–language pathologists are also serving.

There is a current trend to look critically at mild head injury and concussion in student athletes in a more comprehensive and achievement-related way. One in 10 student athletes sustains a behavior-modifying concussion every sports season (Kennedy, 2017). Some of these are short-term (3–5 week) disruptions in their learning. Some are long-term (a year or longer) interference with memory, comprehension, executive functioning, organizing, and learning in high school. In both cases, teachers are ill prepared to understand signs of head injury and often mistake them for obstinate or aggressive behavior, while coaches want their athletes back on the field, and students want to recover quickly. No one wants to test this student athlete for possible special education services, yet that may be the optimum type of support needed for the short or long term. Speech–language pathologists in schools are the most appropriate professionals to serve these youngsters, and some are now being taught to provide coaching exercises to support these students within the general education curriculum (Kennedy, 2017). Soon, we will be learning more about our role in schools expanding to include general education students recovering from sports-related head injuries, as well as our role in preventing that third, frequently more destructive, concussion.

Other students who have not always been well served in our schools are students with high-level autism. These students require specialists and general education teachers to be knowledgeable about their specific needs so they can successfully participate in general education classes. To do so, school teams must provide the necessary supports and systems to deal with anxiety and ensure that structures are in place for the student. School teams designed to understand and design systems of support can ensure the students' success. The speech–language pathologist may need to take the lead in these cases. These students can be successful in schools, but they need something different from a self-contained classroom. They need supports and strategies integrated into their general education program.

Heightened concerns about students with emotional, behavioral, and mental health issues have come to the forefront of American schools and the public. Again, clashes of discipline systems and conflicts in health care and in the engagement between administrators and families to support the needs of these students have created new tensions for the educational system.

One other group worthy of consideration includes students from foreign lands, some of whom come to the United States as refugees, and some of whom come to seek services that are unavailable in their homeland. Under the laws of the United States, all children must be served. Speech–language pathologists may be accustomed to working with long-term English Learners, yet assessing a student who is high school age but has never received any educational services and is now in the United States may require that the speech–language pathologist have a whole different set of skills and understanding and, certainly, cultural competence.

These newly identified groups will continue to tax and expand the skills of speech–language pathologists in schools. But rather than being overwhelmed, speech–language pathologists should think of the opportunities to serve these students and create learning environments that will address their needs.

Testing and Accountability

With the advent of the Common Core State Standards also came a new statewide testing system. The days of excluding students with disabilities from state assessment have been gone for nearly 20 years. The new assessment design is computer adaptive testing (CAT), which is defined as follows on the Smarter Balanced Web site:

> Based on student responses, the computer program adjusts the difficulty of questions throughout the assessment. For example, a student who answers a

question correctly will receive a more challenging item, while an incorrect answer generates an easier question. By adapting to the student as the assessment is taking place, these assessments present an individually tailored set of questions to each student and can quickly identify which skills students have mastered. This approach represents a significant improvement over traditional paper-and-pencil assessments used in many states today, providing more accurate scores for all students across the full range of the achievement continuum. (Smarter Balanced Assessment Consortium, 2016)

This new next-generation assessment system is designed to go beyond paper-and-pencil tests and move to assessing critical thinking through performance tasks and include both formative and summative assessments. What is of critical importance is that speech–language pathologists understand and experience these assessments so that they can help their students and ensure that students have the kinds of learning experiences that will be a part of the assessments that the students take.

Resources and Funding

With advances in educational and medical technology, costs will continue to rise in special education. Currently, local districts and general education funds are needed to subsidize special education at increasingly high levels. This reality creates tension between program administrators and other personnel who are required to manage budgets in the school district. The funding system for special education needs to be overhauled, but in the meantime, cost overages will be blamed on service providers and administrators. The reality is that the program is underfunded. New approaches to special education funding are desperately needed and should be developed at the local and state levels. At the national level, there continues to be bipartisan rhetoric in support of full funding for special education, but in reality, it has never been close. The funding formulas for special education and the levels of actual real dollars need to be tackled, and new solutions need to be generated in the near future. In some states, such as California, new funding models are being used in general education to channel resources to the neediest groups (e.g., foster students, English Learners, low-socioeconomic students), but special education formulas remain unchanged, although dramatic changes are being proposed as of the writing of this text. Recommendations for fiscal changes on a national level can be seen in the Council for Exceptional Children's (2016) report "Federal Outlook for Exceptional Children: Fiscal Year 2016."

Scope of Practice for Speech–Language Pathologists in Education and Health-Care Settings

In 2017, a new and more comprehensive scope of practice for speech–language pathologists in both health care and education was adopted by ASHA. Regulatory agencies and health-care consortiums are strongly urging all certified and licensed professionals to restructure their documents to support intentionally overlapping scopes of practice. The ASHA scope of practice highlights the safe and effective provision of services to all persons with communication disorders. This will affect school-based speech–language pathologists in a number of different ways. Although school systems do not require speech–language pathologists to have ASHA certification to work in educational environments, there will be fewer differences between health-care services and school services. The safe and effective wording supports greater amounts of interprofessional services and increased use of paraprofessionals and support personnel to ensure that less costly ways of providing services are explored as viable alternatives to fully credentialed professionals working in schools. This may be jarring at first, but it is likely to take hold rather quickly in light of the continuing shortage of speech–language pathologists. A new phrase will be heard: "Speech–language pathologists need to work at the top of their license in today's schools." We will be providing direct therapy when only we can provide it. This will ensure that our client and student services are safe and effective. When speech and language services can be safely and effectively provided by others under our supervision, then we will be providing educational or medical services independently or under the supervision of another professional (e.g., video fluoroscopy, scoping, case management, applied behavioral analysis [ABA], concussion monitoring, auditory verbal therapy, mental health protocols). This changes the landscape.

Charting the Next 25 Years of Progress

The next 25 years of the 21st century will provide us an opportunity to ensure that educational improvements for all children include infants, children, and youth with disabilities. "ASHA's Envisioned Future: 2025" defined a vision of what the association will be in 2025, and that gives us a glimpse of what our field anticipates in health care and education (see this document at www.asha.org/About/ASHAs-Envisioned-Future/). Notably, this future deals with a continuum of service providers within the disciplines, interprofessional practice, inclusive service delivery, and evidence-based practices.

To build toward this future, IDEA must expand on its previous support for equality of access and continue to expand and strengthen its support for quality programs and services. Improving educational outcomes for children with disabilities requires a continued focus on the full implementation of IDEA to ensure that each student's educational placement and services are determined on an individual basis, according to the unique needs of each child, and are provided in the least restrictive environment. As results-driven accountability (see Chapter 2) is established, a paradigm shift in service delivery will be realized (Crowley, Washington, & El-Sawaf, 2015). The focus must be on teaching and learning that use individualized approaches to accessing the general education curriculum and that support learning and high achievement for all. In fact, this focus on individualized learning has now expanded to general education and is known as *personalized learning* (ASCD, 2016).

We know that there is no easy or quick fix to the challenges of educating children with disabilities, including communication disabilities. However, we also know that IDEA has been a primary catalyst for the progress we have witnessed. Because of federal leadership, the people of the United States better appreciate the fact that each citizen, including individuals with disabilities, has a right to participate in and contribute meaningfully to society. With continued federal, state, and local partnerships, the nation will similarly demonstrate that improving educational results for children with disabilities and their families is critical to empowering all citizens to maximize their employment, self-sufficiency, and independence in every state and locality across the country. Further, our nation's ability to compete successfully in the global community depends on the inclusion of all citizens. We cannot afford to leave anyone out of our efforts.

Our Predicted Future: Speech-Language Pathologists in Public Schools

The theme throughout this book should be celebrated: The changes that will affect speech–language pathologists working in public schools are the changes that will affect everyone else in public education. To examine the predicted future, four areas should be considered: system, professional, legislative, and research to practice.

System

The educational system is changing rapidly and consistently. Michael Fullan (2001), the foremost authority on change in the educational system, offered these thoughts on educational change:

> Change is a double-edged sword. Its relentless pace these days runs us off our feet. Yet when things are unsettled, we can find new ways to move ahead and to create breakthroughs not possible in stagnant societies. (p. 1)
>
> Remember that a culture of change consists of great rapidity and nonlinearity on the one hand and equally great potential for creative breakthroughs on the other. The paradox is that transformation would not be possible without accompanying messiness. (p. 31)

Although acknowledging that change is a part of life and that conditions change constantly, schools and the organizational institutions that support the schools are slow to embrace new ways. However, the rapid acceleration and necessary response to mandates and problems is not going to slow down anytime soon. The world we live in, and, more important, the world the students will live in, defies stagnancy. Think about the world our students will live in when they are your age—whatever age you are. We cannot afford to not think about them in a world that is globalized, personalized, technology driven, and constantly changing. So, we must update our skills and knowledge and how we do our work constantly so they can be successful in that future.

So Why Change?

Change is necessary to address the pressures, challenges, and needs in the educational system. In responding to change, individuals will be asked to reexamine their roles and how they can contribute to this improvement. New ideas and new ways of approaching emerging issues will present themselves. One example is looking to system supports rather than within student deficits when a student has difficulty in the classroom. Another example is helping students through an RTI model rather than referring for assessment, identifying that student as disabled, and putting the student in a pull-out special education program. A third example is continuing to work on keeping students in the general education classroom so they can receive the core content curriculum by the curriculum experts: general education teachers. Each of these ideas, and many others in this book, are new and are the system's response to the need for change. As the system works through the development of the approaches, it may be, as Fullan (2001) suggested, "messy," but that is what needs to happen to develop better processes to address students' needs. The authors of this book see this context as a prime opportunity for speech–language pathologists to be part of shaping the future.

Professional Shortages

The most significant professional issue that continues to face speech–language pathologists into the next decade will be the consequences of shortages, including doctoral shortages. Persistent vacancies have been reported for many years, and this hardship is becoming more acute. (See Chapter 9 for further discussion.) As we look to the future, again we suggest to "think globally but act locally." The authors and others believe that some of the "big ideas" to be addressed include the following:

1. There is a significant need to increase the supply of speech–language pathologists, especially in high-need areas. High-need areas can be geographic (inner-city, rural, sparsely populated regions [the West]), socioeconomic (poverty areas, culturally diverse), or treatment (autism, augmentative and alternative communication, adolescent services).

2. A change is needed in training institution models so as to accommodate students and potential students who need to support themselves economically while studying communication disorders. We are gradually seeing new models of training. Examples of innovative models include night and evening classes, online courses, and school-based clinic experiences. Interprofessional education also continues to be part of the change in training programs in communication sciences and disorders.

3. Employers need to do everything they can to retain their current speech–language pathologists, including examining compensation and benefit packages, working conditions, and other workplace issues.

4. States and local entities need to work together in ongoing and sustained efforts, including working with other stakeholders to address the systemic issues that have contributed to the shortage and blocked efforts to change the situation.

5. Partnerships with human resources personnel, teachers' unions, and school boards are critical if we are to solve the problem.

6. There should be no separation between efforts to address the shortage in schools and efforts to address health care or other settings.

7. Service delivery models need to be examined on an ongoing basis to ensure that services are being provided in the most efficient manner.

8. Expand the use of speech–language pathology assistants (SLPAs) to provide clinical services through trained paraprofessionals when appropriate. Speech–language pathologists should strive to work at the top of their license.

9. Closely examine opportunities within educational reform to create roles for speech–language pathologists that will streamline their work while capitalizing on their expertise. Again there is the concept of providing supervision to others who can safely and effectively carry out some portions of our current jobs.

10. Examine funding resources for building new programs and attracting and retaining skilled staff.

Roles and Responsibilities

ASHA's (2010a, 2010b) documents on the "Roles and Responsibilities of School-Based Professionals" has contributed to the body of professional guidance on school positions from our national association. Included in these are documents on literacy, response to intervention (RTI), early intervention, attention-deficit disorder, autism spectrum disorders (ASDs), cognitive impairments, audiological screening and services to infants and toddlers, augmentative and alternative communication (AAC), and services to children who are deaf or hard of hearing. ASHA's Evidence Maps (see www.asha.org/Evidence-Maps/) provide clinical evidence needed for a variety of areas.

In addition to the professional documents in the field on roles and responsibilities, legislative requirements will lead to emerging and evolving roles for speech–language pathologists. The area of RTI has been mentioned throughout this text, and this area of practice has been led in many districts by speech–language pathologists who have taken leadership roles to guide system change in their places of employment. In addition, the advent of the common core has provided speech–language pathologists with areas to expand their influence, including helping teachers with the implementation of speaking and listening standards, providing assistance for requirements in mathematics for explaining thoughts and problem solving, and considering the use of questioning as a teaching technique.

Speech–language pathologists will increase their scope of practice and their service delivery models by expanding their influence as consultants and also as developers of "extenders"—those who can support and provide opportunities for learning to students with communication disabilities.

Because of the expansive training and knowledge base that speech–language pathologists bring to the educational work setting, they are often leaders in assuming new roles. Bridging into curriculum issues, for example, is a natural for speech–language pathologists who have expertise in language and can easily conduct task analyses for differentiating instruction for struggling learners. At the same time, some speech–language pathologists feel that their duty is to the "identified" students on their caseloads. In a world of RTI and inclusive settings, speech–language pathologists in particular will continue to expand and redefine their roles.

When taking on new roles, however, speech–language pathologists will find it equally important to evaluate, on an ongoing basis, existing duties and responsibilities to see which are no longer of value to the system or the students. New roles and responsibilities emerge to address needs presented in the system. This also means that some skill sets and actions either will no longer be needed or will need to be reshaped. Sometimes, trying to hang on to all of the old ways of doing things while adding on new responsibilities creates an untenable working situation for the professional. As we grow, we also will need to let go.

The ASHA workload model (ASHA, 2002a, 2002b) continues to be integrated into the speech–language pathologist's work in schools. The workload approach has also gained popularity in other special education arenas, as it makes sense to consider all the duties one has to complete, not just how many students are identified on a caseload. Managing and recognizing all of the duties and responsibilities of the speech–language pathologist works well under the workload model. This method will continue to receive attention and acceptance, even as psychologists, administrators, and others apply the principles of this approach to their own workloads.

Legislative

This text is replete with the history of legislative efforts to ensure that children from all walks of life and circumstances are afforded an opportunity to receive an education. Our nation's belief that education is the key to sustaining our position as a world leader is the foundation of all legislative and judicial decisions in this area. The legislative battles have involved movements that support children who are members of a protected class, as well as those who are not from privileged backgrounds. While the movement to CCSS and the previous iterations of IDEA and ESEA have guided our nation toward a more centered approach to education, the future approach is less certain. ESSA sends more decision making back to the states in terms of accountability decisions and standards. The current administration supports less federal involvement—again, recommending movement of decision making and funding back to states. Even while these trends are seen, the courts are taking stronger action to solidify mandates and expectations, as in the *Endrew F* ruling.

The reauthorization of IDEA is long overdue but may continue to be delayed, especially in an uncertain environment around federal involvement. School districts across the nation have seen the growth of charter schools in their communities, often feeling like these models take away funding and support from public education. Vouchers and school choice have not previously received support at the federal level, but this may be changing. What federal support for vouchers means for students with disabilities, and those who provide services to them, is yet to be seen and will develop over the next 10 years. What is clear is that trends for options other than traditional schools have a stronghold in the United States.

Watching and listening to the arguments of those who are critical of public education are wise activities for those who work in schools. Being a watchdog for legislative changes that may challenge the rights of children and their families is a worthwhile habit. The converging demands of parents and attorneys, legislative mandates, and judicial directives create a dynamic environment requiring vigilance, active participation, and advocacy.

Research to Practice

The heart of the future work of speech–language pathologists in schools is definitely in developing a greater sophistication with curriculum, assessment, and prereferral interventions. The accountability environment of schools sets forth this context and therefore establishes the framework in which improvement needs to occur. Speech–language pathologists need to stay current not only within the evolving practice within their discipline but also within general education curriculum and instruction, special education, reading, psychology, and health care, because children with various medical conditions will be attending school. The future, in fact, will find extremes that in many ways will seem to conflict, specifically between the extremes in the diagnoses and the specialized treatments for students, but at the same time will mandate that all students continue to achieve or make progress toward common curriculum goals. In addition, specialists will have the mandates to prepare students for postsecondary options, including college or work, while at the same time to have experiences with mainstream peers.

If we examine the trends in the research base of all of the disciplines that contribute to education, we can begin to predict where the fields will intersect. As mentioned previously, education research and practice within curriculum and instruction are moving in the direction of looking at the whole child, which must include mental and physical health and living conditions, such as home language and socioeconomic status, in addition to learning needs and styles. As professionals, we must examine and promote ways to change the educational environment to meet students' needs as they relate to the curriculum and classroom instruction rather than remove the student from a nonsupportive environment. In this promotion of the whole child, engaging, differentiating strategies, thinking maps, and other ways of accommodating learner differences is an excellent place to start for speech–language pathologists, audiologists, and other special educators to work collaboratively with teachers.

There are several areas of research to practice that will create a new future in the work of speech–language pathologists and audiologists, many of which have been described in this text. Notably, the areas of autism spectrum disorder (ASD), technological advances in augmentative and alternative communication (AAC), assistive technology and audiology, and early childhood interventions will see advancements that will require adjustments in how speech–language pathologists provide services. Three other practice areas are noteworthy for the changes expected in the future: adolescent literacy, English Learners, and assessment.

Speech–Language Pathologists' Future Watch: Expanded Practice and Professionalism

The work of speech–language pathologists and other educators is complex and important. As the authors view the future through myriad influences creating the change, we predict that speech–language pathologists will expand their practice and professionalism in the following ways:

- Speech–language pathologists should increase their use of and ability to explain their use and choice of evidence-based practice (EBP).
- They should develop their specializations in specific areas, such as ASD, fluency, literacy, AAC and assistive technology (AT), auditory processing, voice, phonology, concussion management, working with adults in the community, and so on.
- They should shift the distribution of how their time is spent by increasing collaboration and consultation with teachers, parents, and paraprofessionals to train others in intervention methods for communication impairments and decrease the amount of time spent in direct service provided to students. The change will reflect not only a maximization of expertise needed by the educational system in a time of shortages and limited availability of professional staff but also the extension of expertise toward students when many people are knowledgeable about their care.
- Speech–language pathologists should provide increased consultation and leadership to curriculum teams with regard to academic literacy, structuring instructional strategies for struggling learners, including English Learners.
- They should conduct more training for paraprofessionals, including speech–language pathology assistants (SLPAs), teachers, and parents on specific strategies that can be provided by these individuals.
- Speech–language pathologists should be involved in the development and delivery of prereferral intervention programs, including MTSS/RTI programs, and consultation on Tier I and Tier II interventions and delivery of Tier III interventions.
- They should realize an enhanced role in collaborative assessment teams, arena assessments, joint observations, and dynamic procedures to more fully identify students' learning issues in relation to the curriculum requirements of the classroom.
- There should be greater participation in site and district teams and committees on system change initiatives, including the development of MTSS/RTI models, and curriculum accommodations and adaptations.
- They should increase their comfort with the "blurring of the lines" in terms of roles, responsibilities, and delineation of "who does what" and participating fully in tiered interventions, problem-solving models, and system changes designed to address learner needs.

- There will be increased competition between employers for speech–language pathologists, leading to increases in salary supplements, bonuses, and other enticements for employment.
- There should be increased availability of assessment instruments appropriate for bilingual children, including instruments that have been normed on bilingual students.
- Leadership roles will expand within the educational system, extending the impact of the discipline. These roles will include but not be limited to program specialist, curriculum specialist, assistant principal, principal, coordinator, director, consortium director, assistant superintendent, and superintendent. These positions and leadership roles may be within special education or within general education.
- Technology is exploding as a tool for assessment, communication, teaching, and service provision. It supports both teachers and students in numerous and expanding ways.

The possibilities for our expanded practice and professionalism are endless and exciting. Speech–language pathologists are experiencing a wonderful time in school services. At the same time that the field is experiencing critical shortages, the demand for our services and expertise is expanding. It is a challenging time for professionals and for the students in our country. Our goal should be to maximize our training, expertise, and resources to create a system that benefits students and stimulates professionals.

We believe that public schools are the best place to work and that speech–language pathologists are, indeed, making a difference every day for our country's children. In his discussion of "The Schools We Need," Fullan (2003) stated,

> The best case for public education has always been that it is a common good. Everyone, ultimately, has a stake in the caliber of schools, and education is everyone's business. The quality of the public education system relates directly to the quality of life that people enjoy (whether as parents, employers, or citizens), with a strong public education system as the cornerstone of a civil, prosperous, and democratic society.
>
> As the main institution for fostering social cohesion in an increasingly diverse society, publicly funded schools must serve all children, not simply those with the loudest and most powerful advocates. This means addressing the cognitive and social needs of all children, with an emphasis on including those who may have not been well served in the past. (p. 3)

Speech–Language Pathologists "I"s on the Future

I-Nouns
- Information
- IDEA
- Involvement
- Instruction
- Intervention
- Improvement
- Influence
- Innovation

I-Adjectives
- Interprofessional
- Inspirational
- Intriguing
- Invigorating
- Important

As we cast our eyes on the future, it seems that the "I"s have it—many "I" words "fit the bill" for the future watch for speech–language pathologists. As you proceed in your speech-language pathology career, see what "I"s will be in your future.

Closing Thoughts

We said this before, and we will say it again: Being a speech–language pathologist in public schools is exciting, energizing, and rewarding. Educational reforms will continue, enabling speech–language pathologists and those concerned about children—all children—to be dramatically involved in creating a system that works for children with communication disorders. Allington and McGill-Franzen (2000) commented,

> So I guess the answer to what sort of schools will we have in the 21st century can be best stated as "It will depend." It will depend on the decisions we as a society make about what it means to teach and what it means to learn and to be literate, and whether schools are seen as important in achieving the ideals of a just, democratic society. (p. 151)

The future depends on the work of many, including speech–language pathologists, who do, indeed, make a difference for America's children.

To Screen or Not to Screen . . .
That Is the Question

Barbara J. Moore, EdD, CCC-SLP, BCS-CL
Director, Special Services, East Side Union High School District, San Jose, CA

Beth A. Nishida, MA
*Executive Director, SELPA/Special Education, Norwalk-LaMirada
Unified School District, CA*

In 1975, Congress passed Public Law 94-142, the Education for All Handicapped Children Act (EAHCA), which mandated educational services for children with disabilities in this country. Since that time, special education has continually evolved. Some of these changes may have seemed subtle, but they were extremely important, like changing the name of the law to the Individuals With Disabilities Education Act (IDEA) in 1990. Other changes have seemed dramatic and have raised high levels of controversy, such as the inclusion of students with significant disabilities in general education programs, or including students with disabilities in statewide testing. Each change has been rooted in the fight to provide a free appropriate public education (FAPE) to students with disabilities. Additionally, the climate of special education has made us increasingly aware of our legal obligations and critical of our practices under the law. The reauthorizations of 1990, 1997, and 2004 all brought sweeping change to how special educators operate in schools, creating the need to examine what we do and why we do it. In some cases, these practices are held near and dear by some individuals who provide service to students with disabilities.

Child Find

In 1975, school districts in many parts of our country were denying educational services to children with disabilities. These circumstances led to a federal mandate for special education in the United States. To ensure that such denial would not occur, procedural safeguards, or rights and protections, were guaranteed to parents and children. Among these procedural safeguards were requirements regarding evaluation and identification of children as having a disability. Key to these rights and protections is parent consent for assessment. In order to ensure that all children with disabilities who might not be in school were located and provided with an education, requirements for "search and serve" or "child find" were put into the law.

In 2000, the U.S. Department of Education (2000) reported to the Congress that the original intent of special education, to locate and provide access to children with disabilities, was met. Previously, in 1997, the focus of IDEA shifted from access to services, to a focus on educational results (IDEA, 1997, § 601[c]). Many things changed between 1975 and 1997, and certainly between 1997 and 2017, but one of the most noteworthy is in how we "search" for, or locate and find, students with disabilities. In 1975, one of the easiest ways to find children who might have disabilities was to conduct massive classroom screenings of all children in certain groups, such as those entering kindergarten, or those at certain grade levels. This usually involved conducting a short battery of sample test items with students to check their articulation, vocabulary, language development, and pre-academic skills. In 1975, some children who did not appear to be school-ready would be sent home to mature for another year, while others would be tested to determine whether they needed special education services. Over 40 years later, the experience of young children entering and in school is much different.

In 2017, many children have some sort of preschool experience prior to entering kindergarten. While there is still a great disparity in skills between children entering school for a variety of reasons, there is no "screening" for academic readiness. It is also rare to find speech–language pathologists who feel compelled to screen kindergarten classes for children who might need services. There are several reasons for this. One is because mass screening is extremely time-consuming, with seemingly little actual benefit in terms of identification. Since many children have attended preschool, most children with speech and/or language difficulties would have been referred at that level. As educators, we also understand that even children with no prior school experience need opportunities to enter school, learn the routine, and have time to learn, adjust, and mature in the educational environment. Children need to be given time to adjust to the learning environment of school, so conducting a screening of their skills early on in their school experience would be meaningless. At all grade levels, teachers and other support staff have a greater understanding of accommodations, modifications, and techniques for adjusting the academic curriculum so that children can be successful. The focus on literacy has resulted in a greater focus on individualized needs that can be addressed in the general education classroom. One final reason that speech–language pathologists no longer conduct mass screenings is that most of them do not need to go in search of students for their caseloads.

Child Find continues to be a mandate under the IDEA, but school systems have different ways of conducting Child Find than existed in 1975. The 2004 reauthorization of IDEA brought into practice models for response to intervention (RTI), which is now part of newer frameworks of Multi-Tiered System of Supports (MTSS). Several components are key to RTI/MTSS models, including effective Tier I instruction, use of data, and functioning instructional support teams (ISTs) (also known as problem-solving teams). When individual students are having difficulties in school, these students are referred to the school's MTSS problem-solving team or instructional support team.

(Note, in some places, the terminology *child study team* [CST] or *student study team* [SST] is still used. However, such terms have more recently been abandoned in favor of terms that reflect solving problems and looking for instructional solutions rather than searching for in-child problems.) This process is a general education function and is designed to help teachers, students, and families by identifying methods of helping the student. If interventions are not successful, and a student continues to struggle, then the student may be referred for special education assessment to determine whether she or he is a child with a disability requiring special education. (See discussion on RTI/MTSS in Moore & Montgomery [2018].) Key to this process is considering all areas that might be impacting the student.

Evaluation Procedures

IDEA is very specific in the procedures that must be followed for evaluation. The *Code of Federal Regulations* (C.F.R., 2006; *Electronic Code of Federal Regulations*, n.d.) (Authority: 20 U.S.C. § 1414[b][1]-[3], 1412[a][6][B]) requires that:

- No single procedure is used as the sole criterion for determining whether a child is a child with a disability and for determining an appropriate educational program for the child (34 C.F.R. § 300.304 [b][2]).
- The child is assessed in all areas of suspected disability, including, if appropriate, health, vision, hearing, social and emotional status, general intelligence, academic performance, communicative status, and motor abilities (34 C.F.R. § 300.304 [c][v][4]).
- In evaluating each child with a disability, the evaluation is sufficiently comprehensive to identify all of the child's special education and related services needs, whether or not commonly linked to the disability category in which the child has been classified (34 C.F.R. § 300.304 [c][v][6]).

> §300.305 (a) *Review of existing evaluation data.* As part of an initial evaluation (if appropriate) and as part of any reevaluation under this part, the IEP Team and other qualified professionals, as appropriate, must—
>
> (1) Review existing evaluation data on the child, including—
>> (i)   Evaluations and information provided by the parents of the child;
>> (ii) Current classroom-based, local, or State assessments, and classroom-based observations; and
>> (iii) Observations by teachers and related services providers; and
>
> (2) On the basis of that review, and input from the child's parents, identify what additional data, if any, are needed to determine—
>> (i)(A) Whether the child is a child with a disability, as defined in §300.8, and the educational needs of the child;

Concerns About Screening as a Prereferral Activity

Even though speech–language pathologists in schools have, for the most part, abandoned the practice of mass screenings of groups of children, a practice of prereferral screening of individual children is still utilized in some places. Speech–language pathologists may conduct a screening as a result of a request by an individual teacher for them to "check" a child or as a result of an IST recommendation. Many speech–language pathologists believe screening is a very efficient practice. They view it as a way to prevent having to conduct a full assessment on an individual child, especially if the referral is inappropriate. They feel they can quickly determine whether the child appears to require the services of a speech–language pathologist or whether the concern that the teacher has brought to their attention is developmental. The problem with this rationale, and practice, is that they are contrary to the MTSS/RTI practice and the requirements described above for evaluation to determine eligibility.

Screening has been an accepted practice for many years in our field and is outlined in the ASHA Preferred Practice Patterns (ASHA, 2004b) and other ASHA documents (2004a, 2010a, 2010b). Screening is also an approved activity for speech–language pathology assistants. Technically, screening is to be used to determine whether further assessment is warranted, but in the context of schools, screening is often used to check whether the child might potentially qualify for services before conducting further evaluation. The problem is that once that has been done, the team has begun conducting an evaluation, most often without parental consent. This practice is contrary to requirements for evaluation.

The practice of screening for the purpose of determining whether or not the child should have additional evaluation is problematic for several reasons. By conducting a screening in this way, a single assessor has predetermined eligibility, violating the requirements for parental consent, the requirements for assessing in all areas of suspected disability, and the requirements for a multidisciplinary team assessment. If the student is recommended for further evaluation as a result of the screening, no other issues may be considered, possibly missing areas of need. If the student is not recommended for further evaluation, then the speech–language pathologist alone has made the determination of eligibility, absent parental and multidisciplinary team participation. One other problem is that when assessments are conducted, a meeting is required to review the evaluation, and this generally does not occur when a screening is done.

Speech–language pathologists may believe that nothing is wrong with going into a classroom and listening to a child, at the teacher's request. The belief holds because they are not administering any formal tests, they are listening to the child at the teacher's request, and they are protecting themselves from time-consuming, inappropriate referrals. The C.F.R. requires that assessments be administered by trained and qualified professionals (§300.304 [c][1][iv]). When a speech–language pathologist goes into a classroom and singles out a given child, and uses his or her trained ear and knowledge skill set to listen to the child, she or he has just conducted an assessment (i.e., data collection and the gathering of evidence) and evaluation (i.e., bringing meaning to that data through interpretation, analysis, and reflection). Even though this assessment may not be a formal one and no formal tests were administered, it can be considered an evaluation because of the knowledge base and expertise of the speech–language pathologist and because the results are potentially being used to determine eligibility status. Additionally, in this scenario, the assessment (albeit a screening) has been done without parental consent or following the other requirements identified above. Violating these requirements can be considered a violation of the child's due process rights and could lead to legal problems for the school district.

Legal Concerns

As early as 1986, a ruling regarding screening held that a school district was conducting an assessment when it used procedures for one student that it did not use for everyone in that child's class (*Forest Park* [MI] *School District*, 352 IDELR 182 [OCR 1986]). In this case, the procedures were used without consent from the parent. That case has implications for speech–language pathologists, as well as for other special education assessors. The outcome of this case suggests that general consultation about student difficulties is acceptable, but when the specialist interacted with the student in an attempt to determine whether more assessment was warranted, the evaluation, in essence, had already begun.

A 1996 9th Circuit Court of Appeals case reinforced the importance of parental consent and not having dual tracks for determining eligibility (*Pasatiempo v. Aizawa*, 103 F.3d 796 [9th Cir. 1966]). In this case, the state of Hawaii defended its use of a dual-track system of evaluation, depending on the suspicion of the school's screening committee as to whether or not the child had a disability. The 9th Circuit Court found that it is not in the purview of the school to make this determination prior to evaluation and that parents cannot be denied their procedural rights to consent. In essence this case emphasized that (a) there need to be procedures in place, (b) the procedures need to be systematic, (c) parents need to give consent prior to assessment, and (d) this consent needs to be informed consent. This case can be interpreted to apply to this discussion about screening, in that if screening is used as part of the procedures to determine whether a child has a disability, then such procedures need to be identified. A 2011 decision by the Office of Administrative Hearing (OAH) found in favor of the school district when the speech–language pathologist had the parent sign a consent for a screening, which included a Preschool Intake Form, a Preschool Language Scale (PLS-4), and a language sample. On the basis of the results of the screening, the speech–language pathologist recommended a comprehensive assessment. In this case, the parent asserted that she wanted speech–language services for her child but did not want additional assessment, just services. Having consent and also the credible testimony of the speech–language pathologist that she did not represent to the parent that the screening would be adequate to determine whether the child needed services was key to the judge's finding in the district's favor (*Panama-Buena Vista Union School District v. Parent on Behalf of Student*, OAH Case No. 2011070635).

Using Effective Procedures

Changing legal requirements, as well as increased due process cases, have forced school personnel to continually examine their practices. The good news is that by analyzing our practices, it may be possible to solve more than one problem at once. Consider for a moment, a long-time complaint of many speech–language pathologists in schools, that "they [teachers, administrators, parents, etc.] don't know what I do!" Many researchers and school-based experts on service delivery have suggested that the best way to solve this problem is by not separating ourselves from the functions of the classroom or school (Ehren, 2000; Montgomery & Moore, 2011; Moore & Montgomery, 2018; Wallach, 2008). In other words, the more we are involved with the issues and concerns of teachers and principals, related to student need, the greater the opportunity they have to learn about our skill set and knowledge base. By extending this line of thinking to utilization of the IST process for consideration of all students with learning problems and suspected disabilities, it is possible to see how ongoing discussion and participation by the speech–language pathologist can help the team understand how speech and language issues impact the child's academic achievement. For example, the speech–language pathologist can help the team understand how concerns about phonemic awareness and reading concerns in children may be related to their suspected phonological impairment. Through utilizing the school's problem-solving process to address student need, the goal to avoid inappropriate referrals can be achieved. We may also be able to increase team members' general awareness of the role of the speech–language pathologist, and how speech and language issues impact academics.

Local Decisions

Whether or not to utilize screening as a part of the protocol for prereferral is a local decision that should be addressed with the special education administration at the school district and local governing agencies. If it is decided to utilize screening as a prereferral practice, then parental consent should be obtained. This is critical, as a single child is being identified as suspected of having a disability, rather than a group of children. Failure to obtain parental consent could be construed as denial of due process procedures. Should further speech and language evaluation not be conducted as a result of the screening results, and the parent had not been informed or consent received, the district could be responsible for the cost of that evaluation and services if the parent sought private evaluation and services.

Speech–language pathologists may be reluctant to use the IST as a process for determining whether a student should receive a comprehensive speech and language evaluation, due to dysfunction of the IST at their school site. However, the speech–language pathologist may find that helping the school solve those problems may be more productive for students and staff in the long run. The benefits of an effective IST process may eventually outweigh the work required to revamp the system so that it is responsive to many needs.

In the long run, the answer on whether to screen or not to screen lies at the local level. Screening is a permissive activity. Mass screenings, as they are completed with large groups of children, do not require parental consent. However, any time an individual child is singled out, parental consent should be obtained.

In looking at updated procedures for Child Find, speech–language pathologists should utilize the IST process of the school, which is designed to be a problem-solving vehicle for teachers, students, and parents. Through this system, team members can learn about developmental milestones for speech and language, how to provide accommodations and modifications, implications for literacy concerns with children suspected of having a speech or language disorder, and how to look at the whole child, not just one presenting issue. Additionally, through the IST, the coordination of interventions available through the MTSS or RTI at the school will be recommended and tracked. By using the IST process, the student's other strengths and needs can be considered. Additionally, when the speech–language pathologist participates in this process, his or her input has the advantage of training IST members in speech and language issues that potentially impact school performance and what types of concerns would warrant an appropriate referral.

Finally, it is noted that the *Code of Federal Regulations* (§300.302) does find that screening for instructional purposes is not considered an evaluation:

> The screening of a student by a teacher or specialist to determine appropriate instructional strategies for curriculum implementation shall not be considered to be an evaluation for eligibility for special education and related services. (Authority: 20 U.S.C. § 1414[a][1][E])

Before deciding whether to screen or not to screen, speech–language pathologists should examine what the purpose of the screening is. If it is to save time and to prevent inappropriate referrals, the problems may outweigh the perceived benefit. Speech–language pathologists need to understand that legally there is no such thing as an individual screening or just popping into a teacher's classroom to listen to a child. The expertise utilized to perform that task constitutes that act an assessment. Speech–language pathologists are strongly encouraged to participate in MTSS/RTI efforts at their school as part of the evolving methods for ensuring that children are provided interventions and also provided protections.

With mandates to consider how the child's disability affects his or her ability to progress in the general education curriculum, utilizing the procedures set forth for assisting students seems to be natural. But most importantly, the increasing world of litigation in special education makes examination of our practices critical. Whatever practice your local agency decides to follow, make sure that you have addressed the required components of multidisciplinary assessment, receiving informed parental consent and assessing in all areas of suspected disability.

Authors' Note

This article was originally published in the *CSHA Magazine* in 2002. The basic information remains sound advice, according to the authors. We have updated it to reflect current application of law and practice (February 11, 2017).

References

American Speech–Language–Hearing Association. (1999). *Guidelines for the roles and responsibilities of the school-based speech–language pathologist.* Rockville, MD: Author.

American Speech–Language–Hearing Association. (2001). *Scope of practice in speech–language pathology.* Rockville, MD: Author.

American Speech–Language–Hearing Association. (2004a). *Admission/discharge criteria in speech–language pathology* [Guidelines]. Retrieved from www.asha.org/policy/GL2004–00046.htm

American Speech–Language–Hearing Association. (2004b). *Preferred practice patterns for the profession of speech–language pathology* [Preferred Practice Patterns]. Retrieved from www.asha.org/policy

American Speech–Language–Hearing Association. (2010a). *Roles and responsibilities of speech–language pathologists in schools* [Position Statement]. Retrieved from www.asha.org/policy

American Speech–Language–Hearing Association. (2010b). *Roles and responsibilities of speech–language pathologists in schools* [Professional Issues Statement]. Retrieved from www.asha.org/policy/PI2010-00317/

Ehren, B. J. (2000). Maintaining a therapeutic focus and sharing responsibility for student success: Keys to in-classroom speech–language services. *Language, Speech, and Hearing Services in Schools, 31,* 219–229.

Electronic Code of Federal Regulations. (n.d.). Retrieved from www.ecfr.gov/cgi-bin/text-idx?tpl=/ecfrbrowse/Title34/34cfr300_main_02.tpl

Individuals With Disabilities Education Act of 1990, 20 U.S.C. § 1400 *et seq.* (1990) (amended 1997).

Individuals With Disabilities Education Improvement Act of 2004, 20 U.S.C. § 1400 *et seq.* (2004).

Montgomery, J., & Moore, B. (2011, November). *Listen, learn, lead: Expanding to integrated models of service delivery.* Paper presented at the ASHA Annual Convention, San Diego, CA.

Moore, B. J., & Montgomery, J. K. (2018). *Speech–language pathologists in public schools: Making a difference for America's children* (3rd ed.). Austin, TX: PRO-ED.

Panama-Buena Vista Union School District v. Parent on Behalf of Student, OAH Case No. 2011070635.

Pasatiempo v. Aizawa, 103 F.3D 796 (9th Cir. 1996). Retrieved from http://caselaw.lp.findlaw.com/scripts/getcase.pl?navby=search&case=data2…9417092.htm

U.S. Department of Education. (2000). *Twenty-second annual report to Congress on the implementation of the Individuals With Disabilities Education Act.* Washington, DC: Author.

REFERENCES

Adams, M. J. (1999). *Beginning to read: Thinking and learning about print.* Cambridge, MA: MIT Press.

The Advocacy Institute. (2013). *ESEA flexibility: Issues for students with disabilities.* Retrieved from www.advocacyinstitute.org/ESEA/AdvocacyInstitute-ESEA.Flexibility.Issues.for.SWDS.pdf

Alexander, K. L., Entwisle, D. R., & Steffel Olson, L. (2007, April). Lasting consequences of the summer learning. *American Sociological Review, 72,* 167–180.

Allington, R. L., & McGill-Franzen, A. (2000). Looking back, looking forward: A conversation about teaching reading in the 21st century. *Reading Research Quarterly, 35,* 136–153.

American Civil Liberties Union. (2014, May). Brown *at 60: Is full equality within our grasp? A conversation on zero tolerance, segregation, and the promise of justice. U.S. National Archives.* Retrieved from www.aclu.org/brown-60-full-equality-within-our-grasp

American Occupational Therapy Association, American Physical Therapy Association, & American Speech–Language–Hearing Association. (2014). *Workload approach: A paradigm shift for positive impact on student outcomes.* Retrieved from www.asha.org/uploadedFiles/ASHA/Practice_Portal/Professional_Issues/Caseload_and_Workload/APTA-ASHA-AOTA-Joint-Doc-Workload-Approach-Schools.pdf

American Psychiatric Association. (2013). *Diagnostic and statistical manual of mental disorders* (5th ed.). Washington, DC: Author.

American Psychological Association. (2010). *Publication manual of the American Psychological Association* (6th ed.). Washington, DC: Author.

American Speech–Language–Hearing Association. (1991). *Guidelines for speech–language pathologists serving persons with language, socio-communication, and/or cognitive-communication impairments* [Guidelines]. Retrieved from www.asha.org/policy

American Speech–Language–Hearing Association. (1993*). Definitions of communication disorders and variations* [Relevant Paper]. Retrieved from www.asha.org/policy/RP1993-00208/

American Speech–Language–Hearing Association. (1996). Inclusive practices for children and youths with communication disorders [Position statement]. *ASHA, 38*(Suppl. 16), 35–44.

American Speech–Language–Hearing Association. (1998a). *Students and professionals who speak English with accents and nonstandard dialects: Issues and recommendations* [Technical Report]. Available from www.asha.org/policy

American Speech–Language–Hearing Association. (1998b). *User's guide: National treatment outcome data collection project.* Rockville, MD: Author.

American Speech–Language–Hearing Association. (1999). *Guidelines for the roles and responsibilities of the school-based speech–language pathologist.* Rockville, MD: Author.

American Speech–Language–Hearing Association. (2000a). *IDEA and your caseload: A template for eligibility and dismissal criteria for students ages 3–21.* Rockville, MD: Author.

American Speech–Language–Hearing Association. (2000b). *Roles and responsibilities of speech–language pathologists with respect to reading and writing in children and adolescents.* Rockville, MD: Author.

American Speech–Language–Hearing Association. (2000c). *What does it mean to be certified?* Retrieved from www.asha.org/Certification/AboutCertificationGenInfo/

American Speech–Language–Hearing Association. (2000d). *National data report 1999–2000: National Outcomes Measurement System.* Rockville, MD: Author.

American Speech–Language–Hearing Association. (2001). *2001 Omnibus survey results.* Rockville, MD: Author.

American Speech–Language–Hearing Association. (2002a). *A workload analysis approach for establishing speech–language caseload standards in the school* [Guidelines]. Retrieved from www.asha.org/policy

American Speech–Language–Hearing Association. (2002b*). A workload analysis approach for establishing speech–language caseload standards in the school* [Position Statement]. Retrieved from www.asha.org/policy/PS2002–00122.html

American Speech–Language–Hearing Association. (2004a). *Admission/discharge criteria in speech–language pathology* [Guidelines]. Retrieved from www.asha.org/policy/GL2004–00046.htm

American Speech–Language–Hearing Association. (2004a). *Admission/discharge criteria in speech–language pathology* [Guidelines]. Retrieved March 5, 2016, from http://www.asha.org/policy/GL2004–00046.htm

American Speech–Language–Hearing Association. (2004b). *Code of fair testing practices in education.* Washington, DC: Joint Committee on Testing Practices. Retrieved from www.asha.org/policy/RP2004-00195/

American Speech–Language–Hearing Association. (2004c). *Preferred practice patterns for the profession of speech–language pathology.* Retrieved from www.asha.org/policy/PP2004–00191.htm

American Speech–Language–Hearing Association. (2004d). *Knowledge and skills needed by speech–language pathologists and audiologists to provide culturally and linguistically appropriate services* [Knowledge and Skills]. Retrieved from www.asha.org/policy

American Speech–Language–Hearing Association. (2004e). *Preferred practice patterns for the profession of speech–language pathology* [Preferred Practice Patterns]. Retrieved from www.asha.org/policy

American Speech–Language–Hearing Association. (2005a). *Early literacy.* Rockville, MD: Author.

American Speech–Language–Hearing Association. (2005b). *Evidence-based practice in communication disorders* [Position Statement]. Retrieved from www.asha.org/policy

American Speech–Language–Hearing Association. (2005c). *Roles and responsibilities of speech–language pathologists with respect to augmentative and alternative communication: Position statement* [Position Statement]. Retrieved from www.asha.org/policy/PS2005-00113.htm

American Speech–Language–Hearing Association. (2006a). *2006 schools survey: Caseload characteristics.* Rockville, MD: Author.

American Speech–Language–Hearing Association. (2006b). *Preferred practice patterns for the profession of audiology.* Retrieved from www.asha.org/policy/PP2006-00274/

American Speech–Language–Hearing Association. (2007). *Language, speech, and hearing contacts in state education agencies.* Retrieved from www.asha.org/advocacy/state/info

American Speech–Language–Hearing Association. (2008a). *Core knowledge and skills in early intervention speech–language pathology practice.* Retrieved from www.asha.org/policy

American Speech–Language–Hearing Association. (2008b). *Roles and responsibilities of speech–language pathologists in early intervention* [Guidelines]. Retrieved from www.asha.org/policy/GL2008-00293.htm

American Speech–Language–Hearing Association. (2008c). *Roles and responsibilities of speech–language pathologists in early intervention* [Technical Report]. Retrieved from www.asha.org/policy

American Speech–Language–Hearing Association. (2010a). *Roles and responsibilities of speech–language pathologists in schools* [Position Statement]. Retrieved from www.asha.org/policy/PS2010-00318/

American Speech–Language–Hearing Association. (2010b). *Roles and responsibilities of speech–language pathologists in schools* [Professional Issues Statement]. Retrieved from www.asha.org/policy/PI2010-00317/

American Speech–Language–Hearing Association. (2010c). *Code of ethics* [Ethics]. Retrieved from www.asha.org/Code-of-Ethics/

American Speech–Language–Hearing Association. (2011*). The clinical education of students with accents* [Professional Issues Statement]. Retrieved from www.asha.org/policy/PI2011-00324.htm

American Speech–Language–Hearing Association. (2012). *2012 schools survey report: SLP caseload characteristics.* Retrieved from www.asha.org/research/memberdata/schoolssurvey

American Speech–Language–Hearing Association. (2013a). *Forum on strategizing solutions to personnel shortages in speech–language pathology.* Retrieved from www.asha.org/slp/slppersonnelforum/#_ga=1.222075292.509329459.1419034974

American Speech–Language–Hearing Association. (2013b). *Speech–language pathology assistant scope of practice [Scope of Practice].* Retrieved from www.asha.org/policy/SP2013-00337

American Speech–Language–Hearing Association. (2014a). *2014 schools survey: SLP caseload characteristics.* Retrieved from www.asha.org/research/memberdata/schoolssurvey

American Speech–Language–Hearing Association. (2014b). *PACE: Performance Assessment of Contributions and Effectiveness of speech–language pathologists.* Retrieved from www.asha.org/Advocacy/state/Performance-Assessment-of-Contributions-and-Effectiveness

American Speech–Language–Hearing Association. (2016a). *Speech–language pathologists: Language experts and literacy resource* [Literacy Gateway (Reading and Writing)]. Retrieved from www.asha.org/publications/literacy

American Speech–Language–Hearing Association. (2016b). *Speech–language pathology assistant scope of practice*. Retrieved from www.asha.org/policy/SP2013–00337/#sec1.7.1

American Speech–Language–Hearing Association. (2016c). *Scope of practice in speech–language pathology* [Scope of practice]. Retreived from www.asha.org/policy

American Speech–Language–Hearing Association. (n.d.-a). *Perceived needs and market trends*. Retrieved www.asha.org/Careers/recruitment/schools/Needs-Trends

American Speech–Language–Hearing Association. (n.d.-b). *Cognitive referencing*. Retrieved from www.asha.org/SLP/schools/prof-consult/Cognitive-Referencing

American Speech–Language–Hearing Association. (n.d.-c). *Cultural competence* [Practice Portal]. Retrieved from www.asha.org/Practice-Portal/Professional-Issues/Cultural-Competence

American Speech–Language–Hearing Association. (n.d.-d). *Forum on strategizing solutions to personnel shortages in speech–language pathology*. Retrieved from www.asha.org/slp/slppersonnelforum/#_ga=1.222075292.509329459.1419034974

American Speech–Language–Hearing Association. (n.d.-e). *Perceived needs and market trends*. Retrieved from www.asha.org/Careers/recruitment/schools/Needs-Trends

American Speech–Language–Hearing Association. (n.d.-f). *Roles and responsibilities of speech–language pathologists in schools*. Retrieved from www.asha.org/policy/PI2010–00317

American Speech–Language–Hearing Association. (n.d.-g). *When supervisor and supervisee disagree*. Retrieved from www.asha.org/practice/ethics/roundtable/supervisee

American Speech–Language–Hearing Association. (n.d.-h). *Autism*. Retrieved from www.asha.org/Practice-Portal/Clinical-Topics/Autism

American Speech–Language–Hearing Association. (n.d.-i). *Augmentative and alternative communication (AAC)*. Retrieved from www.asha.org/public/speech/disorders/AAC

American Speech–Language–Hearing Association. (n.d.-j). *Evidence-based practice glossary*. Retrieved from www.asha.org/Research/EBP/Evidence-Based-Practice-Glossary

American Speech–Language–Hearing Association. (n.d.-k). *Strategic pathway to excellence*. Retrieved from www.asha.org/uploadedFiles/ASHA-Strategic-Pathway-to-Excellence.pdf

American Speech–Language–Hearing Association. (n.d.-l). *Dynamic assessment*. Retrieved from www.asha.org/practice/multicultural/issues/Dynamic-Assessment.htm

American Speech–Language–Hearing Association. (n.d.-m). *Early intervening services*. Retrieved from www.asha.org/Advocacy/federal/idea/04-law-early-services

American Speech–Language–Hearing Association. (n.d.-n). *Issues in ethics: Speech–language pathology assistants*. Retrieved from www.asha.org/Practice/ethics/Speech-Language-Pathology-Assistants

American Speech–Language–Hearing Association. (n.d.-o). *Frequently asked questions: Speech–language pathology assistants (SLPAs)*. Retrieved from www.asha.org/associates/SLPA-FAQs.htm#_ga=1.194756009.509329459.1419034974

Americans With Disabilities Act of 1990, 42 U.S.C. § 12101 *et seq.* (1990).

Apel, K. (1999). An introduction to assessment and intervention with older students with language-learning impairments: Bridges from research to clinical practice. *Language, Speech, and Hearing Services in Schools, 30,* 228–230.

Apel, K., & Swank, L. (1999). Second chances: Improving decoding skills in the older student. *Language, Speech, and Hearing Services in Schools, 30,* 231–242.

Arizona Department of Education. (2012). *Procedures from referral to determination of eligibility*. Retrieved from www.azed.gov/special-education/files/2012/02/evaluation-aztas-6–13–12.pdf

Armbruster, B. A., & Osborn, J. (2001). *Put reading first*. Washington, DC: National Institute for Literacy.

Association of California School Administrators. (2006). *Handbook of goals and objectives related to state of California content standards*. Sacramento, CA: Author.

Association of Supervision and Curriculum Development. (2016). *Education leaders identify top 10 components of personalized learning*. Retrieved from www.ascd.org/news-media/Press-Room/News-Releases/Education-Leaders-Identify-Top-10-Components-of-Personalized-Learning.aspx

August, D., & Shanahan, T. (2006). *Developing literacy in second-language learners: A report of the national literacy panel on language-minority children and youth*. Mahwah, NJ: Lawrence Erlbaum. Retrieved from www.cal.org/projects/archive/nlpreports/Executive_Summary.pdf

Bain, B. A., & Dollaghan, C. A. (1991). The notion of clinically significant change. *Language, Speech, and Hearing Services in Schools, 22,* 264–270.

Barrett, A. E., & Turner, R. J. (2005). Family structure and mental health: The mediating effects of socio-economic status, family process, and social stress. *Journal of Health and Social Behavior, 46,* 159–169.

Batsche, G. (2013). Multi-Tiered Systems of Support: A single system for ALL students. *The Special EDge, 26*(3), 3–5. Retrieved from www.calstat.org/publications/pdfs/summer_2013-spedge-english.pdf

Batsche, G., Elliott, J., Graden, J. L., Grimes, J., Kovaleski, J. F., Prasse, D., . . . Tilly, W. (2005). *Response to intervention: Policy considerations and implementation.* Alexandria, VA: National Association of State Directors of Special Education.

Bellini, P. I., & Pina, D. D. (2010). *One step at a time: Changing preschool delivery models.* Retrieved from www.asha.org/events/convention/handouts/2010/2225-iafrate-bellini-patricia

Bellini, S., & Akullian, J. (2007). A meta-analysis of video modeling and video self-modeling interventions for children and adolescents with ASD. *Exceptional Children, 73,* 261–228.

Best social services jobs: Speech–language pathologist. (2014). *U.S. News & World Report.* Retrieved from http://money.usnews.com/careers/best-jobs/speech-language-pathologist

Bettelheim, B., & Zelan, K. (1982). *On learning to read: The child's fascination with meaning.* New York, NY: Vintage.

Bevilacqua, S., & Norlin, J. W. (Eds.). (2004). *Autism methodologies: Best practices and legal trends.* Horsham, PA: LRP.

Biancarosa, G., & Snow, C. E. (2004). *Reading next—A vision for action and research in middle and high school literacy: A report from Carnegie Corporation of New York.* Washington, DC: Alliance for Excellent Education. Retrieved from https://www.carnegie.org/media/filer_public/b7/5f/b75fba81–16cb-422d-ab59–373a6a07eb74/ccny_report_2004_reading.pdf

Biemiller, A. (1999). *Language and reading success.* Cambridge, MA: Brookline.

Blackstone, S. W. (Ed.). (2000). AAC approaches for infants and toddlers. *Augmentative Communication News, 12*(6), 1–8.

Board of Education of Hendrick Hudson Central School District v. Rowley, 458 U.S. 176 (1982).

Bondy, A. S., & Frost, L. A. (1994). The Picture Exchange Communication System. *Focus on Autistic Behavior, 9,* 1–19.

Bourque Meaux, A., & Powell, R. (2010). *Articulation, phonology, and language: A closer look at SLP caseloads.* Presented at the ASHA Annual Convention. Retrieved from www.asha.org/Events/convention/handouts/2010/2146-Bourque-Meaux-Ashley

Boyle, C. A., Boulet, S., Schieve, L., Cohen, R. A., Blumberg, S. J., Yeargin-Allsopp, M., Visser, S., & Kogan, M. D. (2011). Trends in the prevalence of developmental disabilities in U.S. children, 1997–2008. *Pediatrics.* Retrieved from www.cdc.gov/ncbddd/developmentaldisabilities/features/birthdefects-dd-keyfindings.html

Brannen, S. J., Cooper, E. B., Dellegrotto, J. T., Disney, S. T., Eger, D. L., Ehren, B. J., . . . Whitmire, K. (2000). *Developing educationally relevant IEPs: A technical assistance document for speech–language pathologists.* Rockville, MD: American Speech–Language–Hearing Association.

Brown v. Board of Education, 347 U.S. 483 (1954).

Browning-Wright, D., & Cafferata, G. (2013). *The BIP desk reference: A teacher and behavior intervention team's guide to developing and evaluating behavior intervention plans for behaviors that interfere with the learning of student and/or peers* (Rev.). Retrieved from www.pent.ca.gov/dsk/BIPdeskreference2013.pdf

California Department of Education. (2009). *Determining specific learning disability eligibility using response to instruction and intervention (RtI2).* Retrieved from www.cde.ca.gov/sp/se/sr/documents/sldeligibltyrti2.doc

California Department of Education. (2016a). *Multi-Tiered Systems of Support.* Retrieved from www.cde.ca.gov/ci/cr/ri/

California Department of Education. (2016b). *Definition of MTSS.* Retrieved from www.cde.ca.gov/ci/cr/ri/mtsscomprti2.asp

California Department of Education. (n.d.). *NCLB FAQ for special education teachers.* Retrieved from www.cde.ca.gov/nclb/sr/tq/nclbspecedfaq.asp

California Statewide Special Education Task Force. (2015). *Special Education Task Force submits recommendations to improve outcomes for students with disabilities, establish one coherent system of education.* Retrieved from www.cde.ca.gov/nr/ne/yr15/yr15rel18.asp

Carbajal, P., Homer, E., Kelly, B., Priola, K., & Rizk, J. (2009). *St. Tammany Parish School SLP's report: 10 years of dysphagia in the schools.* Presented at the ASHA Annual Convention, New Orleans, LA.

Cassidy, J., & Cassidy, D. (2007). What's hot, what's not for 2007. *Reading Today, 24*(4), 1, 10.

Catts, H. W., Fey, M. E., Ellis Weismer, S., & Bridges, M. S. (2014). The relationship between language and reading abilities. In J. B. Tomblin & M. A. Nippold (Eds.), *Understanding individual differences in language development across the school years* (pp. 144–165). New York, NY: Psychology Press/Taylor & Francis.

Cedar Rapids Community School District v. Garret F., 526 U.S. 66, 119 S.Ct. 992, 143 L.Ed.2d 154 (1999).

Center for Special Education Finance. (1999, September). *Frequently asked questions.* Retrieved from http://csef.air.org/.html

Centers for Disease Control and Prevention. (2015). *ALARM guidelines.* Retrieved from www.cdc.gov/ncbddd/autism/hcp-recommendations.html

Centers for Disease Control and Prevention. (2016). *Key findings: Trends in the prevalence of developmental disabilities in U.S. children, 1997–2008.* Retrieved from www.cdc.gov/ncbddd/developmentaldisabilities/features/birthdefects-dd-keyfindings.html

Centers for Disease Control and Prevention. (n.d.-a). *Autism spectrum disorder (ASD) data and statistics.* Retrieved from www.cdc.gov/ncbddd/autism/data.html

Centers for Disease Control and Prevention. (n.d.-b). *Screening and diagnosis.* Retrieved from www.cdc.gov/ncbddd/autism/screening.html

Cirrin, F. M., & Gillam, R. B. (2008). Language intervention practices for school-age children with spoken language disorders: A systematic review. *Language, Speech, and Hearing Services in Schools, 39,* S110–S137.

Cirrin, F., Schooling, T., Nelson, N., Diehl, S., Flynn, P., Staskowski, M., . . . Adamczyk, D. (2010). Evidence-based systematic review: Effects of different service delivery models on communication outcomes for elementary school-age children. *Language, Speech, and Hearing Services in Schools, 41,* 233–264.

Cochran-Smith, M. (2004). *Walking the road: Race, diversity, and social justice in teacher education.* New York, NY: Teachers College Press.

Code of Federal Regulations Commentary, pp. 46626–46628.

Cohn, A. (2001). *Positive behavioral supports: Information for educators.* Retrieved from www.nasponline.org/resources/factsheets/pbs_fs.aspx

Colby, S. L., & Ortman, J. M. (2015). *Projections of the size and composition of the U.S. population: 2014 to 2060; Current population reports (P25-1143).* Washington, DC: U.S. Census Bureau.

Cole, L. (1983). Implications of the position on social dialects. *ASHA, 25*(9), 25–27.

Colorado Department of Education. (2016). *Multi-Tiered System of Supports.* Retrieved from www.cde.state.co.us/mtss#sthash.fR5qwglX.dpuf

Common Core State Standards. (n.d.-a). *Application to students with disabilities.* Retrieved from www.corestandards.org/assets/application-to-students-with-disabilities.pdf

Common Core State Standards. (n.d.-b). Retrieved from www.corestandards.org

Cornett, B. (2012, October). *ASHA changing health care landscape summit: Executive summary.* Retrieved from www.asha.org/uploadedFiles/ASHA/Practice/Health-Care-Reform/Healthcare-Summit-Executive-Summary-2012.pdf#search=%22Health%22

Council for Exceptional Children. (1997). A history of special education. *Teaching Exceptional Children, 29*(5), 5–50.

Council for Exceptional Children. (2016). Federal outlook for exceptional children: Fiscal year 2016. Retrieved from www.cec.sped.org/~/media/Files/Policy/Current%20Sped%20Issues%20Home/Federal%20Outlook%202016%20FINAL.pdf

Courtade, G., & Browder, D. M. (2011). *Aligning IEPs to the Common Core State Standards.* Verona, WI: Attainment Company.

Crais, E. R. (2000). Ecologically valid communication assessment of infants and toddlers. In L. R. Watson, E. Crais, & T. L. Layton (Eds.), *Handbook of early language impairment in children: Assessment and treatment* (pp. 1–37). Albany, NY: Delmar.

Creaghead, N. A. (1999). Evaluating language intervention approaches: Contrasting perspectives. *Language, Speech, and Hearing Services in Schools, 30,* 335–338.

Crooke, P. J., Olswang, L., & Winner, M. G. (2016, July–September). Thinking socially: Teaching social knowledge to foster social behavioral change. *Topics in Language Disorders, 36*(3), 284–298.

Crooke, P. J., & Winner, M. G. (2015). Research to frameworks to practice: Social Thinking's® layers of evidence. Retrieved from www.socialthinking.com/-/media/Files/Articles/Research-to-Frameworks-to-Practice-Social-Thinkings-Layers-of-Evidence.ashx?la=en

Cross, F. (2016). *Teacher shortage areas nationwide listing 1990–1991 through 2016–2017.* Washington, DC: U.S. Department of Education.

Crowley, C. J., Washington, T., & El-Sawaf, D. (2015). *Innovative approaches to address disproportionate referrals to SPED in the nation's largest school district.* Paper presented at the ASHA Annual Convention, Denver, CO.

Cypress-Fairbanks Independent School District v. Michael F., No. 96-20221 (5th Cir. 1997).

Daniel R. R. v. State Board of Education (5th Cir. 1989).

Danielson, L., & Rosenquist, C. (2014). Introduction to the TEC special issue on data-based individualization. *TEACHING Exceptional Children, 46*(4), 6–12.

Davis-McFarland, E. (2008). Family and cultural issues in a school swallowing and feeding program. *Language, Speech, and Hearing Services in Schools, 39,* 199–213.

Deal ex rel. Deal v. Hamilton County Board of Education, 42 IDELR 109 (6th Cir. 2004).

Delaney, A. M., Meyers, A. D., Ruth, R. A., Faust, R. A., & Talavera, F. (2012, January 31). *Newborn hearing screening.* Retrieved from http://emedicine.medscape.com/article/836646-overview

Delano, M. E. (2007). Video modeling interventions for individuals with autism. *Remedial and Special Education, 28*(1), 33–42.

Diehl, S. F. (2003). Prologue: Autism spectrum disorders: The context of speech–language pathologist intervention. *Language, Speech, and Hearing Services in Schools, 34*(3), 177–179.

Diehl, S. (2016, November). *Children with ASD making connections: Reading it and meaning it no matter what the genre.* Presented at the ASHA Annual Convention, Philadelphia, PA.

Dill, V. (2015). Homeless—and doubled up. *Educational Leadership, 72,* 42–47.

Dodd, J. (2014a). Taking measure. *The ASHA Leader, 19,* 56–59.

Dodd, J. (2014b). Writing goals in light of the CCSS: How SMART are your goals? *CSHA Magazine,* 44.

Dodd, J., & Gorey, M. (2014, February). AAC intervention as an immersion model. *Communication Disorders Quarterly, 35,* 103–107.

Dodd, J., Schaefer, A., & Rothbart, A. (2015, August). Conducting an augmentative and alternative communication assessment as a school-based speech–language pathologist: A collaborative experience. *SIG 16 Perspectives on School-Based Issues, 16,* 105–117.

Dollaghan, C. (2004, April). Evidence-based practice: Myths and realities. *The ASHA Leader, 12,* 4–5.

Donovan, S., & Cross, C. (2002). *Minority students in special and gifted education.* Washington, DC: National Academy Press.

Doorey, N. (2014, March). The common core assessments: What you need to know. *Educational Leadership, 71*(6), 57–60.

Doug C. v. State of Hawaii Department of Education, 720 F.3d 1038 (9th Cir. 2013), No. 12-15079 D.C., No. 1:11-cv-00441KSC. Retrieved from www.wrightslaw.com/law/caselaw/2013/9th.doug.c.v.hawaii .pdf

Duff, M. C., & Stuck, S. (2012). Pediatric brain injury: Misconceptions, challenges, and a call to reconceptualize our role in the schools. *Perspectives on School-Based Issues, 13*(3), 87.

DuFour, R., Dufour, R., Eaker, R., & Karhanek, G. (2004). *Whatever it takes: How professional learning communities respond when kids don't learn.* Bloomington, IN: Solution Tree.

Early Childhood Technical Assistance Center. (2016). *Outcomes measurement: Outcomes FAQ.* Retrieved from http://ectacenter.org/eco/pages/faqs.asp#ChildOutcomes

Education, 20 U.S.C. § 1414 (a)–(c), § 1401 (3), § 1401 (30), § 1414 (b)(1)–(3), § 1412 (a)(6)(B), § 1415 (b)(1), § 1415 (d)(2)(A) (2011).

Education, 34 C.F.R. § 300.111 (a), § 300.111 (c)(1)(2), § 300.226 (b), § 300.300, § 300.300 (a)(1)(i), § 300.300 (a)(4)(c)(i), § 300.300 (a)(ii), § 300.301, § 300.301 (c)(1)(i), § 300.301 (d)(2), § 300.302, § 300.304, § 300.304 (b)(3)(c)(iv), § 300.304 (4), § 300.304 (c)(6), § 300.305, § 300.3052 (e), § 300.306 (2), § 300.307 (a)(2), § 300.308, § 300.308 (3)(b), § 300.309 (a)(1), § 300.309 (a)(2)(i), § 300.310 (a), § 300.320 (b)(1), § 300.321 (a)(2), § 300.43 (a)(1), § 300.502 (c), § 300.503 (a)(1), § 300.504 (a)(1), § 300.506 (b), § 300.506 (b), § 300.550, § 300.9, § 613 (f)(1), § 613 (f)(5), § 613 (2) (2012).

Education Counsel LLC. (2010, March). *The Obama administration's "blueprint" for ESEA reauthorization: Outline of key points.* from www.educationcounsel.com/files/Elementary_and_Secondary_ Education_Acts.pdf

Education for All Handicapped Children Act, P.L. 94–142 (1975).

Education of the Handicapped Act, P.L. 91-230 (1970).

Educational Audiology Association. (2002). *Early detection and intervention of hearing loss: Roles and responsibilities of educational audiologists.* Retrieved from www.edaud.org/position-stat/4-position-01-02.pdf

Educational Audiology Association. (2009). *Recommended professional practices for educational audiology.* Retrieved from www.edaud.org/position-stat/6-position-05–09.pdf

Educational Audiology Association. (2014, March). *Hearing loss prevention resource guide.* Retrieved from www.edaud.org/position-stat/10-position-03–14.pdf

Ehren, B. J. (2000). Maintaining a therapeutic focus and sharing responsibility for student success: Keys to in-classroom speech–language services. *Language, Speech, and Hearing Services in Schools, 31,* 219–229.

Ehren, B. (2007). External evidence in adolescent reading comprehension and intervention. *Perspectives on Language Learning and Education, 14*(1), 13–16.

Ehren, B. J. (2009, May). Response-to-intervention: SLPs as linchpins in secondary schools. *The ASHA Leader.* Retrieved from www.asha.org/Publications/leader/2009/090505/f090505a.htm

Ehren, B., Montgomery, J., Rudebusch, J., & Whitmire, K. (2006). *Responsiveness to intervention: New roles for speech–language pathologists.* Retrieved from www.asha.org/members/slp/schools/prof-consult/NewRolesSLP.htm

Elbin, R. J., Covassin, T., Gallion, C., & Kontos, A. P. (2015, January). Factors influencing risk and recovery from sport-related concussion: Reviewing the evidence. *Perspectives on Neurophysiology and Neurogenic Speech and Language Disorders, 25,* 4–16.

Elementary and Secondary Education Act of 1974, P.L. 93–380.

Elementary and Secondary Education Act of 2001, P.L. 107–110.

Endrew F. by Joseph F. v. Douglas County School Disttrict RE-1, 580 U.S. Part 2 (2017)

Espinosa, L. M. (2013, August). *PreK–3rd: Challenging common myths about dual language learners: An update to the seminal 2008 report* (Policy to Action Brief, No. 10). New York, NY: Foundation for Child Development.

Every Student Succeeds Act of 2015, P.L. 114-95. Retrieved from https://congress.gov/114/plaws/publ95/PLAW-114publ95.pdf

Fagan, P., Friedman, H., & Fulfrost, H. (2007). *Ten most common IEP mistakes—and how to avoid them.* Presented at the Special Education Symposium 2006–2007, Anaheim, CA.

Family Educational Rights and Privacy Act, P.L. 93-380, § 513 (1974). (The Education Amendments of 1974).

Federal Interagency Forum on Child and Family Statistics. (2013). *America's children: Key national indicators of well-being, 2013.* Washington, DC: U.S. Government Printing Office.

Fergus, E. (2010a). Common causes of disproportionality. *California Department of Education Special Education Newsletter.* Retrieved from www.calstat.org/publications/article_detail.php?a_id=128&nl_id=19

Fergus, E. (2010b, October). *Distinguishing difference from disability: The common causes of racial/ethnic disproportionality in special education.* Tempe, AZ: The Equity Alliance at ASU.

Ferguson, M. L. (1991). Collaborative consultative service delivery: An introduction. *Language, Speech, and Hearing Services in Schools, 22,* 147.

Fey, M. (1999, Winter). Speech–language pathology and the early identification and prevention of reading disabilities. *Perspectives,* 13–17.

Fey, M. E., Richard, G. J., Geffner, D., Kamhi, A. G., Medwetsky, L., Paul, D., . . . Schooling, T. (2011). Auditory processing disorder and auditory/language interventions: An evidence-based systematic review. *Language, Speech, and Hearing Services in Schools, 42,* 246–264.

Fjordbak, B. S. (2011, August). Protecting student athletes: Growing number of states pass concussion-related legislation. *The ASHA Leader, 16,* 1–9.

Flahive, M. (2006, July). *Counseling? But I work in schools!* Presented at the ASHA Schools Conference, Phoenix, AZ.

Flasher, L. V., & Fogle, P. T. (2004). *Counseling skills for speech–language pathologists and audiologists.* Clifton Park, NY: Thompson Delmar Learning.

Flippin, M., Reszka, S., & Watson, L. (2010). Effectiveness of the Picture Exchange Communication System (PECS) on communication and speech for children with autism spectrum disorders: A meta-analysis. *American Journal of Speech–Language Pathology, 19,* 178–195.

Flynn, P. (2010). New service delivery models: Connecting SLPs with teachers and curriculum. *The ASHA Leader, 15,* 22.

Flynn, P. (2013, October). Effective service delivery in middle and high schools. *SIG 16 Perspectives on School-Based Issues, 14,* 68–71.

Flynn, P., Ireland, M., & Hall-Mills, S. (2011, November). *State consultants and school based SLPs improving services to students.* Presented at the ASHA Annual Convention, San Diego, CA.

Folmer, R., Griest, S., & Martin, W. (2002). Hearing conservation education programs for children: A review. *Journal of School Health, 72*(2), 51–57.

Freeman, Y., Freeman, D., & Mercuri, S. (2003). Supporting older bilingual students: Keys for success. *NYSABE Journal, 14,* 1–18.

Friend, M., & Bursuck, W. D. (2002). *Including students with special needs: A practical guide for classroom teachers* (3rd ed.). Boston, MA: Allyn and Bacon.

Friend, M., & Bursuck, W. D. (2012). *Including students with special needs: A practical guide for classroom teachers* (7th ed.). New York, NY: Pearson.

Fuchs, D., Fuchs, L. S., & Vaughn, S. (2014). What is intensive instruction and why is it important? *TEACHING Exceptional Children, 46,* 14.

Fullan, M. (2001). *Leading in a culture of change.* San Francisco, CA: Jossey-Bass.

Fullan, M. (2003). *The moral imperative of school leadership.* Thousand Oaks, CA: Corwin Press.

Furr, A. B., Motteler, E., & Helling, C. (2009). *Developing AAC competence in children with complex communication needs.* Retrieved from www.ncatp.org/Resources/Developing_AAC_Competence_in_Children_with_Complex_Communication_Needs.pdf

Gamm, S. (2007). *Disproportionality in special education: Where and why overidentification of minority students occurs.* Horsham, PA: LRP.

Garcia, E. E., Jensen, B. T., & Scribner, K. P. (2009). The demographic imperative. *Education Leadership, 66,* 8–13.

Gerber, M. M., & Durgunoglu, A. Y. (Eds.). (2004). Reading risk and intervention for young English learners: Introduction to special issue. *Learning Disabilities Research and Practice, 19,* 199–201.

German, D. (1992). Word-finding intervention for children and adolescents. *Topics in Language Disorders, 13*(1), 33–50.

Gierut, J. A. (2001). Complexity in phonological treatment: Clinical factors. *Language, Speech, and Hearing Services in Schools, 32,* 229–241.

Gillam, R., Baker, E., & Williams, L. (2012, November). *How much is enough? Dosage in child language intervention.* Paper presented at the ASHA Annual Convention, Atlanta, GA.

Gillam, S. L., & Gillam, R. B. (2006). Making evidence-based decisions about child language intervention in schools. *Language, Speech, and Hearing Services in Schools, 37*(4), 304–315.

Golden, D. C. (n.d.). *IDEA '04 assistive technology definition revision.* Retrieved from www.asha.org/Advocacy/federal/idea/04-law-assist-tech

Goldsworthy, C. L. (1996). *Developmental reading disabilities: A language-based treatment approach.* San Diego, CA: Singular.

Goldsworthy, C., & Peretti, R. (2012). *Sourcebook of phonological awareness activities: Curriculum relevant literature* (Vol. 4). Independence, KY: Delmar Cengage Learning.

Goldsworthy, C., & Peretti, R. (2013). *Sourcebook of phonological awareness activities: Curriculum relevant literature* (Vol. 4). Clifton Park, NY: Delmar Cengage Learning.

Goss v. Lopez, 419 U.S. 565 (1975).

Gray, C., & Garand, J. (1993). Social Stories: Improving responses of students with autism with accurate social information. *Focus on Autistic Behavior, 8*(1), 1–10.

Gray, C., & White, A. L. (2002). *My social stories book.* New York, NY: Jessica Kingsley.

Gutiérrez-Clellen, V. F., & Peña, E. (2001). Dynamic assessment of diverse children: A tutorial. *Language, Speech and Hearing Services in Schools, 32,* 212–224.

Gutstein, S. E., Burgess, A. F., & Montfrot, K. (2007). Evaluation of the relationship development intervention program. *Autism, 11,* 397–411.

Hall, D. (2013, February). *A step forward or step back? State accountability in the Waiver Era.* Washington, DC: The Education Trust.

Handicapped Children's Protection Act, P.L. 99–372 (1986) (Attorneys' Fees Bill).

Hardman, M. L., Drew, C. J., & Egan, M. W. (2011). *Human exceptionality: School, community, and family* (10th ed.). Belmont, CA: Wadsworth Cengage Learning.

Harris, A. (n.d.). *Visual support for students with autism.* John Hopkins School of Education. Retrieved from www.education.jhu.edu/pd/newhorizons/journals/specialedjournal/harris

Harry, B., & Klingner, J. (2006). *Why are so many minority students in special education? Understanding race and disability in schools.* New York, NY: Teachers College Press, Columbia University.

Harry, B., & Klingner, J. (2007). Discarding the deficit model. *Educational Leadership, 64*(5), 16–21.

Hart, B., & Risley, T. R. (1995). *Meaningful differences in the everyday experience of young American children.* Baltimore, MD: Brookes.

Haynes, W., & Johnson, C. (2008). *Understanding research and evidence-based practice in communication disorders: A primer for students and practitioners.* Boston, MA: Pearson Education.

Haynes, W. O., & Pindzola, R. H. (2012). *Diagnosis and evaluation in speech pathology* (8th ed.). Boston, MA: Pearson Education.

Health Insurance Portability and Accountability Act, P.L. 104–191 (1996, 2003).

Herer, G. R. (2007). Universal newborn screening. In S. Schwartz (Ed.), *Choices in deafness: A parents' guide to communication options* (3rd ed.). Bethesda, MD: Woodbine House.

Herer, G. R. (2015). *Early detection and intervention.* Seminar at Chapman University, Orange, CA.

Herer, G. R., Knightly, C. A., & Steinberg, A. G. (2007). Hearing: Sounds and silences. In M. L. Batshaw (Ed.), *Children with disabilities* (6th ed.). Baltimore, MD: Paul H. Brookes.

Higher Education Opportunity Act, P.L. 110–315 (2008).

Homer, E. (2008, April). Establishing a public school dysphagia program: A model for administration and service provision. *Language, Speech, and Hearing Services in Schools, 39,* 177–191.

Homer, E. (2009, October). Issues of management of swallowing and feeding disorders in the school setting. *SIG 13 Perspectives on Swallowing and Swallowing Disorders (Dysphagia), 18,* 80–85.

Homer, E. M., Bickerton, C., Hill, S., Parham, L., & Taylor, D. (2000). Development of an interdisciplinary dysphagia team in the public schools. *Language, Speech and Hearing Services in Schools, 31,* 62–75.

Honig v. Doe, 484 U.S., 305 (1988).

Hoskins, B., & Noel, K. (2011). *Conversations framework: A program for adolescents and young adults.* Chippewa Falls, WI: Cognitive Press.

Hosp, J. L. (2006, May). Implementing RTI: Assessment practices and response to intervention. *Communiqué, 34*(7). Retrieved from www.nasponline.org/publications/cq/cq347rti.aspx

Howard, T. C. (2010). *Why race and culture matter in schools: Closing the achievement gap in America's classrooms.* New York, NY: Teachers College Press.

Hudley, A. H. C., & Mallinson, C. (2011). *Understanding English language variation in U.S. schools.* New York, NY: Teachers College Press.

Huebner, T. A. (2010). What research says about year-round schooling. *Education Leadership, 67,* 82–84.

Illinois State Board of Education. (2012). *Frequently asked questions about special education eligibility and entitlement within a response to intervention (RtI) framework.* Springfield, IL: Author. Retrieved from www.isbe.net/SPEC-ED/pdfs/faq_sped_entitlement_rti.pdf

Individuals With Disabilities Education Act of 1990, 20 U.S.C. § 1400 *et seq.* (1990) (amended 1991).

Individuals With Disabilities Education Act of 1990, 20 U.S.C. § 1400 *et seq.* (1990) (amended 1997).

Individuals With Disabilities Education Improvement Act of 2004, 20 U.S.C. § 1400 *et seq.* (2004).

Institute of Educational Sciences and National Center on Educational Statistics. (n.d.). *Early Childhood Longitudinal Program: Kindergarten class of 2010–11* (ECLS-K: 2011). Retrieved from http://nces.ed.gov/ecls/kindergarten2011.asp

Interdisciplinary Council on Developmental and Learning Disorders. (2000). *ICDL clinical practice guidelines: Redefining the standards of care for infants, children, and families with special needs.* Bethesda, MD: ICDL Press.

I.R. by E.N. v. Los Angeles Unified School District, No. 13-56211 (Ninth Circuit Court of Appeals 2015). Retrieved from http://caselaw.findlaw.com/us-9th-circuit/1718616.html

Ireland, M., Hall-Mills, S., & Millikin, C. (2013). Appropriate implementation of severity ratings, regulations, and state guidance: A response to "Using norm-referenced tests to determine severity of language impairment in children: Disconnect between U.S. policy makers and test developers" by Spaulding, Szulga, & Figueria (2012). *Language, Speech, and Hearing Services in Schools, 44,* 320–323.

Jakubowitz, M. (2013). *Telepractice.* Paper presented at the third annual conference of the Orange County Childhood Language Center, Orange, CA.

Joffe, V. L., & Nippold, M. A. (2012). Progress in understanding adolescent language disorders. *Language, Speech, and Hearing Services in Schools, 43,* 438–444.

Johnson, D. W., & Johnson, R. T. (1989). *Cooperation and competition: Theory and research.* Edina, MN: Interaction Books.

Justice, L. M. (2006a). Evidence-based practice, response to intervention, and the prevention of reading difficulties. *Language, Speech, and Hearing Services in Schools, 37*(4), 284–297.

Justice, L. M. (2006b). *Communication sciences and disorders: An introduction.* Upper Saddle River, NJ: Pearson Education.

Justice, L. (2007, March). Evidence based intervention approaches for three emergent literacy domains. *SIG 1 Perspectives on Language Learning and Education, 14,* 9–12.

Justice, L., Dollaghan, C., & Gillam, R. (2010, November). *Evidence-based practice and empirically-supported practices in child language disorders.* Presented at the ASHA Annual Convention, Philadelphia, PA.

Kaderavek, J. N. (2010). *Language disorders in children: Fundamental concepts of assessment and intervention.* Upper Saddle River, NJ: Pearson Education.

Kagan, S. (1994). *Cooperative learning.* San Clemente, CA: Kagan.

Kaloi, L. (n.d.). *Is a 504 plan right for my child? National Center for Learning Disabilities.* Retrieved August 8, 2014, from www.ncld.org/students-disabilities/iep-504-plan/is-504-plan-right-for-my-child

Kamhi, A. G. (2006). Prologue: Combining research and reason to make treatment decisions. *Language, Speech, and Hearing Services in Schools, 37*(4), 255–256.

Kamhi, A., & Catts, H. (Eds.). (2012). *Language and reading disabilities.* Boston, MA: Allyn and Bacon.

Kamil, M. (2003). *Adolescents and literacy: Reading for the 21st century.* Retrieved from www.all4ed.org/publications/AdolescentsAndLiteracy.pdf

Karger, J. (n.d.). *Access to the general curriculum for students with disabilities: A discussion of the interrelationship between IDEA 2004 and NCLB.* Washington, DC: National Center on Accessing the General Curriculum. Retrieved from http://aim.cast.org/learn/historyarchive/backgroundpapers/interrelationship_idea04_nclb#.VVYGWcLbLIV

Kari H. v. Franklin Special School District, 23 IDELR 538 (6th Cir. 1995).

Kena, G., Aud, S., Johnson, F., Wang, X., Zhang, J., Rathbun, A., Wilkinson-Flicker, S., & Kristapovich, P. (2014). *The condition of education 2014* (NCES 2014-083). Washington, DC: U.S. Department of Education, National Center for Education Statistics. Retrieved from http://nces.ed.gov/pubsearch

Kennedy, M. R. T. (2017). *Coaching college students with executive function problems.* New York, NY: Guilford.

Kennedy, M. R. T., Krause, M. O., & O'Brien, K. (2014). Psychometric properties of the college survey for students with brain injury: Individuals with and without traumatic brain injury. *Brain Injury, 28*(13–14), 1748–1757. doi:10.3109/02699052.2014.955883

Kevin T. v. Elmhurst Community School District, No. 205, U.S. Dist. Court for the Northern District of Illinois (2002).

Kimble, C. (2013). Speech–language pathologists' comfort levels in English language learner service delivery. *Communication Disorders Quarterly, 35,* 21–27.

Kleyn, T., & Menken, K. (2009). The difficult road for long-term English learners. *Educational Leadership, 66.* Retrieved from www.ascd.org/publications/educational_leadership/apr09/vol66/num07/The_Difficult_Road_for_Long-Term_English_Learners.aspx

KnowledgeWorks. (2015). *Forecast 4.0.* Retrieved from www.knowledgeworks.org/future-learning/forecast-trailer

KnowledgeWorks. (2016). *The shifting paradigm of teaching: Personalized learning according to teachers.* Retrieved from www.knowledgeworks.org/sites/default/files/u1/teacher-conditions.pdf

Koegel, R. L., Robinson, S., & Koegel, L. K. (2009). Empirically supported intervention practices for autism spectrum disorders in school and community settings. In W. Sailor, G. Dunlap, G. Sugai, & R. Horner (Eds.), *Handbook of positive behavior support* (pp. 149–176). New York, NY: Springer.

Kraemer, R., Coltisor, A., Kalra, M., Martinez, M., Savage, B., Summers, S., & Varadharajan, S. (2013). The speech–language assessment of English language learning students: A non-standardized approach. *SIG 16 Perspectives on School-Based Issues, 14,* 95–101.

Krueger, C. (2012, May 1). *Assistive technology.* Lecture given at California State University Long Beach, CSD 481A.

Kuhn, D. (2006). Speedy Speech: Efficient service delivery for articulation errors. *ASHA Perspectives on School Based Issues, Division 16, 7*(4), 11–14.

Kurjan, R. M. (2000). The role of the school-based speech–language pathologist serving preschool children with dysphagia: A personal perspective. *Language, Speech, and Hearing Services in Schools, 31*(1), 42–49.

Langdon, H. W. (2000). Diversity. In E. Pritchard Dodge (Ed.), *The survival guide for school-based speech–language pathologists* (pp. 367–397). San Diego, CA: Singular.

Langdon, H. W. (2002, April). Language interpreters and translators bridging communication with clients and families. *The ASHA Leader, 7,* 14–15.

Langdon, H. W., & Cheng, L.-R. L. (2002). *Collaborating with interpreters and translators.* Greenville, SC: Thinking.

Langenfeld, K., Thurlow, M., & Scott, D. (1997). *High stakes testing for students: Unanswered questions and implications for students with disabilities* (National Center on Educational Outcomes Synthesis 26). Retrieved from http://cehd.umn.edu/nceo/onlinepubs/Synthesis26.htm

La Paro, K. M., Justice, L., Skibbe, L. E., & Pianta, R. C. (2004). Relations among maternal, child, and demographic factors and the persistence of preschool language impairment. *American Journal of Speech–Language Pathology, 13,* 291–303.

Larson, V. L., & McKinley, N. L. (1995). *Language disorders in older students: Preadolescents and adolescents.* Eau Claire, WI: Thinking.

Larson, V. L., & McKinley, N. L. (2003). *Communication solutions for older students.* Greenville, SC: Thinking.

Larson, V. L., & McKinley, N. L. (2007). *Communication solutions for older students* (pp. 133–134). Austin, TX: PRO-ED.

Larson, V., McKinley, N. L., & Boley, D. (1993). Service delivery models for adolescents with language disorders. *Language, Speech and Hearing Services in Schools, 24,* 36–42.

Law, J., Garrett, Z., & Nye, C. (2003, July). Speech and language therapy interventions for children with primary speech and language delay or disorder. *Cochrane Database of Systematic Reviews,* Art. No. CD004110.

Law, J., Garrett, Z., & Nye, C. (2004). The efficacy of treatment for children with developmental speech and language delay/disorder: A meta-analysis. *Journal of Speech, Language, and Hearing Research, 47,* 924–943.

Learning Point Associates. (2007). *Understanding the No Child Left Behind Act: Reading* (Quick Key Series 1). Naperville, IL: Author.

Lewis, N., Castilleja, N., Moore, B. J., & Rodríguez, B. (2010, July). Assessment 360: A panoramic framework for assessing English language learners. *Perspectives on Communication Disorders and Sciences in Culturally and Linguistically Diverse Populations, 17*(2), 35–56.

Lichtenstein, S., & Klotz, M. (2007). Deciphering the federal regulations on identifying children with specific learning disabilities. *Communiqué, 36*(3). Retrieved from www.nasponline.org/publications/cq/mocq363regs.aspx

Lidz, C. S., & Peña, E. (1996). Dynamic assessment: The model, its relevance as a nonbiased approach, and its application to Latino American preschool children. *Language, Speech, and Hearing Services in Schools, 27,* 367.

Lidz, C. S., & Peña, E. D. (2009). Response to intervention and dynamic assessment: Do we just appear to be speaking the same language? *Seminars in Speech and Language, 30*(2), 121–134.

Lieberman, L. J., & Houston-Wilson, C. (2002). *Strategies for inclusion: A handbook for physical education.* Champaign, IL: Human Kinetics.

Loeb, D., & Gillam, R. (2010). Principles for school-age language intervention: Insights from a randomized controlled trial. *The ASHA Leader, 15,* 10–13.

Losen, D. J., & Orfield, G. (Eds.). (2002). *Racial inequity in special education.* Cambridge, MA: Harvard Education Press.

Louisiana Department of Education. (n.d.). *Speech–language–hearing manual.* Unpublished manuscript.

Luterman, D. (2017). *Counseling persons with communication disorders and their families* (6th ed.). Austin, TX: PRO-ED.

Lyon, G. R. (1998). *Overview of reading and literacy initiatives: Testimony provided to the Committee on Labor and Human Resources, United States Senate.* Bethesda, MD: National Institute of Child Health and Human Development.

Manasse-Cohick, N. (2011). *The role of speech–language pathologists in concussion education.* Presented at the ASHA Annual Convention, San Diego, CA.

Manthey, G. (2007). Modifying instruction so intervention isn't needed. *Leadership, 36*(4), 20.

Margolis, R. H. (2004, August). Boosting memory with informational counseling: Helping patients understand the nature of disorders and how to manage them. *The ASHA Leader, 9,* 10–28.

Marian, V., Faroqi-Shah, Y., Kaushanskaya, M., Blumenfeld, H. K., & Sheng, L. (2009, October). Bilingualism: Consequences for language, cognition, development, and the brain. *The ASHA Leader, 14,* 10–13. Retrieved from http://leader.pubs.asha.org/article.aspx?articleid=2289533

Masterson, J., Apel, K., & Wasowicz, J. (2002). *Spelling evaluation for language and literacy–SPELL* [Computer software]. Evanston, IL: Learning by Design.

Masterson, J., Apel, K., & Wasowicz, J. (2006). *Spelling evaluation for language and literacy–2 (SPELL-2)* [Computer software]. Evanston, IL: Learning by Design.

Maxwell, L. A. (2014, May). 60 years after *Brown,* school diversity more complex than ever. *Education Week.* Retrieved from www.edweek.org/ew/articles/2014/05/14/31brown-overview.h33.html

McCardle, P., Mele-McCarthy, J., Cutting, L., Leos, K., & D'Emilio, T. (2005). Learning disabilities in English language learners: Identifying the issues. *Learning Disabilities Research and Practice, 20*(1), 1–5.

McGinty, A., & Justice, L. M. (2006). Classroom-based versus pull-out language intervention: An examination of the experimental evidence. *EBP Briefs, 1*(1), 1–25.

McLaughlin, M. J., Pullin, D., & Artiles, A. (2001). Challenges for the transformation of special education in the 21st century: Rethinking culture in school reform. *Journal of Special Education Leadership, 14*(2), 51–62.

McNulty, R. J., & Gloeckler, L. C. (2011, February). *Fewer, clearer, higher Common Core State Standards implications for students receiving special education services.* Retrieved from www.leadered.com/pdf/Fewer_Clearer_Higher_CCSS_Special_Education_2014.pdf

McWhirt by McWhirt v. Williamson County School, 23 IDELR 509 (6th Cir. 1994).

Mealings, M., Douglas, J., & Olver, J. (2012). Considering the student perspective in returning to school after TBI: A literature review. *Brain Injury, 26,* 1165–1176.

Meline, T., & Kauffman, C. (2010). A speech–language pathologist's dilemma: What is the best choice for service delivery in schools? *EBP Briefs, 5*(4), 1–14.

Merritt, D. D., & Culatta, B. (1998). *Language intervention in the classroom.* San Diego, CA: Singular.

Mesibov, G. B., & Shea, V. (2009, November). The TEACCH program in the era of evidence-based practice. *Journal of Autism and Developmental Disorders.* doi:10.1007/s10803-009-0901-6. Retrieved from www.interactingwithautism.com/pdf/treating/184.TEACCH%20program%20in%20the%20era%20of%20evidenced%20based.pdf

Methaney, G. (2013, January–February). Promise and potential of new assessment system. *Leadership, 42,* 17.

Michelman, B. (2012, Spring). The never-ending story of ESEA reauthorization. *Policy Priorities, 18*(1). Retrieved from www.ascd.org/publications/newsletters/policy_priorities/vol18/num01/The_Never-Ending_Story_of_ESEA_Reauthorization.aspx

Miller, K. (2015, April). Thinking anew: Trends in the education of students who are deaf or hard of hearing and their implications. *SIG 9 Perspectives on Hearing and Hearing Disorders in Childhood, 25,* 37–44.

Miller, L. (1989). Classroom based language intervention. *Language, Speech, and Hearing Services in Schools, 20,* 153–169.

Mills v. D.C. Board of Education, 348 F. Supp. 866 (D.D.C. 1972).

Mills, W. D. (2005). *Response-to-intervention and instructional consultation teams: The SLP's role* (Slide No. 48, 98-102). Seminar presented at the ASHA Annual Convention, San Diego, CA. Retrieved from http://convention.asha.org/2005/handouts/293_Mills_ W.% 20 David_072063_010906093936 .ppt

Milner, H. R., IV. (2012). *Start where you are, but don't stay there: Understanding diversity, opportunity gaps, and teaching in today's classrooms.* Cambridge, MA: Harvard Education Press.

Mire, S. P., & Montgomery, J. K. (2009). Early intervening for students with speech sound disorders: Lessons from a school district. *Communication Disorders Quarterly, 30,* 155–166.

M. L. by C. D. and S. L. v. Federal Way School District, No. 02-35547 (9th Cir. 2003).

Montana Office of Public Instruction. (2004). *Assistive technology: A special education guide to assistive technology.* Helena, MT: Author. Retrieved from www.opi.mt.gov/PDF/SpecED/guides/AssistiveTech Guide.pdf

Montgomery, J. K. (1992). Clinical forum: Implementing collaborative consultation; Perspectives from the field. *Language, Speech, and Hearing Services in Schools, 23,* 363–364.

Montgomery, J. K. (1999). Accents and dialects: Creating a national professional statement. *Topics in Language Disorders, 19,* 78–89.

Montgomery, J. K. (2000). *Inclusive practices in the middle school.* Presented at Hewes Middle School, Tustin Unified School District, Tustin, CA.

Montgomery, J. K. (2004). *Funnel toward phonics.* Greenville, SC: Super Duper.

Montgomery, J. K. (2014). *Service delivery models: Effective, efficient, intensive.* Online presentation for Chapman University Communication Sciences and Disorders Program, Orange, CA.

Montgomery, J. K., & Bonderman, I. R. (1989). Serving preschool children with severe phonological disorders. *Language, Speech, and Hearing Services in Schools, 20,* 76–84.

Montgomery, J., Dunaway, C., & Taps, J. (2005). Interview with Claudia Dunaway and Jennifer Taps. *Communication Disorders Quarterly, 27*(1), 55–58.

Montgomery, J., & Kahn, N. (2005). *What's your story? Evidence narrative strategies for adolescents.* Greenville, SC: Super Duper Publications.

Montgomery, J., & Kahn, N. (2007). *Ten steps to writing better essays.* Greenville, SC: Super Duper.

Montgomery, J., & Moore, B. (2011, November). *Listen, learn, lead: Expanding to integrated models of service delivery.* Presented at the ASHA Annual Convention, San Diego, CA.

Montgomery, J. K., & Moore-Brown, B. J. (2005, May). *Response to intervention: An alternative to special education.* Paper presented at the ASHA Telephone Seminar, Rockville, MD.

Moore, B. J. (2010). *Documentation for SLPs and audiologists in schools* [Audio program]. Rockville, MD: ASHA.

Moore, B. J. (2012, April). Five common documentation questions—answered. *The ASHA Leader, 17,* 22–24. Retrieved from www.asha.org/Publications/leader/2012/120403/Five-Common-Documentation-Questions-Answered.htm

Moore, B. (2013). Documentation issues in speech–language pathology and audiology. In R. Lubinski & M. Hudson (Eds.), *Professional issues in speech–language pathology and audiology* (4th ed.). Clifton Park, NY: Cengage/Delmar.

Moore, B. (2014a, May). *Common Core State Standards and students with severe cognitive disabilities* [Webinar for PresenceLearning].

Moore, B. (2014b, July). *The legally defensible SLP.* Presented at the North Carolina Exceptional Children Division Summer Institute, Greensboro, NC.

Moore, B. J., & Montgomery, J. K. (2008). *Making a difference for America's children: Speech–language pathologists in public schools* (2nd ed.). Austin, TX: PRO-ED.

Moore, B. J., & Nishida, B. (2014, Fall). Cultivating the landscape of Common Core State Standards (CCSS). *CSHA Magazine, 44,* 12–13, 34.

Moore-Brown, B. (1998). When supervisor and supervisee disagree: Ethics Roundtable. *ASHA Magazine, 40,* 54.

Moore-Brown, B. (2000, March). *Skills and competencies needed by the school-based speech–language pathologist in the 21st century: Implications of educational trends.* Paper presented at the Speech–Language Pathologists of Area Education Agency 6, Marshalltown, IA.

Moore-Brown, B. (2001, October). Public school talk: Supervision of paraprofessionals in a school setting: Oversight and insight. *SIG 11 Perspectives on Administration and Supervision, 11,* 16–18.

Moore-Brown, B. (2004, March). Becoming proficient in the lessons of No Child Left Behind. *Perspectives on School Based Issues, 5*(1), 7–10.

Moore-Brown, B. (2006). *Lessons from due process: Being prepared and legally defensible.* National CEU Online Seminar. Retrieved from www.nationalceu.com/Product.aspx?ProductID=11

Moore-Brown, B. (2007). E-ticket service delivery: Effective, efficient, economical and evidence-based. *Perspectives on School Based Issues, Division 16, 8*(1), 11–14.

Moore-Brown, B., Huerta, M., Uranga-Hernandez, Y., & Peña, E. (2006). Using dynamic assessment to evaluate children with suspected learning disabilities. *Intervention in School and Clinic, 41*(4), 209–217.

Moore-Brown, B. J., & Montgomery, J. K. (2001). *Making a difference for America's children: Speech–language pathologists in public schools.* Greenville, SC: Thinking.

Moore-Brown, B. J., Montgomery, J. K., Bielinski, J., & Shubin, J. (2005). Responsiveness to intervention: Teaching before testing helps avoid labeling. *Topics in Language Disorders, 25,* 148–167.

Moore-Brown, B., & Nishida, B. (2002). To screen or not to screen. . . . That is the question. *CSHA Magazine, 31*(4), 39–41.

Moore-Brown, B., Nishida, B., & Laverty-Reeves, R. (2003). *Best practices: Management of speech–language caseloads in California public schools.* Retrieved from www.csha.org/positionpapers

Morrisette, M. L., & Geriut, J. A. (2002). Lexical organization and phonological change in treatment. *Journal of Speech, Language and Hearing Research, 45,* 153–159.

Mullen, R. (2000). Data report available for K–6 schools component of NOMS. *ASHA Special Interest Division 16, 1*(3), 18.

A multitiered system of supports with response to intervention and universal design for learning: Putting it all together. (2015, Spring). *The Special EDge.* Retrieved from www.calstat.org/publications/pdfs/EDge_spring_2015_insert_final_.pdf

Musgrove, M. (2012). *Dear Colleague letter.* Office of Special Education and Rehabilitative Services. Retrieved from www2.ed.gov/policy/speced/guid/idea/memosdcltrs/preschoollre22912.pdf

National Association for the Education of Young Children. (2005). *Screening and assessment of young English-language learners: Supplement to the NAEYC position statement on early childhood curriculum, assessment, and program evaluation.* Washington, DC: Author.

National Autism Center. (2009). *Findings and conclusions: National Standards Project, Phase 1.* Randolph, MA: Author.

National Autism Center. (2015). *Findings and conclusions: National Standards Project, Phase 2.* Randolph, MA: Author.

National Center and State Collaborative. (n.d.). *Commitment to communicative competence.* Retrieved from www.ncscpartners.org/Media/Default/PDFs/Resources/Parents/NCSC-Communicative-Competence-9–10–13.pdf

National Center for Education Statistics. (2014). *The condition of education 2014.* Retrieved from nces.ed.gov/pubs2014/2014083.pdf

National Center for Education Statistics. (2015). *Early childhood longitudinal study, kindergarten class of 2010–2011.* Washington, DC: Author. Retrieved from https://nces.ed.gov/ecls/kindergarten2011.asp

National Center for Education Statistics, U.S. Department of Education. (2016). *The condition of education 2016* (NCES 2016-144). Washington, DC: Author.

National Center for Learning Disabilities. (n.d.). *Issue brief: Multi-tiered system of supports: Aka response to intervention (RTI).* Retrieved from www.ncld.org/wp-content/uploads/2011/05/MTSS-brief-in-LJ-template.pdf

National Center on Intensive Intervention. (2013). *Data based individualization: A framework for intervention.* Retrieved from www.intensiveintervention.org/sites/default/files/DBI_Framework.pdf

National Center on Response to Intervention. (2010, March). *Essential components of RTI: A closer look at response to intervention.* Washington, DC: U.S. Department of Education, Office of Special Education Programs, National Center on Response to Intervention.

National Center on Student Progress Monitoring. (n.d.). Retrieved from www.studentprogress.org

National Commission on Excellence in Education. (1983). *A nation at risk: The imperative for educational reform.* Retrieved from www2.ed.gov/pubs/NatAtRisk/appenda.html

National Dissemination Center for Children With Disabilities. (2004, January). *Severe/multiple disabilities: Disability fact sheet—No. 10.* Retrieved September 1, 2007, from www.nichcy.org/pubs/factshe/fs10.pdf

National Dissemination Center for Children With Disabilities. (2010, October). *IDEA's definition of "highly qualified."* Retrieved from http://nichcy.org/schools-administrators/hqt/idea

National Education Association. (2007). *Truth in labeling: Disproportionality in special education.* Washington, DC: Author. Retrieved from www.nea.org/assets/docs/HE/EW-TruthInLabeling.pdf

National Education Association. (2008). *Disproportionality: Inappropriate identification of culturally and linguistically diverse children* [NEA policy brief]. Retrieved from www.nea.org/assets/docs/HE/mf_PB02_Disproportionality.pdf

National Education Association. (n.d.-a). *Are you a "highly qualified" paraprofessional?* Retrieved from www.nea.org/home/19102.htm

National Education Association. (n.d.-b). *Research spotlight on block scheduling.* Retrieved from www.nea.org/tools/16816.htm

National Institutes of Health. (1993). *Consensus statement on early identification of hearing impairment in infants and young children.* Bethesda, MD: Author.

National Joint Committee for the Communication Needs of Persons With Severe Disabilities. (2002). *Access to communication services and supports: Concerns regarding the application of restrictive "eligibility" policies* [Technical report]. Retrieved from www.asha.org/policy/TR2002-00233

National Joint Committee on Learning Disabilities. (2008). *Adolescent literacy and older students with learning disabilities.* Retrieved from www.asha.org/policy/TR2008-00304.htm

National Joint Committee on Learning Disabilities. (2010). *Comprehensive assessment and evaluation of students with learning disabilities.* Retrieved from www.ldonline.org/about/partners/njcld

National Literacy Act of 1991, P.L. 102-73, 102nd Cong. (1991).

National Reading Panel. (2000). *Teaching children to read: An evidence-based assessment of the scientific research literature on reading and its implications for reading instruction.* Washington, DC: U.S. Department of Health and Human Services.

National Reading Panel. (2006). *Teaching children to read: An evidence-based assessment of the scientific literature on reading and its implication for reading instruction.* Retrieved from www.nichd.nih.gov/publications/pubs/nrp/Documents/report.pdf

National Research Council. (2001). Educating children with autism: Committee on Educational Interventions for Children With Autism. In C. Lord & J. P. McGee (Eds.), *Division of Behavioral and Social Sciences and Education.* Washington, DC: National Academy Press.

National Research Council. (2002). Minority students in special and gifted education. In M. S. Donovan & C. T. Cross (Eds.), *Committee on Minority Representation in Special Education, Division of Behavioral and Social Sciences and Education.* Washington, DC: National Academy Press.

National Research Council & Institute of Medicine. (2000). *From neurons to neighborhoods: The science of early childhood development* (J. P. Shonkoff & D. A. Phillips, Eds.). Washington, DC: National Academy Press.

National School Boards Association. (2014, January). *Individuals With Disabilities Education Act (IDEA): Early preparation for reauthorization.* Retrieved from www.nsba.org/sites/default/files/reports/Issue%20Brief-Individuals%20with%20Disabilities%20Education%20Act.pdf

Nelson, N. W. (1992). Targets of curriculum-based language assessment. In W. Secord & J. Damico (Eds.), *Best practices in school speech–language pathology: Descriptive nonstandardized language assessment* (pp. 73–85). San Antonio, TX: Psychological Corporation.

Nelson, N. W., & Hoskins, B. (1997). *Strategies for supporting classroom success* [Audiotape set]. San Diego, CA: Singular.

Neuman, S. B. (2009). *Changing the odds for children at risk: Seven essential principles of educational programs that break the cycle of poverty.* Westport, CT: Praeger.

New America Foundation. (2012, March). *Individuals With Disabilities Education Act overview. Federal Education Budget Project.* Retrieved from http://febp.newamerica.net/background-analysis/individuals-disabilities-education-act-overview

New America Foundation. (2014a, April). *Federal, state, and local K-12 school finance overview. Federal Education Budget Project.* Retrieved from http://febp.newamerica.net/background-analysis/school-finance

New America Foundation. (2014b, April). *No Child Left Behind overview. Federal Education Budget Project.* Retrieved from http://febp.newamerica.net/background-analysis/no-child-left-behind-overview

New America Foundation. (2014c, April). *Individuals With Disabilities Education Act: Cost impact on local school districts. Federal Education Budget Project.* Retrieved from http://febp.newamerica.net/background-analysis/individuals-disabilities-education-act-cost-impact-local-school-districts

New York State Education Department. (2010). *Minimum requirements of a response to intervention program (RtI): Use of RtI in the determination of a learning disability.* Retrieved from www.p12.nysed.gov/specialed/RTI/guidance/LD.htm

No Child Left Behind Act of 2001, 20 U.S.C. 70 § 6301 *et seq.* (2002).

Nolet, V., & McLaughlin, M. J. (2000). *Accessing the general curriculum including students with disabilities in standards-based reform.* Thousand Oaks, CA: Corwin Press.

North Central Regional Educational Laboratory and the Metiri Group. (2003). *enGauge 21st century skills.* Retrieved from http://pict.sdsu.edu/engauge21st.pdf

Oberti v. Board of Education of Borough of Clementon School District, No. 92-5462 (3rd Cir. 1993).

Office for Civil Rights, § 104.4 [a] (1999).

Office of Special Education and Rehabilitative Services. (1999, March). *IDEA '97.* Retrieved from www .ed.gov/offices/OSERS/IDEA/IDEA.pdf

Office of Special Education Programs. (2000). *Twenty-five years of progress in educating children with disabilities through IDEA.* Retrieved from www.ed.gov/policy/speced/leg/idea/history.pdf

Office of Special Education Programs. (n.d.). *IDEA dispute resolution processes comparison chart.* Retrieved from www.directionservice.org/cadre/exemplar/artifacts/MD-7%20IDEA%20Dispute%20 Resolution%20Processes%20Comparison%20Chart.pdf

Olsen, L. (2010). *Reparable harm: Fulfilling the unkept promise of educational opportunity for California's long term English learners.* Retrieved from www.californianstogether.org/reparable-harm-fulfilling-the-unkept-promise-of-educational-opportunity-for-californias-long-term-english-learners

Ortiz, A. A., & Yates, J. R. (2002). Considerations in the assessment of English language learners referred to special education. In A. J. Artiles & A. A. Ortiz (Eds.), *English language learners with special education needs.* Washington, DC: Center for Applied Linguistics.

O'Toole, T. J. (2000). Legal, ethical, and financial aspects of providing services to children with swallowing disorders in the public schools. *Language, Speech, and Hearing Services in Schools, 31,* 56–61.

Patient Protection and Affordable Health Care Act, P.L. 111–148, 111th Cong. (2010).

Paul, R., & Roth, F. P. (2011, July). Characterizing and predicting outcomes of communication delays in infants and toddlers: Implications for clinical practice. *Language, Speech, and Hearing Services in Schools, 42,* 331–340.

Peña, E. (2000). Measurement of modifiability in children from culturally and linguistically diverse backgrounds. *Communication Disorders Quarterly, 21*(3), 87–97.

Peña, E. D. (2012, April). *Language assessment and treatment in ELL children: Current recommendations.* Presented at the California Speech–Language–Hearing Association Annual Convention, San Francisco, CA.

Pennsylvania Association for Retarded Children (PARC) v. Commonwealth of Pennsylvania, 334 F. Supp. 1257 (E.D. PA 1972).

Polmanteer, K., & Turbiville, V. (2000). Family responsive individualized family service plans for speech–language pathologists. *Language, Speech, and Hearing Services in Schools, 31*(1), 4–14.

Poolaw v. Bishop, 67 F.3d 830 (9th Cir. 1995).

Positive Behavioral Interventions and Supports. (n.d.). *PBIS and the law.* Retrieved August 31, 2014 from www.pbis.org/school/pbis-and-the-law

Posny, A. (2007, March). *Director of OSEP, to Catherine D. Clarke, director of Education and Regulatory Advocacy, ASHA.* Retrieved from www.ed.gov/policy/speced/guid/idea/letters/2007-1/clarke030807 disability1q2007.pdf

Power-deFur, L., & Flynn, P. (2012). Unpacking the standards for intervention. *Perspectives on School-Based Issues, 13,* 11–16.

Pransky, K. (2009). There's more to see. *Education Leadership, 66*(7), 74–78.

Prelock, P. A. (2000a, July). An intervention focus for inclusionary practice. *Language, Speech, and Hearing Services in Schools, 31,* 296–298.

Prelock, P. A. (2000b). Multiple perspectives for determining the roles of speech–language pathologists in inclusionary classrooms. *Language, Speech, and Hearing Services in Schools, 31,* 213–218.

Prelock, P. A. (2001). Understanding autism spectrum disorders: The role of speech–language pathologists and audiologists in service delivery. *The ASHA Leader, 6,* 4–7.

Prelock, P. A., Beatson, J., Bitner, B., Broder, C., & Ducker, A. (2003, July). Interdisciplinary assessment of young children with autism spectrum disorder. *Language, Speech, and Hearing Services in Schools, 34,* 194–202.

Preschool Amendments to the Education of the Handicapped Act, P.L. 99–457, 99th Cong. (1986). Retrieved from www.gpo.gov/fdsys/pkg/STATUTE-100/pdf/STATUTE-100-Pg1145.pdf

President's Commission on Excellence in Special Education. (2002, July). *A new era: Revitalizing special education for children and their families.* Retrieved from http://ectacenter.org/~pdfs/calls/2010/ earlypartc/revitalizing_special_education.pdf

Prizant, B. (2015). *Uniquely human: A different way of seeing autism.* New York, NY: Simon & Schuster.

Prizant, B. M., Wetherby, A. M., Rubin, E., & Laurent, A. C. (2010). The SCERTS model. In K. Siri & T. Lyons (Ed.), *Cutting-edge therapies for autism: 2010–2011*. New York, NY: Skyhorse.

Prizant, B., Wetherby, A., Rubin, E., Laurent, A., & Rydell, P. (2006). *The SCERTS model: A comprehensive educational approach for children with autism spectrum disorders*. Baltimore, MD: Paul H. Brookes.

R.B. v. Napa Valley Unified School Dist. R.B., by and through her guardian ad litem, F.B., and F.B, plaintiff(s), v. Napa Valley Unified School District, defendant, No. 05–16404, U.S. Court of Appeals (9th Cir. 2007). Retrieved from http://caselaw.findlaw.com/us-9th-circuit/1432896.html#sthash.LrNruoz0.dpuf

Rehabilitation Act Amendments of 1992, Pub. L. No. 102–569, § 508, 106 Stat. 4430 (1992).

Rehabilitation Act of 1973, 29 U.S.C. § 794, Section 504 (1973).

Reynhout, G., & Carter, M. (2006). Social stories for children with disabilities. *Journal of Autism and Developmental Disorders, 36*(4), 445–469.

Richard, G. (2008, September). Autism spectrum disorders in the schools assessment, diagnosis, and intervention pose challenges for SLPs. *The ASHA Leader, 13*, 26–28.

Riquelme, L. F. (2013, November). Evolving expressions of culture. *The ASHA Leader, 18*, 52–55.

Ritzman, M. J., & Sanger, D. (2007). Principals' opinions on the role of speech–language pathologists serving students with communication disorders involved in violence. *Language, Speech, and Hearing Services in Schools, 38*, 1–13.

Rooney, R. (2009). *ECO COSF 101: What is a functional outcome?* Presented at the ASHA Annual Convention, New Orleans, LA.

Rooney Moreau, M., & Fidrych-Puzzo, H. (1994). *The story grammar maker: A guide for improving speaking, reading and writing skills within your existing program*. Easthampton, MA: Discourse Skills Productions.

Rosa-Lugo, L. I., Rivera, E., & Rierson, T. K. (2010). The role of dynamic assessment within the response to intervention model in school-age English language learners. *SIG 16 Perspectives on School-Based Issues, 11*, 99–106. Retrieved from http://sig16perspectives.pubs.asha.org/article.aspx?articleid=1768676#_ga=1.187356716.509329459.1419034974

Roseberry-McKibbin, C. (2007). *Language disorders in children: A multicultural and case perspective*. Boston, MA: Allyn and Bacon.

Roseberry-McKibbin, C. (2008). *Increasing language skills of students from low-income backgrounds: Practical strategies for professionals*. San Diego, CA: Plural.

Roseberry-McKibbin, C. (2012, July). *The impact of poverty and homelessness on children's oral and literate language: Practical implications for service delivery*. Paper presented at the ASHA Schools Conference, Milwaukee, WI.

Rosenbek, J. C. (1984). Treating the dysarthric talker. *Seminars in Speech and Language, 5*(4), 359–384.

Roth, F. P., Dougherty, D. P., Paul, D. R., & Adamczyk, D. (2010). *RTI in action: Oral language activities for K–2 classrooms*. Rockville, MD: American Speech–Language–Hearing Association.

Roth, F. P., & Worthington, C. K. (2000). *Treatment resource manual for speech–language pathology* (2nd ed.). San Diego, CA: Singular Thomson Press.

Roth, F. P., & Worthington, C. K. (2013). *Treatment resource manual for speech–language pathology* (5th ed.). Clifton Park, NY: Cengage Learning.

RtI, RtI2, MTSS: Establishing clarity. (2013, Summer). *The Special EDge, 26*(3). Retrieved from www.calstat.org/publications/pdfs/summer_2013-spedge-english.pdf

Rudebusch, J. (2008). *The source for RTI: Response to intervention*. East Moline, IL: LinguiSystems.

Rudebusch, J. (2012, March). From Common Core State Standards to standards-based IEPs: A brief tutorial. *SIG 16 Perspectives on School-Based Issues, 13*, 17–24.

Rudebusch, J., & Wiechmann, J. (2011, August). How to fit response to intervention into a heavy workload. *The ASHA Leader, 16*(10), 10–13.

Sacramento City School Dist. v. Rachel H., 14 F.3d 1398 (9th Cir. 1994).

Samuels, C. A. (2016, February 23). ESSA spotlights strategy to reach diverse learners. *Education Week*. Retrieved from www.edweek.org/ew/articles/2016/02/24/essa-spotlights-strategy-to-reach-diverse-learners.html

Sandall, S., Hemmeter, M. L., Smith, B. J., & McLean, M. E. (2005). *DEC recommended practices: A comprehensive guide for practical application in early intervention/early childhood special education*. Longmont, CO: Sopris West.

San Diego City Schools. (2004–2005). *Articulation differences and disorders manual*. San Diego, CA: Author. Retrieved from www.csha.org/pdf/CSHAArticulationManual.pdf

Sanger, D., & Moore-Brown, B. (2000, November). *Advancing the discussion on communication and violence*. Presented at the ASHA Annual Convention, Washington, DC.

Sanger, D., Moore-Brown, B., & Alt, E. (2000). Advancing the discussion on communication and violence. *Communication Disorders Quarterly, 22*(1), 43–48.

Schaffer v. Weast (State of Maryland; U.S. Supreme Court 54 U.S. 04-698) (2005).

Scherer, M. (2009). In the neighborhood. *Educational Leadership, 66*, 7.

Schmitt, M. B., & Justice, L. (2011). Schools as complex host environments: Understanding aspects of schools that may influence clinical practice and research. *The ASHA Leader, 16*, 8–11. Retrieved from http://leader.pubs.asha.org/article.aspx?articleid=2279098

Schooling, T., Venediktov, R., & Leech, H. (2010). *Evidence-based systematic review: Effects of service delivery on the speech and language skills of children from birth to 5 years of age*. Rockville, MD: ASHA.

Secord, W. A. (1999). *School consultation: Concepts, models, and procedures*. Flagstaff, AZ: Northern Arizona University.

Secord, W. A., & Damico, J. S. (1998, Summer). *Let's get practical: 49 ways to work with teachers in the classroom*. Presented at the summer schools conferences on Achieving Successful Outcomes in Schools of the American Speech–Language–Hearing Association, Washington, DC.

Shepard, S., & Sheng, L. (2009). Vocabulary intervention for elementary and secondary school students who are English language learners: A review of research. *EBP Briefs, 4*(4), 1–13.

Shipley, K. G., & McAfee, J. G. (2009). *Assessment in speech–language pathology: A resource manual* (4th ed.). Clifton Park, NY: Delmar Cengage Learning.

Shorter, T. N. (2004). *Understanding HIPPA: A guide to school district privacy obligations*. Horsham, PA: LRP.

Silliman, E., & Scott, C. (2006). Language impairment and reading disability: Connections and complexities; Introduction to the special issue. *Learning Disabilities Research and Practice, 21*, 1–7.

Singer, B. D., & Bashir, A. S. (1999). What are executive functions and self-regulation and what do they have to do with language learning disorders? *Language, Speech, and Hearing Services in Schools, 30*, 265–273.

Singer, B. D., & Bashir, A. S. (2004). EmPOWER: A strategy for helping students with language disorders learn to write expository text. In E. Silliman & L. C. Wilkinson *(Eds.), Language and literacy learning* (pp. 239–272). New York, NY: Guilford.

Slavin, R. E. (1990). *Cooperative learning: Theory, research, and practice*. Englewood Cliffs, NJ: Prentice Hall.

Smarter Balanced Assessment Consortium. (2016). *Testing technology*. Retrieved from www.smarterbalanced.org/smarter-balanced-assessments/computer-adaptive-testing

Snow, C. E., Burns, M. S., & Griffin, P. (Eds.). (1998). *Preventing reading difficulties in young children*. Washington, DC: National Academy Press.

Snow, K. (2017). *People first language*. Retrieved from www.disabilityisnatural.com/people-first-language.html

Special education: A service, not a place. (2013). *The Special EDge, 27*(1). Retrieved from www.calstat.org/publications/pdfs/edge_autumn2013.pdf

Speech–language pathologist overview. (2016). *U.S. News and World Report*. Retrieved from http://money.usnews.com/careers/best-jobs/speech–language-pathologist

Statewide Special Education Task Force. (2015). *Conceptual framework for Special Education Task Force: Successful educational evidenced based practices*. Retrieved from www.smcoe.org/assets/files/about-smcoe/superintendents-office/statewide-special-education-task-force/EBP%20-%20Final%203.2.15.pdf

Stone, C. A., Silliman, E. R., Ehren, B. J., & Wallach, G. (Eds.). (2014). *Handbook of language and literacy: Development and disorders* (2nd ed.). New York, NY: Guilford.

Sturm, J. (2012, November). *Providing effective differentiated writing instruction for students with developmental disabilities*. Presented at the ASHA Annual Convention, Atlanta, GA.

Sturm, J. (2015). *First author writing curriculum*. Volo, IL: Don Johnston.

Taps, J. (2006, December). An innovative educational approach for addressing articulation differences. *Perspectives on School-Based Issues, 7*(4), 7–11.

Taps, J. (2008, October). RtI services for children with mild articulation needs: Four years of data. *Perspectives on School-Based Issues, 9*(3), 104–110.

Taps, J. (2009). Efficient articulation services: One group at a time. *California Speech–Language–Hearing Association Magazine, 38*(4), 11–14.

Texas Speech–Language–Hearing Association. (n.d.). *Linguistically diverse populations: Considerations and resources for assessment and intervention.* Retrieved from www.txsha.org/Diversity_Issues/cld_document.asp

Texas Woman's University. (2016). *Project INSPIRE: Least restrictive environment (LRE), inclusion and mainstreaming.* Retrieved from www.twu.edu/inspire/least-restrictive.asp

Thiemann-Bourque, K. (2010). Navigating the transition to middle school: Peer network programming for students with autism. *The ASHA Leader, 15,* 12–15.

Thordardottir, E. (2006, August 15). Language intervention from a bilingual mind. *ASHA Leader,* 6–7, 20–21.

Thrasher, A., Burke, H., Klaer, M., & Schaller, S. (2012). *Video modeling and peer play in young children with autism: Story of friendship.* Presented at the ASHA Annual Convention, Atlanta, GA.

Throneburg, R. N., Calvert, L. K., Sturm, J. J., Paramboukas, A. A., & Paul, P. A. (2000). A comparison of service delivery models: Effects on curricular vocabulary skills in the school setting. *American Journal of Speech–Language Pathology, 9,* 10–20.

Thurlow, M. (2015). Stepping up for the next challenge. *The Special EDge, 29*(1), 10–12.

Tomlinson, C. A. (2006). Differentiating instruction: Why bother? *Middle Ground, 9*(1), 11–15.

Toner, M., & Helmer, D. (2006). *Language and learning in school-age children and adolescents: When language is normal but reading isn't: Possible solutions.* Poster board presentation at the ASHA Annual Convention, Miami Beach, FL.

Torgeson, J. K. (1998). Catch them before they fall: Identification and assessment to prevent reading failure in young children. *American Educator, 22*(1–2), 32–39.

Torres, I. G. (2013, February). Know what you don't know. *The ASHA Leader, 18,* 38–41.

Troia, G. (2005). Responsiveness to intervention: Roles of SLPs in the prevention and identification of learning disabilities. *Topics in Language Disorders, 25,* 106–119.

Trukstra, L. S., & Byom, L. J. (2010). Executive functions and communication in adolescents. *The ASHA Leader, 15,* 8–11.

Turnbull, H. R., III. (1993). *Free appropriate public education: The law and children with disabilities* (4th ed.). Denver, CO: Love.

Ujifusa, A. (2016, May 31). Proposed ESSA rules aim to walk fine line on accountability. *Education Week.* Retrieved from www.edweek.org/ew/articles/2016/06/01/proposed-essa-rules-aim-to-walk-fine.html

Ukrainetz, T. A. (2006). *Contextualized language intervention: Scaffolding K–12 literacy achievement.* Greenville, SC: Thinking.

Ukrainetz, T. (Ed.). (2015). *School-age language intervention: Evidence-based practices.* Austin, TX: PRO-ED.

Ukrainetz, T., Proctor-Williams, K., Baumann, B., Allen, M., Hoffman, L. M., & Justice, L. (2008, November). *How much is enough? The intensity evidence in language intervention.* Presented at the ASHA Annual Convention, Chicago, IL.

Union v. Smith, 15 F.3d 1519, Union School District v. B Smith 2-7 Union School District. Retrieved from http://openjurist.org/15/f3d/1519/union-school-district-v-b-smith-2-7-union-school-district

U.S. Department of Commerce. (1993). *We the American children.* Washington, DC: U.S. Government Printing Office.

U.S. Department of Education. (2010). *Guidelines for educators and administrators for implementing Section 504 of the Rehabilitation Act of 1973: Subpart D.* Retrieved from https://doe.sd.gov/oess/documents/sped_section504_Guidelines.pdf

U.S. Department of Education. (2013). *2013 annual reports to Congress on the Individuals With Disabilities Education Act (IDEA).* Retrieved from www2.ed.gov/about/reports/annual/osep/2013/index.html

U.S. Department of Education. (2014, June). *New accountability framework raises the bar for state special education programs.* Washington, DC: The Education Trust. Retrieved from www.ed.gov/news/press-releases/new-accountability-framework-raises-bar-state-special-education-programs

U.S. Department of Education. (n.d.-a). Prior written notice. Retrieved from http://idea.ed.gov/download/modelform2_Prior_Written_Notice.pdf

U.S. Department of Education. (n.d.-b). Protecting students with disabilities. Retrieved from www2.ed.gov/about/offices/list/ocr/504faq.html

U.S. Departments of Education and Health and Human Services. (2015, May). *Draft policy statement on inclusion of children with disabilities (executive summary).* Retrieved from www2.ed.gov/policy/speced/guid/idea/memosdcltrs/inclusion-policy-executive-summary-draft-5–15–2015.pdf

Valdez, F., & Montgomery, J. K. (1996). Outcomes from two treatment approaches for children with communication disorders in Head Start. *Journal of Children's Communication Development, 18*, 65–71.

Van Kleeck, A. (1998). Preliteracy domains and stages: Laying the foundations for beginning reading. *Journal of Children's Communication Development, 20*(1), 33–51.

Van Kleeck, A. (2014). Distinguishing between casual talk and academic talk beginning in the preschool years: An important consideration for speech–language pathologists. *American Journal of Speech Language Pathology, 23*(4), 1–18. doi:10.1044/2014_AJSLP-14–0032

Vicker, B. (2009). The 21st century speech language pathologist and integrated services in classrooms. *The Reporter, 14*(2), 1–5, 17.

Villa, R. A., & Thousand, J. S. (2003). Making inclusive education work. *Educational Leadership, 61*(2), 19–23.

Villa, R. A., Thousand, J. S., & Nevin, A. I. (2013). *A guide to co-teaching: New lessons and strategies to facilitate student learning* (3rd ed.). Thousand Oaks, CA: Corwin Press.

Virginia Department of Education. (2009). *RtI and the special education eligibility process frequently asked questions.* Retrieved from www.doe.virginia.gov/instruction/virginia_tiered_system_supports/response_intervention/special_ed_eligibility_faq.pdf

Virginia Department of Education. (2011). *Speech–language pathology services in schools: Guidelines for best practice.* Richmond, VA: Author.

Vygotsky, L. S. (1978). *Mind in society: The development of higher mental processes.* Cambridge, MA: Harvard University Press.

Wallach, G. W. (2008). *Language intervention for school-age students: Setting goals for academic success.* St. Louis, MO: Mosby Elsevier.

Warren, S. F., Fey, M. E., & Yoder, P. J. (2007). Differential treatment intensity research: A missing link to creating optimally effective communication interventions. *Mental Retardation and Developmental Disabilities Research Reviews, 13*, 70–77.

Wesley, P., Dennis, B., & Fenson, C. (2007). *PFI model of on-site consultation to enhance quality in early childhood programs.* Adapted from original sources: Bergan, 1977, 1995; Bergan & Kratochwill, 1990; Caplan, 1970; Caplan & Caplan, 1999.

WestEd. (2014, May). *Taking a closer look at English learner subgroups whose achievement stalls out.* San Francisco, CA: *Regional Educational Laboratory West.*

Wetherby, A. (2000, July). *Understanding and enhancing communication and language.* Paper presented at two-day institute at Northern Arizona University, Flagstaff, AZ.

The White House. (2015). *Fact sheet: Congress acts to fix No Child Left Behind.* Retrieved from www.whitehouse.gov/the-press-office/2015/12/03/fact-sheet-congress-acts-fix-no-child-left-behind

Whitmire, K. (2000). Action: School services; Dysphagia services in schools. *Language, Speech, and Hearing Services in Schools, 31*, 99–103.

Whitmire, K. (2002). The evolution of school-based speech–language services: A half century of change and a new century of practice. *Communication Disorders Quarterly, 23*(2), 68–76.

Whitmire, K., Karr, S., & Mullen, R. (2000). Action: School services. *Language, Speech, and Hearing Services in Schools, 31*, 402–406.

Whitmire, K., Rivers, K., Mele-McCarthy, J., & Staskowski, M. (2014, January). Building an evidence base for speech–language services in the schools: Challenges and recommendations. *Communication Disorders Quarterly, 35*(2), 84–92.

Wieder, S., & Greenspan, S. (2003). Climbing the symbolic ladder in the DIR model through floor time/interactive play. *Autism, 7,* 425–435.

Wiig, E. H., & Secord, W. A. (2006). Clinical measurement and assessment: A 25-year retrospective. *The ASHA Leader, 11*(2), 10–11, 27. Retrieved from http://leader.pubs.asha.org/article.aspx?articleid=2288237

Will, M. (1986). *Educating students with learning problems: A shared responsibility.* Washington, DC: U.S. Department of Education.

Winner, M. G. (n.d.). *Social thinking models.* Retrieved from www.socialthinking.com/home

Winner, M., & Crooke, P. (2011). Thinking about thinking: Social communication for adolescents with autism. *The ASHA Leader, 16,* 8–11.

Wipple, W. (2014). *Key principles of early intervention and effective practices: A crosswalk with statements from discipline specific literature.* Regional Resource Center Program Mountain Plains. Retrieved from http://ectacenter.org/~pdfs/topics/eiservices/KeyPrinciplesMatrix_01_30_15.pdf

Wolter, J. A., DiLollo, A., & Apel, K. (2006). A narrative therapy approach to counseling: A model for working with adolescents and adults with language-literacy deficits. *Language, Speech, and Hearing Services in Schools, 37,* 168–177.

Woods, J. (2008). Providing early intervention services in natural environments. *The ASHA Leader, 13*(4), 14–17.

Wrightslaw. (n.d.). *IDEA 2004: Highly qualified special education teachers.* Retrieved from www.wrightslaw.com/idea/tchr.hq.require.htm#require

Wyatt, T., & Weddington, G. (2010, November). *Going beyond language: Closing the gap for African American students.* Paper presented at the ASHA Annual Convention, Philadelphia, PA.

Yoshinaga-Itano, C. (2014, March). *Universal newborn hearing screening: The evolution of a public health revolution; The anatomy of the implementation of a universal newborn screening program in Colorado and across states* [Presentation video]. CREd Library. doi:10.1044/cred-pvid-implscid2p8

Zipoli, R. P., & Kennedy, M. (2005). Evidence-based practice among speech–language pathologists: Attitudes, utilization, and barriers. *American Journal of Speech–Language Pathology, 14*(3), 208–220.

Zirkel, P. A. (2011). Autism litigation under the IDEA: A new meaning of "disproportionality"? *Journal of Special Education Leadership, 2,* 92–103.

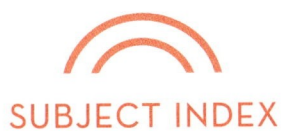

SUBJECT INDEX

In this index, *f* denotes figure and *t* denotes table.

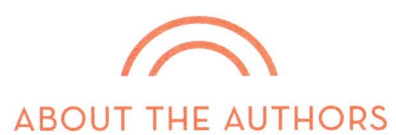

ABOUT THE AUTHORS

Dr. Barbara J. Moore, CCC-SLP, is the director of special services for the East Side Union School District in San Jose, California. An American Speech–Language–Hearing Association (ASHA) board-certified specialist in child language, she has served in several leadership roles in professional associations, including treasurer for the American Board of Child Language and Language Disorders (2016–2017), ASHA vice president of planning (2011–2013), president of the California Speech–Language–Hearing Association (1997–1999), and president of the Council of State Speech–Language–Hearing Association Presidents (2000–2001). She lectures widely on issues related to special education, response to intervention, and school-based speech–language services. Dr. Moore holds a bachelor's degree in communicative disorders and linguistics from California State University, Fullerton; a master's degree in communication disorders from Whittier College; and a doctorate in education leadership from the University of Southern California.

Judy K. Montgomery, PhD, CCC-SLP, is a professor of communicative sciences and disorders at Chapman University in Irvine, California, and a board-certified specialist in child language, with 24 years of experience in the public schools as a speech–language pathologist, K–8 principal, and director of special education. She is the executive director of the Childhood Language Center in Santa Ana, California, and the former president of ASHA, the California Speech–Language–Hearing Association, and the U.S. Society for Augmentative and Alternative Communication. Her research interests include evidence-based practice, vocabulary interventions, and collaborative service delivery models. She enjoys sharing knowledge with fellow professionals and has written numerous books, has authored a standardized test (*Montgomery Assessment of Vocabulary Acquisition*), and is the editor of *Communication Disorders Quarterly*.